Developmental Psychopathology and Wellness

Genetic and Environmental Influences

Developmental Psychopathology and Wellness

Genetic and Environmental Influences

Edited by

James J. Hudziak, M.D.

Professor, Departments of Psychiatry, Medicine, and Pediatrics
Director of Child and Adolescent Psychiatry
Thomas M. Achenbach Chair in Developmental Psychopathology
Director of the Vermont Center for Children, Youth, and Families
University of Vermont College of Medicine, Burlington, Vermont

Professor and Endowed Chair on Genetics of
Childhood Behaviour Problems, Biological Psychology
Vrije Universiteit, Amsterdam, the Netherlands

Adjunct Professor of Psychiatry
Dartmouth School of Medicine

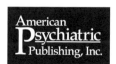

American Psychiatric Publishing, Inc.

Washington, DC
London, England

Note: The authors have worked to ensure that all information in this book is accurate at the time of publication and consistent with general psychiatric and medical standards, and that information concerning drug dosages, schedules, and routes of administration is accurate at the time of publication and consistent with standards set by the U.S. Food and Drug Administration and the general medical community. As medical research and practice continue to advance, however, therapeutic standards may change. Moreover, specific situations may require a specific therapeutic response not included in this book. For these reasons and because human and mechanical errors sometimes occur, we recommend that readers follow the advice of physicians directly involved in their care or the care of a member of their family.

Manufactured in the United States of America on acid-free paper
12 11 10 09 08   5 4 3 2 1
First Edition

Typeset in Adobe's Janson and Myriad.

American Psychiatric Publishing, Inc.
1000 Wilson Boulevard
Arlington, VA 22209-3901
www.appi.org

Library of Congress Cataloging-in-Publication Data
Developmental psychopathology and wellness : genetic and environmental influences / edited by James J. Hudziak. — 1st ed.
    p. ; cm.
    Includes bibliographical references and index.
    ISBN 978-1-58562-279-5 (alk. paper)
    1. Child psychopathology—Genetic aspects. 2. Child psychopathology—Environmental aspects. 3. Adolescent psychopathology—Genetic aspects.
4. Adolescent psychopathology—Environmental aspects. I. Hudziak, James J.
    [DNLM: 1. Psychopathology. 2. Adolescent Development. 3. Adolescent.
4. Child Development. 5. Child. 6. Mental Disorders—etiology.
WS 350 D4888 2008]
    RJ499.D4833 2008
    618.92′89042—dc22

                                                                2007049666

British Library Cataloguing in Publication Data
A CIP record is available from the British Library.

To my wife, Theresa, and our children,
Vicenta, Sam, Maddie, and Emma.
Thank you for the wonderful environment.

CONTENTS

Part 1

BASIC PRINCIPLES OF DEVELOPMENTAL PSYCHOPATHOLOGY

Part 2

GENERAL CONCEPTS OF GENE–ENVIRONMENT INTERACTION ON CHILD DEVELOPMENT

Part 3

DISORDER-BASED EXAMPLES OF THE STUDY
OF GENE–ENVIRONMENT INTERACTION

Part 4

THE FUTURE OF THE STUDY OF
DEVELOPMENTAL PSYCHOPATHOLOGY
IN GENETICS AND CLINICAL SETTINGS

CONTRIBUTORS

Thomas M. Achenbach, Ph.D.
Professor of Psychiatry and Psychology, Department of Psychiatry, University of Vermont, Burlington, Vermont

Adrian Angold, M.R.C.Psych.
Center for Developmental Epidemiology, Duke University Medical Center, Durham, North Carolina

Meike Bartels, Ph.D.
Assistant Professor, Department of Biological Psychology, Vrije Universiteit, Amsterdam, the Netherlands

Dorret I. Boomsma, Ph.D.
Department of Biological Psychology, Vrije Universiteit, Amsterdam, the Netherlands

John N. Constantino, M.D.
Associate Professor of Psychiatry and Pediatrics, Department of Psychiatry, Division of Child Psychiatry, Washington University School of Medicine, St. Louis, Missouri

Stephen V. Faraone, Ph.D.
Departments of Psychiatry and Neuroscience and Physiology, SUNY Upstate Medical University, Syracuse, New York

Nathan A. Gillespie, Ph.D.
NHMRC Postdoctoral Fellow, Virginia Institute of Psychiatric and Behavioral Genetics, Virginia Commonwealth University, Richmond, Virginia

James J. Hudziak, M.D.
Professor, Departments of Psychiatry, Medicine, and Pediatrics; Director, Child and Adolescent Psychiatry; Thomas M. Achenbach Chair in Developmental Psychopathology; Director, Vermont Center for Children, Youth, and Families, University of Vermont College of Medicine, Burlington; Professor and Endowed Chair on Genetics of Childhood Behaviour Problems, Biological Psychology, Vrije Universiteit, Amsterdam, the Netherlands; Adjunct Professor of Psychiatry, Dartmouth School of Medicine

Joan Kaufman, Ph.D.
Department of Psychiatry, Yale University, New Haven, Connecticut

Michelle Luciano, Ph.D.
ARC Postdoctoral Fellow, Queensland Institute of Medical Research, Brisbane, Queensland, Australia

Dana March, M.P.H.
Ph.D. Candidate, Department of Epidemiology and Center for History & Ethics of Public Health, Mailman School of Public Health, Columbia University, New York, New York

Nicholas G. Martin, Ph.D.
Senior Principal Research Fellow, Queensland Institute of Medical Research, Brisbane, Queensland, Australia

Rosalind J. Neuman, Ph.D.
Research Professor of Mathematics in Psychiatry and Professor of Genetics, Department of Psychiatry Division of Child Psychiatry, Washington University School of Medicine, St. Louis, Missouri

Wendy Reich, Ph.D.
Research Associate Professor, Anthropology in Psychiatry (Child), Department of Psychiatry, Division of Child Psychiatry, Washington University School of Medicine, St. Louis, Missouri

Angela M. Reiersen, M.D., M.P.E.
Instructor in Psychiatry, Department of Psychiatry, Division of Child Psychiatry, Washington University School of Medicine, St. Louis, Missouri

David C. Rettew, M.D.
Assistant Professor of Psychiatry and Pediatrics, Director, Pediatric Psychiatry Clinic, University of Vermont College of Medicine, Burlington, Vermont

Michael Rutter, M.D.
Professor, Institute of Psychiatry, Kings College, London, England

Ezra Susser, M.D., Dr.P.H.
Anna Cheskis Gelman and Murray Charles Gelman Professor and Chair, Department of Epidemiology, Mailman School of Public Health, Columbia University and New York State Psychiatric Institute, New York, New York

Richard D. Todd, Ph.D., M.D.
Blanche F. Ittleson Professor of Psychiatry and Professor of Genetics, Director of Child and Adolescent Psychiatry in the Division of Child Psychiatry, Department of Psychiatry, Washington University School of Medicine, St. Louis, Missouri

C.E.M. van Beijsterveldt, Ph.D.
Department of Biological Psychology, Vrije Universiteit, Amsterdam, the Netherlands

Frank C. Verhulst, M.D.
Erasmus University Medical Center, Sophia Children's Hospital, Rotterdam, The Netherlands

Heather E. Volk, Ph.D., M.P.H.
Postdoctoral Fellow, Division of Biostatistics, Department of Preventive Medicine, University of Southern California, Los Angeles, California

Margaret J. Wright, Ph.D.
Senior Research Fellow, Queensland Institute of Medical Research, Brisbane, Queensland, Australia

Gu Zhu, M.P.H., M.D.
Research Officer, Queensland Institute of Medical Research, Brisbane, Queensland, Australia

Disclosure of Competing Interests

The contributors have declared all forms of support received within the 12 months prior to manuscript submittal that may represent a competing interest in relation to their work published in this volume, as follows:

John N. Constantino, M.D.—Dr. Constantino is the author of the Social Responsiveness Scale (SRS), an instrument used in the research described in the chapters to which he has contributed. Although the SRS is commercially distributed and Dr. Constantino received royalties for its sales, no royalties were received for any of his own research using the SRS. The material presented in this book pertaining to the SRS is not designed to promote the instrument, rather to describe scientific understanding that has been derived from use of the instrument in research studies of social development in children.

The following contributors stated that they had no competing interests during the year preceding manuscript submission:

Thomas M. Achenbach, Ph.D.
Adrian Angold, M.R.C.Psych.
Meike Bartels, Ph.D.
Dorret I. Boomsma, Ph.D.
Stephen V. Faraone, Ph.D.
James J. Hudziak, M.D.
Joan Kaufman, Ph.D.
Dana March, M.P.H.
Angela M. Reiersen, M.D., M.P.E.
David C. Rettew, M.D.
Michael Rutter, M.D.
Ezra Susser, M.D., Dr.P.H.
Richard D. Todd, Ph.D., M.D.
Frank C. Verhulst, M.D.
Heather E. Volk, Ph.D., M.P.H.
Margaret J. Wright, Ph.D.

PREFACE

In early March 2007 the American Psychopathological Association (APPA) convened its annual conference with the theme of genetic and environmental influences on developmental psychopathology and wellness. The goal of the conference was to present and discuss the remarkable recent advances made in identifying genetic and environmental influences on the development of emotional-behavioral disorders of children and adolescents. The long-term goal of this work is to advance our understanding of the causes of child psychopathology, with an aim toward improving the way we conceptualize and treat child psychiatric illness. This book is a by-product of that meeting. Each of the scientists who participated in the meeting kindly contributed an up-to-date chapter of their important work. This effort is truly international. Authors in this edition hail from a wide variety of places from around the globe, including England, Australia, the Netherlands, and the United States. I am grateful to each of them for their friendship, excellence, and esprit de corps in ensuring that this book could be completed in such rapid fashion. One of the joys of academic life is to meet and work with wonderful people, and each of the scholars who participated in this process is such a person. To each of you, I publicly state my gratitude. It is my contention that this book is written in such a way that it will be useful to families, clinicians, research scientists, and anyone else who has wondered why some children are always well, why some children sometimes suffer and recover, and why others remain worried or sad throughout their lives.

The book contains 13 chapters divided into four parts: Part 1: Basic Principles of Developmental Psychopathology; Part 2: General Concepts of Gene–Environment Interaction on Child Development; Part 3: Disorder-Based Examples of the Study of Gene-Environment Interaction; and Part 4: The Future of the Study of Developmental Psychopathology in Genetics and Clinical Settings.

PART 1: BASIC PRINCIPLES OF DEVELOPMENTAL PSYCHOPATHOLOGY

Part 1 provides the uninitiated and cognoscenti of developmental psychopathology with a primer and an update on the development of the field and how it has been influenced by advances in genomic medicine. Readers will be treated to chapters by the founders of this field. Sir Michael Rutter contributes a brilliant overview of the history of this young field (with its beginnings in the early 1970s) and more importantly provides readers with a road map for the future of the study of gene–environment interaction by defining the developmental perspective. He finishes by outlining the work ahead. Professor Thomas Achenbach coined the phrase "developmental psychopathology" in 1974 in his book of that same name. In the second chapter, he builds on Rutter's contribution to this volume by detailing the necessity of identifying the contributions of age, gender, informant, and cultural sources of variance on developmental perspective. His chapter is especially focused on the importance of culture in understanding the genetic and environmental influences on children's and families' problems. In addition to identifying the problem of how to measure these sources of influence, he has also provided us with a solution. The final chapter in this section is by Professor Ezra Susser and Dana March, who extend and expand on Rutter and Achenbach's lessons by reminding us all of the importance of social context when considering the measurement of one's experience (good or bad). Susser and March elegantly point out that one's experience matters and that the social context in which that experience occurs can vary widely and lead to different outcomes. The net lessons gleaned from these three outstanding chapters will be to introduce families, clinicians, and scientists to or expand their awareness of the importance of the developmental perspective as providing the basis to understand all complex medical illnesses, of which child psychopathology is only one example.

PART 2: GENERAL CONCEPTS OF GENE–ENVIRONMENT INTERACTION ON CHILD DEVELOPMENT

Part 2 includes three chapters presenting the important concepts of personality and temperament, cognition, and sex. Dr. David Rettew provides an overview of the relations between temperament and developmental psychopathology, including findings from genetics and neurobiology. He argues that the continued study of temperamental traits and their close association to child emotional reactivity and control likely will lead to an understanding of the mechanisms of these relations in a developmentally sensitive perspective. Dr. Margaret Wright, from Professor Nick Martins's group, and colleagues advance the discussion from temperament to personality and cognition. They provide an expert overview of the field and present findings from their molecular genetic investigations on adolescent cognition, temperament, and brain function. Professor Andrian Angold provides a scholarly and important contribution explaining that sex should not be considered as a separate categorical construct, but rather as a developmental process itself. Understanding such a point, he argues, will illuminate sex differences in psychopathology.

PART 3: DISORDER-BASED EXAMPLES OF THE STUDY OF GENE–ENVIRONMENT INTERACTION

Part 3 includes five chapters, beginning with Dr. Joan Kaufman's seminal work on the genetic and environmental modifiers of risk and resilience in maltreated children. Kaufman elegantly describes maltreatment and its relation to other forms of environmental risk, genetic mediation, and reactivity in the presence of maltreatment. She concludes with a terribly important lesson for all of us who care about children's problems: "the negative effects associated with early stress are not inevitable and need not be permanent." As will be evidenced throughout this section, we no longer think of emotional-behavioral illness and wellness as exclusively caused by genetic or environmental factors, but rather their interaction over time. Kaufman's lessons are then extended to the study of anxious depression, attention-deficit/hyperactivity disorder (ADHD), autism and pervasive developmental disorders, and antisocial personality disorders. It is important to our readers to know these lessons have been applied to almost every child psychiatric condition; however, it is simply beyond the scope of this book to address them all. In her chapter on anxious depression, Professor Boomsma and colleagues provide a picture of the genetic architecture of childhood worry from ages 3 to 12. They present data from an extraordinary twin sample of 30,000 pairs that have been followed since birth. Here we learn how genetic and environmental influences vary by the age (and, in some instances, gender) of a child—findings that perhaps give us a clue on how to design interventions for children who worry. Dr. Angela Reiersen (from Professor Richard Todd's group) and colleagues, also using a twin sample, discuss the importance of considering genotypes, environment (in this case, maternal substance use behavior), and co-occurrence of other disorders in a chapter that explores preferential risks (both genetic and environmental) for ADHD and a subtype of ADHD in which children also meet the criteria for an autism spectrum disorder (ASD). The discussion of the genetic epidemiology of ASD is elaborated by Drs. John Constantino and Richard Todd, who detail the possibility that ASD is best conceptualized as existing on a severity continuum in which multiple genes of small effect contribute aspects of the overall syndrome. An individual with a few of these genes may have only mild symptoms or in fact be at an advantage. Further, these authors hypothesize, as the genes of risk accumulate, so does the expression of the syndrome. Here we learn that therapeutic interventions that have been unsuccessful in severely affected persons may be useful in less affected individuals. Lastly, Professor Frank Verhulst presents results from a 14-year longitudinal study on the risk for developing antisocial behavior in adulthood. In this chapter he details the advantages of the developmental perspective by revealing that only some of the findings generated on antisocial behavior in studies that ignore the developmental approach are supported in a longitudinal prospective study. Pathways into and out of antisocial personality are identified and hold important clues for the clinician.

PART 4: THE FUTURE OF THE STUDY OF DEVELOPMENTAL PSYCHOPATHOLOGY IN GENETICS AND CLINICAL SETTINGS

For much of the last decade of my career I have been asked two critical questions about child psychiatric genetics: Where can I learn about this stuff (child psychiatric genetics)? and Does it really matter if I can't use it in the clinic? Part 4 of the present volume is a first pass at providing an answer to both questions. Professor Stephen Faraone, arguably the preeminent molecular geneticist in child psychopathology today, gives us the answer to the first question. He has provided us with an excellent primer on the application of statistical and molecular genetic approaches to developmental psychopathology. In addition, he provides some provocative strategies for learning from our own mistakes and those of other fields to move rapidly forward in our search for genes that influence developmental psychopathology. In the final chapter, Dr. Meike Bartels and I attempt to answer the second question: Does it really matter if I can't use it in the clinic? Here we provide a synthesis of what I have learned over my years in this field as a scientist, teacher, and clinician. The chapter summarizes the gene–environment family-based approach I developed for our clinic. In order to bridge the gap between research findings and clinical practice, we argue that much of what you will find in this book is already clinically useful. Critics may object that our approach is too time consuming, economically unrealistic, or ecologically invalid. However, on the basis of our knowledge of genetic and environmental influences, I ask you to carefully consider the value of a genetically informed family-based approach.

It is my hope that you will find valuable lessons contained in this book. I use them in my daily practice, teaching, and research. At its best, this work is changing the way the fields of child psychiatry and clinical psychology are conceptualized by debunking and demystifying damaging misconceptions about child psychiatric illness. We are leaving behind the era of false dichotomies—of nature versus nurture and genes versus environment—and are entering a period of progress in which relations between nature and nurture—genes and environment—can be better understood.

James J. Hudziak, M.D.

Part 1

BASIC PRINCIPLES OF DEVELOPMENTAL PSYCHOPATHOLOGY

Chapter 1

DEVELOPING CONCEPTS IN DEVELOPMENTAL PSYCHOPATHOLOGY

Michael Rutter, M.D.

CONCEPTUALIZATION OF DEVELOPMENTAL PSYCHOPATHOLOGY

The history of developmental psychopathology as an organizing construct really began with Achenbach's (1974) book *Developmental Psychopathology*. He argued that developmental dimensions should constitute the primary basis for the study of childhood psychopathology and that it is not acceptable to view it as no more than a downward extension of adult mental disorder. However, in making that point, he was at pains to emphasize the crucial importance of scientific strategies to test developmental concepts, and he noted the inadequacy of all the prevailing theories and concepts.

It was during the 1980s that developmental psychopathology paradigms came to be established as a mainstream approach in conceptualization, through the writings of researchers such as Garmezy, Sroufe, Cicchetti, and Rutter. Their views had much in common, but there were some crucial differences. However, some key features unified their proposals. First, they argued for a bringing together of research into child development and into child psychiatry but with the need to do so in particular ways (Rutter and Garmezy 1983; Sroufe and Rutter 1984). Traditionally developmental psychology had tended to focus on developmental universals and/or on trait continuities over time, whereas developmental psychopathology required it also to focus on individual differences, on the growing psychological cohesion that may extend across traits, and on the modifications and changes that occur with altered circumstances. Child psychiatry, by contrast, had tended to concentrate on the causes and course of individual diagnostic conditions. Developmental psychology accepted their importance but argued that a developmental perspective requires somewhat different questions to be asked (Rutter 2005b): To what extent are there age-related variations in susceptibility to stress? Is the development of depression or delinquent activities dependent on prior circumstances at an earlier age? Are there points in development when psychological qualities became relatively stabilized so that, although behavior might change, it was no longer possible for functioning to be totally transformed? Why do some psychopathological patterns (e.g., depression, eating disorders, and schizophrenia) become so much more common during adolescence (Rutter 1979; Rutter 2007c)?

Rutter and Garmezy (1983) noted the pioneering contributions of high-risk longitudinal studies based on the risks associated with schizophrenia and drew attention to the developmental tasks and challenges that extended into adult life. They were forthright in arguing that a lifespan perspective is essential and that developmental psychopathology perspectives apply as much to adult psychiatry as to child psychiatry. They stressed that development has to be viewed in terms of biology and not just early life experiences and argued that, more than anything else, developmental psychopathology constitutes a guide to research strategies. Not only were the "big theories" of development hopelessly inadequate, but it was implausible that any one type of mechanism could account for all aspects of normal and abnormal development. Sroufe and Rutter (1984), arguing along somewhat similar lines, noted that the links between early adaptation and later psychopathology could not be expected to be simple or direct. Individual patterns would need to incorporate both the salient issues of a given developmental period and the transactions among prior adaptation, maturational change, and environmental challenges.

Cicchetti (1984, 1990) similarly emphasized the need to focus on causal processes but went further in insisting that the scientific enterprise had to incorporate genetics and neuroscience as well as psychological studies. One particular contribution of his was the emphasis on the need to recognize the diverse pathways that could lead to the same end point and, conversely, that a single risk feature (whether a gene or an experience) could have a range of disparate effects.

Perhaps more than most reviewers, although still within the tradition of Cicchetti, Rutter (1988) highlighted that developmental psychopathology, by focusing (as a research strategy) on continuities and discontinuities over time (the developmental element) and over the span of behavioral variation (the psychopathological element), was characterized more by the questions it posed than by the specific answers it provided. The unifying feature was the investigation of such continuities and discontinuities to determine causal mechanisms. Thus, emphasis was placed on age as an ambiguous variable, reflecting both variation in experiences and different aspects of maturation (Rutter 1989a). This emphasis led to a recognition that development needed to be considered in its social context and that it was essential to consider indirect, as well as direct, causal chains of connections. This in turn led to the development of "natural experiments" that could pull apart variables that ordinarily go together and, in so doing, pit one explanatory hypothesis against others (Rutter 2007b; Rutter et al. 2001). Contrasts needed also to be made between pervasive and situation-specific disorders, and between a focus on single variables as against behavioral composites.

Up to this point, the concepts of developmental psychopathology have been mainly shared by reviewers and commentators. There are, however, three ways in which concepts have diverged. First, although all writers have implicitly accepted a lifespan view, some have had a main focus on child psychopathology (Achenbach and Edelbrock 1978; Cicchetti and Cohen 2006; Lewis and Miller 1990), whereas others have made the lifespan orientation central (Rutter 1988, 1996; Rutter and Sroufe 2000). Second, some have seemed to wish to place developmental psychopathology outside of biology and medicine by adopting a nineteenth-century concept of medicine as preoccupied with single basic causes for utterly distinct diseases unconnected with dimensional risk (Cummings et al. 2000; Sroufe 1997). Others have seen medicine as providing some of the best examples of developmental psychopathology approaches (see Costello and Angold 1996; Rutter 1996, 2007a).

Third, and most crucially of all, some have placed the history of developmental psychopathology in the writings of theoretical systematizers such as Freud, Piaget, and Erikson (Cicchetti 1984, 1990). For others, such as the present author, the inadequacies of these perspectives constitute the main reason why there was the need for the new approach of developmental psychopathology. The systematizers rejected the need to test their theories empirically; the theories were based on a view of "life" rather than empirical observations to be explained and were manifestly wrong in crucial respects. As Bowlby (1988), for example, commented, psychoanalysis was never more wrong than in its view of developmental processes.

Accordingly, in turning to the pioneers who set the stage for developmental psychopathology, I will accord prime respect to scientists whose research and/or ideas set the scene for developmental psychopathology. Although very few of them used developmental psychopathology terminology, they were the originators (or parents) of what we now call developmental psychopathology.

NORMALITY–PATHOLOGY INTERCONNECTIONS

Let me start with the demonstration of interconnections between normality and pathology. Rapoport's (Rapoport et al. 1978) study of the effects of stimulant medication on both patients and normal participants was critically important. Before her study, the prevailing view was that stimulants had a paradoxical tranquilizing effect on individuals with attention-deficit/hyperactivity disorder (ADHD). Her findings were compelling in showing that, to the contrary, the effects of stimulants on attention were the same in all groups. Of course, that is not to argue that this will always be the case; it is not. Thus, neuroleptics benefit individuals with schizophrenia, but they have no beneficial effects on healthy subjects. Rapoport (1980) also noted a potentially important age difference—namely, that stimulants tend to have a euphoriant effect in adults but a dysphoriant effect on children. Once more the argument was not that there would always be age effects in drug response but, rather, that continuities and discontinuities across the two spans of development and of behavioral variation could be informative.

Hermelin and O'Connor (1970; O'Connor and Hermelin 1987) similarly deserve high credit for their experiments with autistic children and then with blind and with deaf children. Their crucial insight was that the experimental study of children with a severe disorder could throw light on normal psychological processes and vice versa. This led to the cognitive psychology studies of theory of mind by Uta Frith (2003), Simon Baron-Cohen (1995), and others. Incidentally, this same body of research also highlighted the value of examining interconnections between specific cognitive deficits and impairments in social reciprocity, rather than examining the syndrome of autism as a whole.

The first systematic twin study of autism, by Folstein and Rutter (1977), was also important in showing for the first time that the genetic liability to autism extended well beyond the traditional handicapping disorder to milder variants of the same construct—an extension now well documented by numerous other studies (Bailey et al. 1998; Rutter 2005a).

Much early research was preoccupied with identifying the effect of some risk or protective factor in isolation from all others. Sameroff and Chandler (1975) played a seminal role in challenging this concept. They did not deny that effects could be independent, but they noted the frequency of two-way interplay in what they termed *transactional effects*. Bronfenbrenner (1979) developed that theme still further in his nested concept of how social systems interact with one another in a dynamic fashion. It came to be recognized that, just as environments affect individuals, so individuals shape their environments. Four key individuals, together with their research groups, played a major role in developing this theme. First, in an influential paper published in 1968, Bell argued that some of the supposed effects of social-ization experiences might derive from children's effects on their rearing en-vironments, rather than the other way round. Thomas and Chess (1968), in their research on children's temperamental styles, made much the same point. Second, Hugh Lytton and his colleagues showed how appropriate experi-ments could test these postulated two-way effects (Anderson et al. 1986). By using samples of typically developing children and children with behavioral problems, and pairing mothers (for a specific child task) with their own child, with someone else's child with the same behavioral style, and with someone else's child with a different style, investigators could truly differ-entiate parent and child effects. Third, Plomin and Bergeman (1987) showed the importance of parent–child gene–environment correlations. Parental behavior had a passive influence on the rearing environment because parents transmitted both risky genes and risky environments. Child behav-ior had active effects because genetically influenced behaviors played a part in shaping and selecting environments and in evoking particular responses in other people. Fourth, in her now classic long-term follow-up into adult life, Robins (1966) showed how behavior in childhood served to shape adult environments. Antisocial boys behaved in ways that predisposed to environments in adult life that brought new psychopathological risks (stemming from broken relationships, lack of social support, and the like). Champion, Goodall, and Rutter (1995), in a much later study, showed the same in relation to the fostering of both acute life stresses and long-term adversities.

PSYCHOPATHOLOGICAL PROGRESSIONS

Robins's (1966) long-term follow-up study was also pioneering in high-lighting important psychopathological progressions in relation to the child-hood precursors of schizophrenia in adult life. From the beginning of the twentieth century, reports by Bleuler and Kraepelin had noted that about half of all individuals who developed schizophrenic psychoses in adult life had shown abnormal, but nonpsychotic, patterns of behavior in childhood. The 1960s and 1970s took the matter much further through three main re-search strategies.

1. Follow-ups into adult life of children with psychiatric disorders, in which Robins showed the way.
2. Prospective studies of high-risk populations (usually as indexed by be-ing born to a mother with schizophrenia). Mednick and Schulsinger's Copenhagen study (Mednick et al. 1984) pioneered this strategy, and

Erlenmeyer-Kimling's New York study (Erlenmeyer-Kimling et al. 1984) warrants a special mention as one of the best planned and most thorough of the prospective studies.
3. Follow-back studies focusing on the school records of individuals who were identified in adult life as having schizophrenia. Watt's (1974) research set the standard for this approach.

EFFECTS OF EARLY EXPERIENCES

The relevance of children's experiences in and outside the family as possible risk or protective factors in relation to psychopathology had been a crucial part of the philosophy of the mental hygiene movement in the early years of the twentieth century, which constituted a major influence on the establishment of child guidance clinics. However, the conceptualization of those experiences changed radically in the 1950s and 1960s, largely as the result of five key advances.

First, Bowlby (1951), through his World Health Organization report, placed the emphasis firmly on early caregiver–child social relationships instead of discipline or toileting practices. This emphasis had a rather critical reception from academic psychology and an even more hostile response from the psychoanalytic world, but detailed critiques, such as Rutter's (Rutter 1972), concluded that there was substance to Bowlby's claims, even though there were also questions and doubts on some important details. Clinicians dealing with young children came to recognize that Bowlby was definitely on target in his scathing criticisms of the prevailing conditions of residential care for children. With respect to developmental psychopathology, however, Bowlby's most important contribution was his integration of developmental psychology and biology and of human and animal research.

Second, then, were the monkey studies. Harlow (1958, 1961) did much to force the world to recognize that "love" was a crucial element and not just stimulation (Blum 2002), and Hinde did most to tease apart the mechanisms involved in the effects of mother–infant separation (Hinde and McGinnis 1977).

Third, there were the advances in the measurement of both family relationships and stress experiences. The work of Brown (Brown and Harris 1978; Brown and Rutter 1966; Rutter and Brown 1966) stands out in that connection, and that of Ainsworth et al. (1978) does so with respect to her devising of the strange situation to assess individual variations in attachment security. In addition, researchers such as Tizard and colleagues (1975; King et al. 1971) showed that it was possible to measure the qualities of institutional environments.

Fourth, there was the demonstration, through animal studies, of the effects of visual experiences on the development of the visual cortex—the research by Hubel and Wiesel (2004) that led to their Nobel prize—together with the effects of stress on the structure and function of the neuroendocrine system—as shown by Levine and his colleagues (Hennessey and Levine 1979). It became clear that experiences had biological effects that played a part in bringing the environment inside the skin, thereby providing possible mechanisms for long-term effects.

Fifth, there was the research showing the developmental consequences of obstetric complications, in which Pasamanick and Knobloch (1966) put forward their concept of a "continuum of reproductive causality," plus the demonstration of the effects on the fetus of exposure to high levels of maternal alcohol (Jones and Smith 1973; Streissguth et al. 1999). Developmentalists needed to accept that key experiences begin prenatally, and not just at birth.

EPIDEMIOLOGY

The 1950s and 1960s also constituted the time when the epidemiology of psychopathology in childhood and adolescence became established as an essential tool for both the planning of services and the study of risk and protective factors. Lapouse and Monk (1958) led the way in the study of individual behaviors, and the Isle of Wight studies did so with respect to psychopathology (Rutter 1979; Rutter et al. 1970a, 1970b/1981). Among other things, the findings showed the high frequency of the co-occurrence of supposedly separate patterns of disorder.

SOME ACCOMPLISHMENTS OF DEVELOPMENTAL PSYCHOPATHOLOGY RESEARCH

Let me now jump forward in time to the present day and ask how much the research strategies that characterize developmental psychopathology have achieved? Have the conceptual innovations, and the empirical discoveries of the pioneers that I have highlighted, borne fruit? In considering these questions, I will focus on developmental psychopathology concepts and strategies and, as in my brief historical survey, I will ignore whether the individual scientists see themselves as part of developmental psychopathology.

Numerous topics could be discussed, but I am going to highlight and discuss just eight: 1) the acceptance of the relevance of behavior and experiences in childhood for adult mental disorder; 2) the demonstration of the environmental mediation of risks for psychopathology; 3) the evidence that some genetic effects are indirect and, as it were, operate outside the skin; 4) the parallel demonstration that environments get inside the skin through effects on gene expression, on neuroendocrine functioning, and on the brain; 5) the meaning and psychopathological effects of age differences in susceptibility to genetic and environmental influences; 6) the use of brain imaging to investigate risk and protective processes; 7) continuities and discontinuities between normality and disorder; and 8) resilience.

Relevance of Behavior and Experience in Childhood for Adult Mental Disorder

Perhaps the most striking change in concept has been the general acceptance by adult psychiatrists that a developmental perspective is essential for mental disorders in adult life (see Rutter et al. 2006a for a review). Thus, the notion that schizophrenia arises on the basis of a neurodevelopmental impairment is now a mainstream view. Prospective studies have shown clearly the childhood risks associated with language and motor deficits and below-average cognitive functioning; the early adolescence precursors are evident in the psychotic-like features; and the prodromata are seen in late adolescence and early adult life, before overt psychosis appears. Depression in young people is associated with a high risk of major depression in adult life, and ADHD is followed by a substantial increase in psychopathology in adulthood. The feature that surprised many conservative adult psychiatrists is not so much that most mental disorders in early adult life had their onset in childhood, but rather that the childhood condition carrying the highest risk for adult psychopathology is conduct disorder.

So far as experiences in childhood are concerned, the feature most convincingly demonstrated as carrying environmentally mediated risks for disorder in adult life is abuse, physical and sexual, but particularly the latter. However, a wider range of failures in good parenting have also been shown to involve long-term risks.

Demonstration of Environmental Mediation Effects

Genetic findings on gene–environment correlations led to an appreciation that there can be genetic mediation of the risks associated with adverse environments (Plomin and Bergeman 1987) and that, before making any inferences about environmental influences, it is necessary to use research designs that pit the two alternatives against each other (Rutter, submitted). A range of genetic strategies, including the study of discordant monozygotic twins, and investigations of the children of twins, as well as the more familiar twin and adoptee designs, have been developed (see Kendler and Prescott 2006;

Rutter 2007b). In addition, however, a diverse mixture of "natural experiments" has been used to great effect (Rutter 2007b; Rutter et al. 2001). The result has been a convincing demonstration that there are truly environmentally mediated risks. Equally, however, the findings have been important in showing that some of the effects claimed did not involve environmental mediation. That applies, for example, to the supposed effect of the measles-mumps-rubella vaccine in causing an "epidemic" of autism. This effect could be excluded on the basis of risk-reversal findings. Similarly, several genetically sensitive designs showed that the early drinking of alcohol did not cause alcohol dependence; rather, the findings reflected a shared liability.

In keeping with the early evidence on prenatal effects, replicated time series designs have shown associations between prenatal famine and an increased risk of schizophrenia—an effect that seems likely to involve environmental mediation. The physical environment in adolescence has also been shown to be relevant in terms of the evidence that heavy early use of cannabis (but not occasional use and not even heavy use if it starts only in adult life) increases the risk of schizophrenia. It may be concluded that there are indeed environmental risks for psychopathology, but these extend back into the prenatal period and include physical as well as psychosocial hazards.

Genetic Effects Outside the Skin

Early claims in the field of behavioral genetics tended to use terms such as the "gene for" schizophrenia or bipolar disorder, with the misleading implication of a somewhat direct deterministic effect. It is now clear, as a result of gene–environment correlations and interactions, that there are also indirect routes whereby genes influence psychopathology through effects on exposure and sensitivity to environments (Kendler and Prescott 2006; Rutter 2006a; Rutter et al. 2006b). In many circumstances, there is co-action between genes and environments, and it is misleading to conceptualize effects as due to either nature or nurture. Before the development of molecular genetics, which allowed identification of specific genes, and the use of discriminating measures of observed specific environments, researchers relied on "black box" analyses of anonymous genetic and environmental effects. All of that has now changed—particularly as a result of the pioneering research by Caspi and Moffitt using the Dunedin Longitudinal Study (see Caspi and Moffitt 2006; Moffitt et al. 2006). Not only have findings been replicated, but they have been taken further through experimental studies with monkeys (in which the leadership is provided by the group led by Suomi [see Ichise et al. 2006; Suomi 2005]), and experimental brain imaging studies in humans (in which the leadership comes from the group led by Weinberger [see Hariri and Weinberger 2003]).

How Environments Get Under the Skin

For many years, few psychosocial researchers showed much interest in the varied mechanisms by which environments might have long-term effects (see Rutter 1989b), but that has now changed as a result of several rather different areas of research. First, there is the evidence from the outstanding experiments with rats undertaken by Meaney and his group, which have shown that a particular form of archback nursing in the first weeks of life has substantial effects on the pups' behavior and neuroendocrine functioning. Cross-fostering studies have shown that the effects are environmentally mediated, and neurochemical investigations have indicated that the mediation comes about through effects on gene expression. Environments cannot change gene sequences, but they can change gene expression, which is a necessary process for genes to have effects (see Rutter 2006b; Weaver et al. 2004).

Second, the important rat studies undertaken by Greenough and colleagues (Greenough and Black 1992; Greenough et al. 1987) showed the effects of environmental restriction and enhancement on brain structure and function. Interestingly, and importantly, these effects are by no means confined to the infancy period when brain growth peaks but also apply in adulthood.

Third, human brain imaging studies have shown that intensive training, as with taxi drivers learning all routes in London, or with expert musicians, leads to structural brain changes—again in adult life (Elbert et al. 1995; Maguire et al. 2000). Functional brain imaging has similarly shown brain changes as a result of both pharmacological and psychological interventions (Goldapple et al. 2004).

Fourth, evidence from both human and animal studies suggests that there are biological programming effects from environmental influences during sensitive periods of development (see Rutter 2005b for a review). The theoretical point is that the development of somatic systems is designed to be adapted to the environmental circumstances prevailing at the time of the peak development of the relevant systems. A human example is provided by the long-term effects of institutional deprivation, which have been found to be surprisingly persistent and highly sensitive to developmental phase.

Fifth, there is the growing body of evidence on the neuroendocrine effects of both acute and chronic stress experiences (see McEwen and Lasley 2002). In the field of developmental human studies, Gunnar has been a leader (Gunnar and Quevedo 2007), and in animal studies Sapolsky (1998, 2005) stands out as a particularly creative investigator. At present, we lack evidence on the role of the neuroendocrine changes on psychological sequelae, and that stands out as an important research challenge.

Age Differences in Susceptibility

Despite its centrality in developmental psychopathology concerns, age differences in susceptibility have been investigated only to a very limited extent. The early literature had suggested that young organisms were less vulnerable than older ones to the effects of brain injury—the so-called Kennard principle (see Rutter 1982). More recent research has shown that this is not the case. The effects of lateralized brain lesions in infancy do differ from those in later life in having a less differentiated effect on patterns of language/cognitive functions, but the overall effect on cognitive functioning is clearly not less (Varga-Khadem et al. 1992). The nature and degree of brain plasticity does change with age but we know surprisingly little about the mechanisms.

There is growing evidence that drug effects in childhood and adult life are not the same (see, e.g., the relative lack of response of childhood depression to tricyclic medication despite the strong continuity with depression in adult life). Once more, there is good reason to conclude that the topic is both theoretically and practically important, but there is a paucity of research into its mechanisms.

The greater risk effect of cannabis in childhood/adolescence has already been noted, and this is paralleled by similar age differences in effects on cognition as shown in animal studies. But what processes are involved?

Moffitt (1993) opened up new ways of thinking about antisocial behavior through her differentiation between life course–persistent antisocial behavior (which typically begins early and is associated with neurodevelopmental impairment) and an adolescence-limited variety, which is less strongly associated with risk factors both biological and experiential. The validity of this differentiation has been mainly supported by other research, but it is clear that an onset of conduct disorder in childhood does not usually lead to life course–persistent problems (Odgers et al. 2007). Also, it remains uncertain whether the key differentiation lies in neurodevelopmental impairment or ADHD rather than age at onset per se. Clearly, major research questions on age effects remain.

Brain Imaging in Investigating Risk and Protective Processes

The development of structural and functional brain imaging—initially positron emission tomography (PET) and then magnetic resonance imaging (MRI)—has opened up new possibilities to investigate brain–mind interconnections. Thus, studies of individuals with autism have produced evidence of differences in interconnectivity of brain functioning (C. Frith 2003). (Reference has already been made to investigation of responses to treatment and to gene–environment interactions.) In addition, brain imaging carries the potential to differentiate between adverse effects on neural structure and positive compensatory effects—as suggested by a pilot study of Romanian adoptees (Rutter et al. 2007a). When combined with longitudinal studies, brain imaging may also throw light on the brain changes associated with both normal development (Gogtay et al. 2004; Shaw et al. 2006) and the development of psychopathology (Rapoport et al. 2005; Whalley et al. 2005, 2006).

Continuities and Discontinuities Between Normality and Disorder

From the outset, developmental psychopathology has been concerned with the extent to which disorder is on the same continuum as normal variation. Genetic findings have been informative, for example, in showing the need to broaden the concept of autism very substantially, with findings raising queries as to whether the normal population varies in features reflecting a liability to autism (Rutter 2005a). If so, what processes underlie the transition from the normal variation, to the broader phenotype, to seriously handicapping autism? Should a two-hit mechanism be considered? Variations in attachment security have proved to be important correlates of psychopathology, but although social relationships as a whole show strong associations with outcome, attachment insecurity as measured in infancy does not (Grossman et al. 2005). Does this mean that qualitative changes take place with development, or is this primarily a measurement difficulty? Institution-reared children who suffered severe deprivation prior to adoption show rather distinctive social relationship difficulties, as reflected in what has been termed *disinhibited attachment*, but this seems rather different from attachment insecurity as seen in general population samples (Rutter et al. 2007b). Studies of social cognition in autism have proved to be highly informative—with good evidence that theory-of-mind deficits play a substantial role in etiology (Baron-Cohen 1995; U. Frith 2003). But are these deficits qualitatively different from normal variations in theory of mind, or are they variations of what is seen in normal development? Good questions have been posed on the broad issue of continuities and discontinuities between normality and disorder, but definitive answers have proved frustratingly difficult to obtain.

Resilience

The final topic, resilience, had its origins in the observation—most usefully highlighted by Garmezy (1974)—that people varied greatly in their response to stress and adversity. Some become severely impaired, some survive relatively unscathed, and a few appear even to be strengthened through coping successfully with the hazards they face. Masten (2001) has led the way in using longitudinal study approaches, Luthar (2003) has been foremost in bringing together the conceptual issues and empirical findings, and Rutter (2006c) has highlighted the ways in which the topic of resilience goes beyond (but builds on) risk and protective factors approaches. It has to be said that the potential of the resilience concept still requires much better empirical study, but it constitutes a prime example of the developmental psychopathology focus on individual differences in developmental functioning.

CHALLENGES FOR THE FUTURE

There has been space to do no more than touch on a few examples of accomplishments in developmental psychopathology. It may be concluded that much has been achieved by a combination of gains in conceptual understanding and in technologies. In keeping with the whole of science, but especially biomedical science, interdisciplinary collaboration has played a major role in the discoveries, and that will certainly continue to be the case. The particular challenge for clinical scientists is the need to develop experimental medicine in which there can be a two-way interplay between clinical advances and scientific advances, and not just the mechanized application at the bedside of findings deriving from basic science.

The big questions that demand our attention involve five key issues.

1. Given the evidence on the importance of multiphase causal pathways, what are the mechanisms involved in phase transitions—such as those from the precursors and prodromata of schizophrenia to overt psychosis? Or from early physical aggression or disruptive behavior or inattention/overactivity to life course–persistent antisocial behavior and antisocial personality disorder? Or from occasional recreational use of drugs to heavy regular use to drug dependence and abuse?
2. What are the causal processes involved in the direct and indirect pathways from the presence of a susceptibility gene, on through gene expression, to effects on proteins, and from there, in the less well understood pathway, to manifestations of particular phenotypes? What is the importance of gene actions outside the skin through gene–environment correlations and interactions? How do environmental effects get under

the skin? How do genes and environments come together in causal pathways in either normal development or psychopathology?

3. How do the neural changes involved in brain development relate to the alterations in the workings of the mind as they apply across both the span of development and the span from normality to disorder? To what extent do the processes depend on neurotransmitter functions as against the interconnectivity among neural systems? In what ways is neuroendocrine functioning implicated in any of these pathways—such as from environmental adversity to psychological malfunction or in the changing rates and patterns of psychopathology that are seen in adolescence? In considering risk and protective factors, will it be important to extend our study into general bodily functions such as immune responses or sensitivity to dietary features?

4. What are the causal mechanisms involved in individual differences in responses to stress and adversity? In seeking to obtain an understanding of the mechanisms involved in resilience, how should we investigate the processes that lead to steeling rather than sensitization effects? What is the role of personal agency in successful coping with stress and adversity? The development of positive, rather than negative, mental sets or internal working models seems likely to be important, but how do such sets develop and how do they operate?

5. What underlies the age differences we see in rates and patterns of psychopathology and in styles of response to psychosocial hazards or to physical substances? A central tenet of developmental psychopathology is that children are not just little adults, but what are the processes involved in age-indexed variations? Why, for example, do depressive disorders become more frequent in adolescence, and why do they become more common in females during that age period?

Of course, clinical practice in psychiatry or psychology or pediatrics raises a host of issues beyond these, but the importance of developmental psychopathology lies in its role in making us frame particular sorts of questions about development and about psychopathology, and in suggesting what might be useful research strategies to pursue. Developmental psychopathology is not, and should not become, a "big" theory or ideology. Also, it constitutes a central feature in the whole of biology and of medicine, and we need to ensure that we do not cut ourselves off from these broader fields. The pioneers who paved the way to the growth of developmental psychopathology tended to be iconoclasts who challenged set ways of thinking and who refused to accept the given wisdom just because it came from senior figures who held positions of power. We should follow their model and do the same in pursuing our interest in taking developmental psychopathology forward.

REFERENCES

Achenbach TM: Developmental Psychopathology. New York, Wiley, 1974

Achenbach TM, Edelbrock CS: The classification of child psychopathology: a review and analysis of empirical efforts. Psychol Bull 85:1275–1301, 1978

Ainsworth MDS, Blehar MC, Waters E, et al: Patterns of Attachment: A Psychological Study of the Strange Situation. Hillsdale, NJ, Erlbaum, 1978

Anderson KE, Lytton H, Romney DM: Mothers' interactions with normal and conduct-disordered boys: who affects whom? Dev Psychol 22:604–609, 1986

Bailey A, Palferman S, Heavey L, et al: Autism: the phenotype in relatives. J Autism Dev Disord 28:381–404, 1998

Baron-Cohen S: Mindblindness: An Essay on Autism and Theory of Mind. Cambridge, MA, MIT Press, 1995

Bell RQ: A reinterpretation of the direction of effects in studies of socialization. Psychol Rev 75:81–95, 1968

Blum D: Love at Goon Park: Harry Harlow and the Science of Affection. Cambridge, MA, Perseus Publishing, 2002

Bowlby J: Maternal Care and Mental Health. Geneva, Switzerland, World Health Organization, 1951

Bowlby J: A Secure Base: Clinical Implications of Attachment Theory. London, Routledge & Kegan Paul, 1988

Bronfenbrenner U: The Ecology of Human Development: Experiments by Nature and Design. Cambridge, MA, Harvard University Press, 1979

Brown GW, Harris TO: The Social Origins of Depression: A Study of Psychiatric Disorder in Women. London, Tavistock, 1978

Brown GW, Rutter M: The measurement of family activities and relationships: a methodological study. Hum Relat 19:241–263, 1966

Caspi A, Moffitt TE: Gene environment interactions in psychiatry: joining forces with neuroscience. Nat Rev Neurosci 7:583–590, 2006

Champion LA, Goodall GM, Rutter M: Behavioural problems in childhood and stressors in early adult life: a 20-year follow-up of London school children. Psychol Med 25:231–246, 1995

Cicchetti D: The emergence of developmental psychopathology. Child Dev 55:1–7, 1984

Cicchetti D: A historical perspective on the discipline of developmental psychopathlogy, in Risk and Protective Factors in the Development of Psychopathology. Edited by Rolf J, Masten AS, Cicchetti D, et al. Cambridge, UK, Cambridge University Press, 1990, pp 1–28

Cicchetti D, Cohen DJ (eds): Developmental Psychopathology, 2nd Edition. Hoboken, NJ, Wiley, 2006

Costello EJ, Angold A: Developmental psychopathology, in Developmental Science. Edited by Cairns RB, Elder GH Jr, Costello EJ. New York, Cambridge University Press, 1996, pp 168–189

Cummings EM, Davies PT, Campbell SB: Developmental Psychopathology and Family Process: Theory, Research and Implications. New York, Guilford, 2000

Elbert T, Pantev C, Wienbruch C, et al: Increased cortical representation of the fingers of the left hand in string players. Science 270:305–307, 1995

Erlenmeyer-Kimling L, Marcuse Y, Cornblatt B, et al: The New York high risk project, in Children at Risk for Schizophrenia: A Longitudinal Perspective. Edited by Watt NF, Anthony EJ, Wynne LC, et al. New York, Cambridge University Press, 1984, pp 169–189

Folstein S, Rutter M: Infantile autism: a genetic study of 21 pairs. J Child Psychol Psychiatry 18:297–321, 1977

Frith C: What do imaging studies tell us about the neural basis of autism? in Autism: Neural Basis and Treatment Possibilities. Edited by Bock G, Goode J. Chichester, UK, Wiley, 2003, pp 149–176

Frith U: Autism: Explaining the Enigma. Oxford, UK, Blackwell, 2003

Garmezy N: The study of competence in children at risk for severe psychopathology, in The Child in His Family: Children at Psychiatric Risk, Vol 3. Edited by Anthony E, Koupernik C. New York, Wiley, 1974, pp 77–98

Gogtay N, Giedd JN, Lusk L, et al: Dynamic mapping of human cortical development during childhood through early adulthood. Proc Natl Acad Sci U S A 101:8174–8179, 2004

Goldapple K, Segal Z, Garson C, et al: Treatment-specific effects of cognitive behavior therapy. Arch Gen Psychiatry 61:34–41, 2004

Greenough WT, Black JE: Induction of brain structure by experience: substrates for cognitive development, in Developmental Behavior Neuroscience. Edited by Gunnar MR, Nelson CA. Hillsdale, NJ, Erlbaum, 1992, pp 155–200

Greenough WT, Black JE, Wallace CS: Experience and brain development. Child Dev 58:539–559, 1987

Grossman KE, Grossman K, Waters E (eds): Attachment From Infancy to Adulthood: The Major Longitudinal Studies. London, Guilford, 2005

Gunnar M, Quevedo K: The neurobiology of stress and development. Annu Rev Psychol 58:145–173, 2007

Hariri AR, Weinberger DR: Imaging genomics. Br Med Bull 65:259–270, 2003

Harlow HF: The nature of love. Am Psychol 13:673–685, 1958

Harlow HF: The development of affectional patterns in infant monkeys, in Determinants of Infant Behaviour, Vol 1. Edited by Foss BM. London, Methuen, 1961

Hennessey JW, Levine S: Stress, arousal, and the pituitary-adrenal system: a psychoendocrine hypothesis, in Progress in Psychobiology and Physiological Psychology. Edited by Sprague JM, Epstein AN. New York, Academic Press, 1979, pp 133–178

Hermelin B, O'Connor N: Psychological Experiments With Autistic Children. New York, Pergamon, 1970

Hinde RA, McGinnis L: Some factors influencing the effect of temporary mother-infant separation: some experiments with rhesus monkeys. Psychol Med 7:197–212, 1977

Hubel DH, Wiesel TN: Brain and Visual Perception: The Story of a 25-Year Collaboration. New York, Oxford University Press, 2004

Ichise M, Vines DC, Gura T, et al: Effects of early life stress on [11C]DASB positron emission tomography imaging of serotonin transporters in adolescent peer- and mother-reared rhesus monkeys. J Neurosci 26:4638–4643, 2006

Jones KL, Smith DW: Recognition of the fetal alcohol syndrome in early infancy. Lancet 2:999–1001, 1973

Kendler KS, Prescott CA: Genes, Environment, and Psychopathology: Understanding the Causes of Psychiatric and Substance Use Disorders. New York, Guilford, 2006

King RD, Raynes NV, Tizard J: Patterns of Residential Care: Sociological Studies in Institutions for Handicapped Children. London, Routledge & Kegan Paul, 1971

Lapouse R, Monk MA: An epidemiologic study of behavior characteristics in children. Am J Public Health 48:1134–1144, 1958

Lewis M, Miller SM (eds): Handbook of Developmental Psychopathology. New York, Plenum, 1990

Luthar S (ed): Resilience and Vulnerability: Adaptation in the Context of Childhood Adversities. New York, Cambridge University Press, 2003

Maguire EA, Gadian DG, Johnsrude IS, et al: Navigation-related structural change in the hippocampi of taxi drivers. Proc Natl Acad Sci U S A 97:4398–4403, 2000

Masten AS: Ordinary magic. Am Psychol 56:227–238, 2001

McEwen B, Lasley EN: The End of Stress as We Know It. Washington, DC, Joseph Henry Press, 2002

Mednick S, Cudeck AR, Griffith JJ, et al: The Danish high risk project (1962–1982): recent methods and findings, in Children at Risk for Schizophrenia: A Longitudinal Perspective. Edited by Watt NS, Anthony EJ, Wynne LC, et al. Cambridge, UK, Cambridge University Press, 1984, pp 21–42

Moffitt TE: Adolescence-limited and life-course persistent antisocial behavior: a developmental taxonomy. Psychol Rev 100:674–701, 1993

Moffitt TE, Caspi A, Rutter M: Measured gene-environment interactions in psychopathology: concepts, research strategies, and implications for research, intervention, and public understanding of genetics. Perspectives on Psychological Science 1:5–27, 2006

O'Connor N, Hermelin B: Seeing and Hearing and Space and Time. London, Academic Press, 1987

Odgers CL, Caspi A, Broadbent JM, et al: Prediction of differential adult health burden by conduct problem subtypes in males. Arch Gen Psychiatry 64:476–484, 2007

Pasamanick R, Knobloch H: Retrospective studies on the epidemiology of reproductive casualty: old and new. Merrill Palmer Q 12:7–26, 1966

Plomin R, Bergeman CS: The nature of nurture: genetic influence on "environmental" measures. Behav Brain Sci 14:373–427, 1987

Rapoport J: Diagnostic significance of drug response in child psychiatry, in Psychopathology of Children and Youth. Edited by Purcell EF. New York, Josiah Macy Jr Foundation, 1980

Rapoport JL, Buchsbaum MS, Zahn TP, et al: Dextroamphetamine: cognitive and behavioral effects in normal prepubertal boys. Science 199:560–563, 1978

Rapoport JL, Addington AM, Frangou S: The neurodevelopmental model of schizophrenia: update 2005. Mol Psychiatry 10:1–16, 2005

Robins L: Deviant Children Grown Up: A Sociological and Psychiatric Study of Sociopathic Personality. Baltimore, MD, Williams & Wilkins, 1966

Rutter M: Maternal Deprivation Reassessed. Harmondsworth, UK, Penguin Books, 1972

Rutter M: Changing Youth in a Changing Society: Patterns of Adolescent Development and Disorder. London, Nuffield Provincial Hospitals Trust, 1979

Rutter M: Developmental neuropsychiatry: concepts, issues, and prospects. J Clin Neuropsychol 4:91–115, 1982

Rutter M: Epidemiological approaches to developmental psychopathology. Arch Gen Psychiatry 45:486–495, 1988

Rutter M: Age as an ambiguous variable in developmental research: some epidemiological considerations from developmental psychopathology. Int J Behav Dev 12:1–34, 1989a

Rutter M: Pathways from childhood to adult life. J Child Psychol Psychiatry 30:23–51, 1989b

Rutter M: Developmental psychopathology: concepts and prospects, in Frontiers of Developmental Psychopathology. Edited by Lenzenweger MF, Haugaard JJ. New York, Oxford University Press, 1996, pp 209–237

Rutter M: Genetic influences and autism, in Handbook of Autism and Pervasive Developmental Disorders, 3rd Edition. Edited by Volkmar FR, Paul R, Klin A, et al. New York, Wiley, 2005a, pp 425–452

Rutter M: Multiple meanings of a developmental perspective on psychopathology. Eur J Dev Psychol 2:221–252, 2005b

Rutter M: Genes and Behavior: Nature-Nurture Interplay Explained. Malden, MA, Blackwell Publishing, 2006a

Rutter M: The psychological effects of institutional rearing, in The Development of Social Engagement: Neurobiological Perspectives. Edited by Marshall P, Fox N. New York, Oxford University Press, 2006b, pp 355–391

Rutter M: Implications of resilience concepts for scientific understanding. Ann NY Acad Sci 1094:1–12, 2006c

Rutter M: Gene-environment interplay and developmental psychopathological development across adolescence, in Multilevel Dynamics in Developmental Psychopathology. Edited by Masten A. Mahwah, NJ, Erlbaum 2007a

Rutter M: Proceeding from observed correlations to causal inference: the use of natural experiments. Perspectives on Psychological Science 2:377–395, 2007b

Rutter M: Psychopathological development across adolescence. J Youth Adolesc 36:101–110, 2007c

Rutter M, Brown GW: The reliability and validity of measures of family life and relationships in families containing a psychiatric patient. Soc Psychiatry 1:38–53, 1966

Rutter M, Garmezy N: Developmental psychopathology, in Handbook of Child Psychology, 4th Edition, Vol 4: Socialization, Personality, and Social Development. Edited by Mussen PH (series ed), Hetherington EM (volume ed). New York, Wiley, 1983, pp 775–911

Rutter M, Sroufe LA: Developmental psychopathology: concepts and challenges. Dev Psychopathol 12:265–296, 2000

Rutter M, Graham P, Yule W: A Neuropsychiatric Study in Childhood. Clinics in Developmental Medicine 35/36. London, Heinemann/SIMP, 1970a

Rutter M, Tizard J, Whitmore K (eds). Education, Health, and Behaviour (1970b). Melbourne, FL, Krieger, 1981

Rutter M, Pickles A, Murray R, et al: Testing hypotheses on specific environmental causal effects on behaviour. Psychol Bull 127:291–324, 2001

Rutter M, Kim-Cohen J, Maughan B: Continuities and discontinuities in psychopathology between childhood and adult life. J Child Psychol Psychiatry 47:276–295, 2006a

Rutter M, Moffitt TE, Caspi A: Gene-environment interplay and psychopathology: multiple varieties but real effects. J Child Psychol Psychiatry 47:226–261, 2006b

Rutter M, Beckett C, Castle J, et al: Effects of profound early institutional deprivation: an overview of findings from a UK longitudinal study of Romanian adoptees. Eur J Dev Psychol 4:332–350, 2007a

Rutter M, Colvert E, Kreppner J, et al: Early adolescent outcomes for institutionally deprived and non-deprived adoptees. I: disinhibited attachment. J Child Psychol Psychiatry 48:17–30, 2007b

Sameroff AJ, Chandler MJ: Reproductive risk and the continuum of caretaking casualty, in Review of Child Development Research. Edited by Horowitz FD. Chicago, IL, University of Chicago Press, 1975, pp 187–244

Sapolsky RM: Why Zebras Don't Get Ulcers: An Updated Guide to Stress, Stress-Related Diseases, and Coping. New York, WH Freeman, 1998

Sapolsky RM: The influence of social hierarchy on primate health. Science 308:648–652, 2005

Shaw P, Greenstein D, Lerch J, et al: Intellectual ability and cortical development in children and adolescents. Nature 440:676–679, 2006

Sroufe A: Pyschopathology as an outcome of development. Dev Psychopathol 9:251–268, 1997

Sroufe A, Rutter M: The domain of developmental psychopathology. Child Dev 55:17–29, 1984

Streissguth AP, Barr HM, Bookstein FL, et al: The long-term neurocognitive consequences of prenatal alcohol exposure. Psychol Sci 10:186–190, 1999

Suomi SJ: Aggression and social behaviour in rhesus monkeys. Novartis Found Symp 268:216–226, 2005

Thomas A, Chess S, Birch HG: Temperament and Behavior Disorders. New York, New York University Press, 1968

Tizard J, Sinclair I, Clarke RVG: Varieties of Residential Experience. London, Routledge & Kegan Paul, 1975

Vargha-Khadem F, Isaacs E, van der Werf S, et al: Development of intelligence and memory in children with hemiplegic cerebral palsy: the deleterious consequences of early seizures. Brain 115:315–329, 1992

Watt NF: Childhood roots of schizophrenia, in Life History Research in Psychopathology, Vol 3. Edited by Ricks DF, Thomas A, Roff M. Minneapolis, MN, University of Minnesota Press, 1974, pp 194–211

Weaver ICG, Cervoni N, Champagne FA, et al: Epigenetic programming by maternal behavior. Nat Neurosci 7:847–854, 2004

Whalley HC, Simonotto E, Marshall I, et al: Functional disconnectivity in subjects at high genetic risk of schizophrenia. Brain 128:2097–2108, 2005

Whalley HC, Simonotto E, Moorhead W, et al: Functional imaging as a predictor of schizophrenia. Biol Psychiatry 60:454–462, 2006 Feb 7 [Epub ahead of print]

Chapter 2

MULTICULTURAL PERSPECTIVES ON DEVELOPMENTAL PSYCHOPATHOLOGY

Thomas M. Achenbach, Ph.D.

The first college course I taught was on child psychopathology at Yale University. At that time, many years ago, there were several competing theoretical viewpoints, each of which was centered in a particular approach to treatment. The viewpoints included the psychodynamic, behavioral, family systems, and nondirective. Each viewpoint had its own publications that mainly used case illustrations to support its own respective theory. I tried to present each viewpoint objectively. But each viewpoint focused on only a small piece of children's functioning, typically as it was manifested during the course of therapy. Unfortunately, my course was a failure, because I could not make these disparate viewpoints add up to a compelling picture of whole children.

To improve the course and also to establish guidelines for my own research, I concluded that an organizing framework was needed for presenting what could be supported with empirical findings and for advancing knowledge beyond the conventional wisdom of the day. As I was immersed at that time in developmental research related to Jean Piaget's perspective, it seemed evident that the principles, mechanisms, and sequences of development were essential to understanding all aspects of children's functioning, both normal and abnormal. It also seemed evident that abnormal functioning needed to be understood in relation to the normal course of development rather than as something that was categorically different and disconnected from normal development. Of course, it was also possible that some abnormalities might ultimately be found to be categorically outside the normal range.

I concluded that the term *developmental psychopathology* could encompass a more empirically based, comprehensive, and developmentally informed approach to understanding abnormal functioning than what characterized the prevailing approaches. When I was well into my effort to pull all the relevant literature together in a book titled *Developmental Psychopathology*, I had the good fortune to meet Jean Piaget, who invited me to be a visiting fellow at his Centre d'Épistémologie Génétique in Geneva, Switzerland, in 1971.

By the time I went to Geneva, I had learned that Piaget had used the term *developmental psychopathology* in his house journal, *Etudes d'Épistémologie Génétique*. But after arriving in Geneva, I also learned that when one of Piaget's doctoral students wanted to do a dissertation on disturbed children, Piaget said (loosely translated), "What, you are interested in crazy people?" Piaget was definitely not interested in the abnormal. Nevertheless, it was axiomatic for him to view psychopathology from a developmental perspective, because so much of human functioning is predicated on development.

When the first edition of my book *Developmental Psychopathology* was published (Achenbach 1974), the developmental view of psychopathology was not widely shared. In recognition of how uncommon this view was, I began the book with the words, "This is a book about a field that hardly exists yet." By 1982, when the second edition of *Developmental Psychopathology* was published (Achenbach 1982), the view had become more common and was being actively promoted by others (e.g., Rutter and Garmezy 1983). By 1995, the view was common enough to justify a 1,695-page compendium of research on developmental psychopathology edited by Dante Cicchetti and Donald Cohen (1995). And by 2006, the second edition of this compendium filled three volumes totaling nearly 3,000 pages (Cicchetti and Cohen 2006).

GENES, ENVIRONMENT, AND CULTURE

Nearly everything about humans is related not only to development but also to genes, because we are a biological species whose structures, functioning, and developmental course are affected by our DNA. Just as nearly everything is related to development and to genes, nearly everything is also related to the environment. As marvelously explicated by Sir Michael Rutter (2006), genetic influences cannot be adequately understood without understanding their interplay with environmental factors, and vice versa. And, in the twenty-first century, it is especially vital to recognize the importance of those aspects of the human environment that can be lumped under the heading of "culture."

Violent clashes between cultures are painfully obvious throughout the world. But even more widespread are the less dramatic multicultural encounters, frictions, and blendings that result from immigration, electronic communication, and the globalization of commerce, science, and education. Multicultural encounters can spawn both risks and benefits. For the study and treatment of psychopathology, the increasing salience of cultural variations forces us to question the generalizability of our mainly Western concepts. Until recently, much of the professional literature related to psychopathology was written primarily by Westerners from a handful of societies. These Westerners have written mainly about Westerners and for Westerners.

When comparisons with non-Western societies are made, they are often made in terms of a categorical dichotomy that Hermans and Kempen (1998) dubbed "the West versus the Rest." By this, Hermans and Kempen meant that there has been a tendency to view the West as categorically different from the rest of the world. They argued that this dichotomy, as well others such as individualism versus collectivism, falsely represents "cultures as internally homogeneous and externally distinctive" (Hermans and Kempen 1998, p. 1119). Hermans and Kempen (1999) warned against tendencies for these kinds of categorical dichotomies to reify cultures as if they were concrete objects that are categorically distinct from one another.

MULTICULTURAL APPROACHES TO THE STUDY OF PSYCHOPATHOLOGY

How do cultural issues pertain to the study of psychopathology, which mainly concerns differences among individuals? Cultural issues are very pertinent to the study of psychopathology for at least the following reasons:

1. If research, theory, and treatment are based almost exclusively on members of a handful of societies, we cannot know how well they generalize to the rest of the human species.
2. Cross-cultural collaboration in research, training, and treatment requires use of the same standardized assessment instruments, plus evidence that the instruments yield comparable results in different societies.
3. To properly serve the millions of immigrants in today's world, the mental health, education, and welfare systems of the host societies need stan-

dardized assessment instruments that are appropriate for the immigrants but that are also easily used and understood by host society professionals.

Research, theory, training, and treatment can all benefit from assessment instruments that can be similarly applied to diverse groups. To test the ability of particular instruments to assess psychopathology in diverse societies, my colleagues and I have been obtaining data from many societies on the same standardized assessment instruments. These data enable us to identify similarities and differences in both the patterning and prevalence of problems reported by people in different societies. They also enable us to test the effects of age, gender, and other variables on problems across many societies. Such efforts are needed to advance multicultural research on the developmental course of psychopathology.

When testing particular instruments in many societies, we do not assume that any one instrument or one set of items can completely assess everything important about psychopathology in all cultures. There are many ways to define cultures, many groups that can be identified as having different cultures, and many concepts of psychopathology. Consequently, it is unrealistic to expect that all potentially relevant characteristics of all cultural groups can actually be assessed in the same way. Nevertheless, to advance our knowledge of psychopathology, it is essential to apply the same methods to different cultural groups in order to identify both similarities and differences in findings. Otherwise, we will not know whether findings for one cultural group are limited to that group or are generalizable to others.

MULTICULTURAL FINDINGS ON SYNDROMES OF PROBLEMS

To strengthen the empirical basis for developmental research on psychopathology, we have factor analyzed large sets of items that describe rather specific behavioral and emotional problems. We designate the patterns of co-occurring problems as "syndromes" in the original Greek meaning of the word *syndrome*, which refers to characteristics that tend to co-occur (Gove 1971, p. 2320). This research started long ago as an effort to determine whether more syndromes of child psychopathology could be identified than were implied by the DSM-I categories of adjustment reaction of childhood and schizophrenic reaction, childhood type (American Psychiatric Association 1952). Factor analyses of problems reported in child psychiatric case records identified considerably more syndromes than were implied by the two DSM-I categories (Achenbach 1965, 1966).

Subsequent extensions of this research to data obtained directly from parents, teachers, clinicians, observers, test examiners, and children themselves have yielded several syndromes that are similar across data from different informants, as well as some syndromes that are more specific to data from particular informants. To facilitate use of the assessment instruments in research, clinical, and training contexts, we have developed hand-scored and computer-scored profiles that display syndrome scores in relation to norms that are age, gender, and informant specific. To provide crosswalks to DSM diagnoses, we have also developed DSM-oriented scales comprising items identified by international panels of psychiatrists and psychologists as being very consistent with DSM-IV-TR (American Psychiatric Association 2000) diagnostic categories (Achenbach and Rescorla 2000, 2001; McConaughy and Achenbach 2001, 2004).

Although the assessment instruments and the data for the factor analyses originated in the United States, mental health professionals from other societies now use the instruments to assess children and youth in their societies. At this writing, there are translations in more than 80 languages and over 6,000 published reports of use of the instruments in more than 67 societies (Bérubé and Achenbach 2007).

TESTING OF SYNDROMAL PATTERNS IN MULTIPLE SOCIETIES

Researchers in many societies have used the instruments to obtain parent, teacher, and self-ratings of large representative samples of children and youth. This use makes it possible to test the generalizability of the U.S. syndromes to other societies. To conduct such tests, Dr. Masha Ivanova and colleagues have performed confirmatory factor analyses of parent ratings on the Child Behavior Checklist (CBCL), teacher ratings on the Teacher's Report Form (TRF), and self-ratings on the Youth Self-Report (YSR) from many societies (Ivanova et al. 2007a, 2007b, 2007c). An eight-syndrome model derived from ratings of U.S. children and youth was tested in CBCL ratings of more than 58,000 children and youth from 30 societies, TRF ratings of 30,000 students from 20 societies, and YSR ratings by 30,000 youth from 23 societies. Table 2–1 displays the items of the eight-syndrome model. (The TRF Attention Problems syndrome includes subscales for Inattention and Hyperactivity-Impulsivity, which were tested as a model separate from the other syndromes.)

There are many reasons why a complex syndrome model encompassing more than 100 items derived from U.S. parent, teacher, and youth ratings would not generalize to other societies. The vicissitudes of translating col-

TABLE 2–1. Items defining the school-age syndromes, plus items specific to the Child Behavior Checklist/6–18 (CBCL/6–18), Youth Self-Report (YSR), and Teacher's Report Form (TRF) syndrome scales[a]

Anxious/Depressed	Withdrawn/Depressed	Somatic Complaints	Social Problems	Thought Problems
14. Cries a lot	5. Enjoys little	47. Nightmares[c]	11. Too dependent	9. Can't get mind off thoughts
29. Fears	42. Rather be alone	51. Feels dizzy	12. Lonely	18. Harms self
30. Fears school	65. Refuses to talk	54. Overtired	25. Doesn't get along	40. Hears things
31. Fears doing bad	69. Secretive	56a. Aches, pains	27. Jealous	46. Twitching
32. Must be perfect	75. Shy, timid	56b. Headaches	34. Others out to get him/her	58. Picks skin
33. Feels unloved	102. Lacks energy	56c. Nausea	36. Accident-prone	66. Repeats acts
35. Feels worthless	103. Sad	56d. Eye problems	38. Gets teased	70. Sees things
45. Nervous, tense	111. Withdrawn	56e. Skin problems	48. Not liked	76. Sleeps less[c]
50. Fearful, anxious		56f. Stomachaches	62. Clumsy	83. Stores things
52. Feels too guilty		56g. Vomiting	64. Prefers younger kids	84. Strange behavior
71. Self-conscious		**Specific to CBCL**	79. Speech problems	85. Strange ideas
91. Talks or thinks of suicide		49. Constipated[c,d]		100. Trouble sleeping[c]
112. Worries				**Specific to CBCL**
Specific to TRF				59. Sex parts in public[c,d]
81. Hurt when criticized[b,d]				60. Sex parts too much[c,d]
106. Anxious to please[b,c]				92. Sleep talks/walks[c,d]
108. Afraid to make mistakes[b,c]				

TABLE 2–1. Items defining the school-age syndromes, plus items specific to the Child Behavior Checklist/6–18 (CBCL/6–18), Youth Self-Report (YSR), and Teacher's Report Form (TRF) syndrome scales[a] *(continued)*

Attention Problems	Rule-Breaking Behavior	Aggressive Behavior
1. Acts young	2. Drinks alcohol[c]	3. Argues a lot
4. Fails to finish	26. Lacks guilt	16. Mean to others
8. Can't concentrate	28. Breaks rules	19. Demands attention
10. Can't sit still	39. Bad friends	20. Destroys own things
13. Confused	43. Lies, cheats	21. Destroys others' things
17. Daydreams	63. Prefers older kids	22. Disobedient at home[c]
41. Impulsive	67. Runs away[c]	23. Disobedient at school
61. Poor schoolwork	72. Sets fires[c]	37. Gets in fights
78. Inattentive	73. Sex problems[c,d]	57. Attacks people
80. Stares blankly[d]	81. Steals at home[c]	68. Screams a lot
Specific to TRF	82. Steals outside home	86. Stubborn, sullen
2. Odd noises[b,d]	90. Swearing	87. Mood changes
7. Brags	96. Thinks of sex too much	88. Sulks[d]
15. Fidgets[b,d]	99. Uses tobacco	89. Suspicious
22. Difficulty with directions[b,d]	101. Truant	94. Teases a lot
24. Disturbs others[b,d]	105. Uses drugs	95. Temper
49. Difficulty learning[b,d]	106. Vandalism[c,d]	97. Threatens others
53. Talks out of turn[b,d]	**Specific to TRF**	104. Loud
60. Apathetic[b,d]	98. Tardy[b,d]	**Specific to TRF**
67. Disrupts discipline[b,d]		6. Defiant[b,d]
72. Messy work[b,d]		76. Explosive[b,d]
73. Irresponsible[b,d]		77. Easily frustrated[b,d]
74. Shows off		
92. Underachieving[b,d]		
93. Talks too much		
100. Fails to carry out tasks[b,d]		
109. Whining[d]		

[a]Items are designated by the numbers they bear on the CBCL/6–18, YSR, and TRF and summaries of their content. From Achenbach and Rescorla 2001. [b]Not on CBCL. [c]Not on TRF. [d]Not on YSR.

loquial American descriptions of problems into many other languages could cause the basic items to be interpreted differently by parents, teachers, and youths in other societies. Furthermore, the informants' feelings about completing rating forms, their judgments and memories of problems, and their willingness to report problems are apt to vary greatly among different societies. Equally important, factors such as the number of children in families and in school classes, parent and teacher expectations, and the structures of family and school systems could affect informants' reports. In addition to all these possible influences on the findings, there may also be major differences in the actual prevalence and patterning of problems in different societies.

For all of the foregoing reasons, the syndrome model was not expected to be supported in societies as different from the United States as Iran, Ethiopia, the People's Republic of China, Lebanon, and Russia. Yet, to the amazement of the research team, the syndrome model was supported in data from more than 115,000 assessment forms completed by parents, teachers, and youths in all the societies that were analyzed.

The support for the syndrome model in so many societies indicates that the eight syndromes reflect considerable multicultural consistency in the patterns of problems reported by parents, teachers, and youths. The findings do not necessarily mean that the assessed problems are the only ones pertinent to child and adolescent psychopathology. Nor do the findings mean that the syndrome model reflects the only patterns that might be detectable in every society. Nevertheless, the findings do indicate that the syndrome model is generalizable well beyond the U.S. society in which it was developed. The findings justify using the eight syndromes as foci for research, training, and practice in the societies where they have been supported, as outlined in the following sections.

DISTRIBUTIONS OF PROBLEMS IN MANY SOCIETIES

The support for the syndrome model in many societies justifies making rigorous comparisons of scores obtained on the syndromes in those societies. Dr. Leslie Rescorla and colleagues have statistically compared scores on each of the eight syndromes obtained from CBCL, TRF, and YSR ratings in general population samples from the societies in which the confirmatory factor analyses had supported the syndromes (Rescorla et al. 2007a, 2007b, 2007c). They also compared CBCL, TRF, and YSR scores for Total Problems (the sum of ratings on all problem items), Internalizing (the sum of scores on the Anxious/Depressed, Depressed/Withdrawn, and Somatic Complaints syndromes), Externalizing (the sum of scores on the Rule-Breaking Behavior and Aggressive Behavior syndromes), and each of the DSM-oriented scales (Affective Problems, Anxiety Problems, Somatic Problems, Attention Deficit Hyperactivity Problems, Oppositional Defiant Problems, and Conduct Problems). In addition to comparing the scores from each society on each scale, Rescorla and colleagues tested the effects of age, gender, and interactions of society with age and gender on scores for each scale.

Using Cohen's (1988) criteria for the magnitudes of effect sizes in analyses of variance, effect sizes accounting for 1%–6% of the variance are small, and effect sizes accounting for 6%–14% of the variance are medium. The effects of differences among all societies ranged from small to medium on the various scales. Thus there were some definite but mostly modest differences among the mean scale scores obtained in different societies. Figure 2–1 graphically depicts the mean Total Problems scores on the TRF in 21 societies. No interactions of culture with age and gender explained even 1% of the variance. This finding indicated that age and gender effects were quite consistent across diverse cultures. The overall mean in Figure 2–1 is the arithmetical average of the mean scores from the 21 societies.

Gender Differences

Analyses of gender differences revealed some significant gender effects that were very consistent across societies. As an example, Figure 2–2 illustrates the consistency with which teachers rated boys higher than girls on the DSM-oriented Attention Deficit Hyperactivity Problems syndrome in every society except Iran, where the gender difference was negligible. A difference between the Iranian sample and those from the other societies was that, in accord with standard practices in Iran, all the Iranian students attended single-gender schools (n=90 boys schools and 90 girls schools). Although we could hypothesize that teachers might rate girls higher on attention problems when no boys are in the classes than when there are boys for comparison, Rescorla et al. (2007b) found that Iranian parents, unlike parents in the other societies, also rated girls as high as boys on Attention Problems. The Iranian exception to findings of higher Attention Problems scores for boys than girls was thus not limited to teachers' ratings.

Overlapping Distributions of Scores

The statistical and bar graph comparisons of scores from many societies focus on the mean of each distribution of scores. However, it is essential to remember that the scores from each society are broadly distributed around the mean score for each society. In fact, the scores from every society overlap with the scores from every other society. As illustrated in Figure 2–3, even when

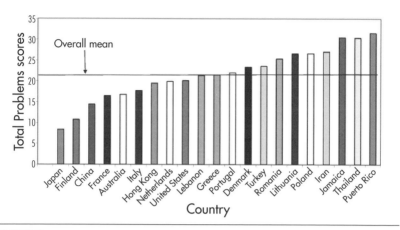

FIGURE 2–1. **Teacher's Report Form Total Problems scores in 21 societies (*N* =30,957).**

The "overall mean" is the arithmetical mean of the 21 mean Total Problems scores. *Source.* Reprinted from Rescorla LA, Achenbach TM, Ginzburg S, et al.: "Consistency of Teacher-Reported Problems for Students in 21 Countries." *School Psychology Review* 36:91–110, 2007. Used with permission.

we divide societies into those with relatively low mean Total Problems scores (>1 standard deviation below the multicultural mean), those with medium Total Problems scores (from –1 to +1 standard deviation from the multicultural mean), and those with relatively high mean Total Problems scores (>1 standard deviation above the multicultural mean), there is much overlap among scores from all three groups of societies. Equally important is that differences between societies accounted for only 4%–14% of the variance in the scale scores. This finding means that individual differences within societies accounted for the remaining 86%–96% of the variance.

CORRELATES OF PROBLEM SCORES IN DIFFERENT SOCIETIES

The use of the same standardized instruments for assessing psychopathology in many societies makes it possible to determine whether correlates of problem scores identified in one society are generalizable to other societies. Findings presented in the previous section indicated that gender differences on certain scales, such as Attention Deficit Hyperactivity Problems, are very consistent across many societies. Other kinds of correlates of the scale scores that have been tested in multiple societies include psychiatric diagnoses, referral for mental health services, genetic factors, socioeconomic

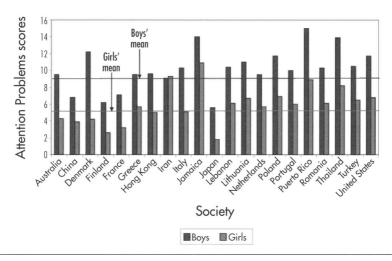

FIGURE 2–2. Teachers' ratings of the DSM-oriented Attention Deficit Hyperactivity Problems scale by gender in 21 societies (*N*=30,957).

Source. Reprinted from Achenbach TM, Rescorla LA: *Multicultural Understanding of Child and Adolescent Psychopathology: Implications for Mental Health Assessment.* New York, Guilford, 2007. Used with permission.

status (SES), developmental course, and long-term outcomes. The main findings are summarized only briefly here, but detailed reviews are available elsewhere (see, e.g., Achenbach and Rescorla 2007b).

Diagnoses and Referral for Mental Health Services

Studies from at least nine societies have reported that children or youth who were referred for mental health services or who qualified for DSM diagnoses obtained significantly higher scores on CBCL, TRF, and/or YSR scales than those who were not referred or did not qualify for diagnoses. The studies of diagnoses have also reported significant associations between particular diagnoses and analogous problem scales. For example, diagnoses of attention-deficit/hyperactivity disorder have been significantly associated with high scores on the Attention Problems scale. Similarly, diagnoses of oppositional defiant disorder and conduct disorder have been significantly associated with high scores on the Rule-Breaking Behavior and Aggressive Behavior scales.

Genetic Factors

More than 160 published studies from societies, including the Netherlands, Norway, Sweden, Taiwan, the United Kingdom, and the United States, have

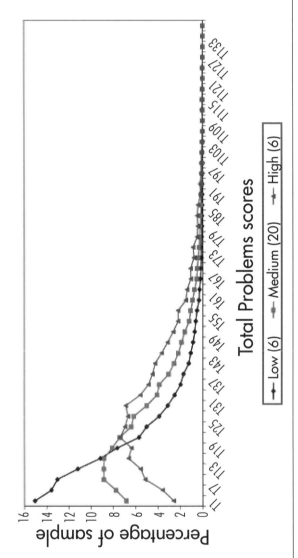

FIGURE 2–3. **Overlapping distribution of Child Behavior Checklist Total Problems scores.**

From societies where mean scores were at least 1 standard deviation below the omnicultural mean ("low-scoring societies"), within 1 standard deviation of the overall mean ("medium-scoring societies"), or at least 1 standard deviation above the overall mean ("high-scoring societies"). Each hash mark on the horizontal axis includes three Total Problems scores (e.g., T1=0, 1, 2).

Source. Reprinted from Achenbach TM, Rescorla LA: *Multicultural Understanding of Child and Adolescent Psychopathology: Implications for Mental Health Assessment.* New York, Guilford, 2007. Used with permission.

reported significant associations of scores on the problem scales with genetic factors (Bérubé and Achenbach 2008). An especially important finding from several societies is higher heritability for the Aggressive Behavior syndrome than for the Rule-Breaking Behavior syndrome. Although the diagnostic category of conduct disorder encompasses both syndromes, the different heritabilities indicate that problems of aggression have different etiologic pathways than do unaggressive violations of social mores.

Socioeconomic Status

With SES measured in terms of parental education and/or occupation, studies in 15 societies have consistently revealed higher problem scores for lower-SES than higher-SES children and youth, even where income differences were relatively small, such as in China and Sweden. Associations between some forms of adult psychopathology and low SES may be attributable to the "downward drift" of disturbed adults who are unable to hold high-level jobs. However, children's behavior does not determine the SES of their families. Consequently, the effects of downward drift can be avoided in longitudinal analyses of SES differences in incidence and remission rates for clinically deviant problem scores from childhood through young adulthood.

Longitudinal analyses of this sort have revealed an elevated incidence of deviant scores on certain scales among lower-SES individuals at multiple developmental periods (Wadsworth and Achenbach 2005). Equally important, among individuals who had deviant scale scores, lower-SES individuals less frequently remitted than higher-SES individuals. Thus, higher incidence and lower remission rates may both contribute to elevated rates of psychopathology among lower-SES individuals, independent of the downward drift that may later result from adult psychopathology.

Developmental Course and Long-Term Outcomes

Longitudinal studies in several societies have revealed long-term predictive relations between initial scores on the CBCL, TRF, and YSR and subsequent measures, diagnoses, and signs of disturbance. The longest study of this type began with a general population sample of 2,076 Dutch 4- to 16-year-olds who were then reassessed periodically over the next 21 years with the CBCL, TRF, and YSR, and later with adult versions of these instruments. Individually administered psychiatric interviews were used to make DSM diagnoses, and data were obtained on signs of disturbance, including suicidal behavior, substance abuse, police contacts, school problems, and use of mental health services.

It was found that child and adolescent scores on several scales significantly predicted adult diagnoses and signs of disturbance. Especially important for the developmental study of psychopathology, some scales predicted different outcomes in adulthood than during childhood and adolescence. For example, childhood scores on the Social Problems and Externalizing scales significantly predicted adult anxiety disorders, after other predictors were controlled for, but these scores have not been found to predict anxiety disorders during childhood (Roza et al. 2003). Studies of outcomes in clinical samples have also revealed significant predictive relations between childhood scale scores obtained at intake into mental health services and outcomes in later developmental periods (e.g., Stanger et al.1996; Visser et al. 2003).

STUDIES OF IMMIGRANTS: COMPARISONS OF TURKISH IMMIGRANT CHILDREN, TURKISH CHILDREN IN TURKEY, AND DUTCH CHILDREN

In addition to advancing the developmental study of psychopathology, the use of the same standardized instruments to assess members of diverse cultural groups can illuminate how the behavioral and emotional problems of immigrants compare with the problems of peers in their home societies and with those of people in the host societies. Increasing demands on host society mental health, education, and welfare systems to serve millions of immigrants argue for assessment instruments that can be used to identify problems that characterize particular cultural groups. Such instruments may also be used to determine whether particular problems are associated with immigration and to help policy makers and practitioners tailor services to the needs of each cultural group.

Comparisons of problems reported for Dutch children, Turkish immigrant children in the Netherlands, and Turkish children in Turkey illustrate how a particular set of standardized assessment instruments can illuminate similarities and differences between cultural groups and can also aid in policy and clinical decisions. Comparisons of CBCLs completed for 2,081 Dutch children, 833 Turkish children living in the Netherlands, and 3,127 Turkish children living in Turkey showed that Turkish children in the Netherlands scored significantly higher than Dutch children on six problem scales, with the largest difference being on the Anxious/Depressed scale (effect size=16%, which meets Cohen's criterion for a large effect) (Bengi-Arslan et al. 1997). Problem scores obtained for Turkish children in Turkey were also significantly higher than scores obtained for Dutch children, especially on the Anxious/Depressed scale. However, the problem scores of Turkish children in Turkey were somewhat lower than the problem scores of Turkish children in the Netherlands. The findings thus showed that Turkish parents in general report more problems than Dutch parents, especially on the Anxious/Depressed syndrome but that factors associated with immigration may increase Turkish problem scores somewhat. The authors of the study suggested that the exceptionally high Anxious/Depressed scores for both groups of Turkish children may reflect children's reactions to childrearing practices characterized by strict demands for obedience, harsh verbal criticism, physical punishment, and threats of punishment by God.

Cross-Informant Comparisons

The importance of obtaining reports from multiple informants is highlighted by problem scores obtained from Dutch teachers' ratings of Turkish students. When students were rated by Dutch teachers, Turkish students' problem scores did not differ significantly from Dutch students' problem scores, after SES was controlled for (Crijnen et al. 2000). However, when Turkish immigrant students were rated by Turkish teachers who instructed them for part of the school day, they obtained much higher Anxious/Depressed scores (effect size=20%) than did the Dutch students rated by Dutch teachers. The authors interpreted this finding as indicating that Turkish teachers, who shared the students' cultural heritage and language, were much more aware of the Turkish students' anxiety and depression than were the Dutch teachers.

Significantly higher scores on the Anxious/Depressed scale and other problem scales have also been found on YSRs completed by Turkish immigrant youths than by Dutch youths (Murad et al. 2003). Thus, Turkish immigrants consistently obtained elevated scores on the Anxious/Depressed scale according to reports by Turkish parents, teachers, and youths, but not according to Dutch teachers of Turkish students.

Importance of Individual Differences

The finding of significantly elevated problem scores for Turkish immigrants in the Netherlands does not mean that all Turkish immigrants have uniformly high scores. As Figure 2–3 shows, individual problem scores are widely distributed, with much overlap among the scores obtained in societies with low, medium, and high mean scores. And, as shown by comparisons of scores from many societies, individual differences *within* societies accounted for much more variance than the differences *between* societies. Research on factors associated with individual differences in problem scores obtained by Turkish immigrants in the Netherlands has shown that higher Anxious/Depressed scores were associated with parental arguments, incarceration of a family member, theft or fire in the home, and family financial or employment problems (Sowa et al. 2000). Thus, even when there is consistent evidence for markedly elevated rates of problems in a particular group, such as on the Anxious/Depressed syndrome for Turkish immigrants in the Netherlands, the individual differences in scores and associated factors argue for evaluating the specific characteristics of individuals in relation to relevant norms. For immigrants, the relevant norms may include those based on representative samples from both their own society of origin and the host society in which they reside. The following sections present practical methods for using multicultural norms to evaluate individuals for research and clinical purposes.

MULTICULTURAL NORMS

To facilitate practical applications of norms from different societies, we have identified societies whose mean Total Problems scores were at least 1 standard deviation below or above the omnicultural mean on the CBCL, TRF, or YSR (Achenbach and Rescorla 2007a). To create norms for the low-scoring societies, we computed averages of the percentage of children from all the low-scoring societies who obtained each score on a scale, such as the Attention Problems syndrome scale. The average percentages of children from low-scoring societies who obtained each score were then used to generate the low-scoring society percentiles for all the scores on the Attention Problems scale. A similar procedure was used to create norms for high-scoring societies.

If a user wishes to compare a child's score on the problem scales with norms for the low-scoring societies, the user clicks the option for the scoring software to display a profile of the child's scale scores in relation to the norms generated from the low-scoring societies, as illustrated in Figure 2–4. In addition to displaying the child's profile of scores in relation to the norms for the low-scoring societies, the software also prints the percentile and standard score (T score) for the child's score on each scale, based on the norms for the low-scoring societies.

If the user wants to display the same child's scale scores in relation to norms for the middle-scoring societies or high-scoring societies, the user merely clicks the respective options. The options for displaying a child's scale scores in relation to low-, middle-, and/or high-scoring societies are helpful for both clinical evaluations of individual children and for research on particular groups. As an example, if we are evaluating a Japanese youth living in the United States, we may want to display his scale scores obtained from a CBCL completed by his mother in relation to the low-scoring norms,

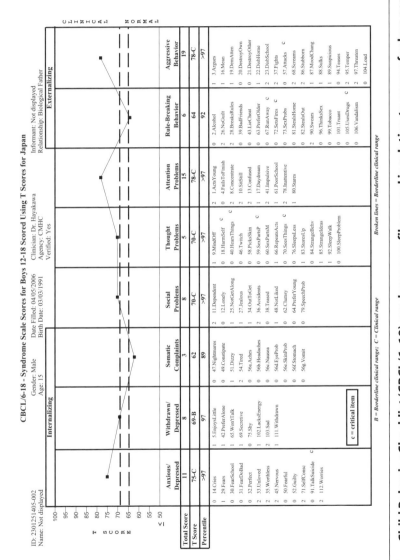

FIGURE 2–4.   Child Behavior Checklist (CBCL/6–18) syndrome profile scored in relation to norms for low-scoring societies.

Source.   Reprinted from Achenbach TM, Rescorla LA: *Multicultural Supplement to the Manual for the ASEBA School-Age Forms and Profiles.* Burlington, University of Vermont Research Center for Children, Youth, and Families, 2007. Used with permission.

because CBCL scores in the sample from Japan were more than 1 standard deviation below the omnicultural mean. However, if the youth has lived in the United States for a long time, we may also want to display the scale scores obtained from his mother's CBCL in relation to the middle-scoring norms, which include the United States.

It is important to note that a particular society's norms may be from the low-scoring group for the CBCL but from the middle- or high-scoring group for the TRF or YSR. Although Japanese normative data for both the CBCL and TRF qualify for the low-scoring group, Japanese youth report enough problems on the YSR to place their normative data in the middle-scoring group. Consequently, when we evaluate a Japanese youth in relation to norms from Japan, we would click the option for the low-scoring norms for CBCLs and TRFs completed by Japanese parents and teachers but select the middle-scoring norms for the YSR completed by the youth. If the youth had U.S. teachers, we would probably want to display the youth's TRF scale scores in relation to the middle-scoring norms, which include the United States.

Cross-Informant Comparisons in Relation to Multicultural Norms

Meta-analyses have yielded correlations averaging only 0.28 between reports of psychopathology by informants who play different roles with respect to the children being assessed (e.g., parents, teachers, mental health workers, observers) (Achenbach et al. 1987). The correlations averaged only 0.22 between children's self-reports and reports by people who knew the children, including parents, teachers, and mental health workers. For adult psychopathology, meta-analyses have yielded a mean correlation of 0.45 between self-reports and collateral reports of diverse problems except substance use (Achenbach et al. 2005). A higher mean correlation of 0.68 was obtained between adult self-reports and collateral reports of substance use, perhaps because judgments of substance use are less inferential than judgments of other kinds of problems. Kappas between diagnoses based on self-reports versus reports by others have been reported to range from only 0.12 to 0.18 (Meyer et al. 2001).

The low to moderate agreement between reports of psychopathology by different informants indicates that no one informant's reports can substitute for reports by others. Instead, comprehensive assessment requires data from other people, as well as from self-reports. For assessing children, it is especially important to obtain data from parent figures and from as many teachers as possible, as well as from children who are old enough to provide self-reports.

To facilitate comparisons of data from multiple informants in relation to multicultural norms, the software that displays profiles of scale scores also displays comparisons between scores obtained from different informants' ratings. As an example, Figure 2–5 displays DSM-oriented scale scores from CBCLs completed by a 15-year-old Japanese youth's mother and father, TRFs completed by three teachers, and the YSR completed by the youth himself. This youth has lived in the United States for a long time and attends an American school. However, because his parents remain immersed in Japanese culture and they completed a Japanese translation of the CBCL, the scales scored from their CBCLs are shown in Figure 2–5 in relation to the low-scoring norms, which include Japan. Because the TRFs were completed by the youth's American teachers, the TRF scale scores are shown in relation to the middle-scoring norms, which include the United States. And because both Japanese and U.S. YSR norms are included in the middle-scoring norms, the YSR scale scores are shown in relation to these norms.

Clinical, Research, and Systems Applications

Twenty-first century clinicians, researchers, and managers of mental health, education, and welfare systems increasingly need to take account of cultural differences, clashes, and blending. As Hermans and Kempen (1998, 1999) have argued, cultures are not concrete entities that are "internally homogeneous and externally distinct." Although individuals may be classified according to their membership in particular cultural groups, individual differences in psychopathology within groups are at least as important as differences between groups. To cope effectively with cultural variations, we need to take account of both the within-group and between-group differences.

The foregoing sections illustrated how assessment of individual children and youth can include comparisons of multi-informant reports with multicultural norms. Effective use of multicultural data for evaluating individuals requires flexible approaches that avoid monolithic assumptions about either differences or similarities between people from different cultural backgrounds. For purposes of research and systems management, the same standardized assessment instruments can be used as are used for clinical assessment. The use of the same assessment instruments can facilitate applications of research findings to clinical assessment of individuals and to documentation of needs and outcomes for people served by mental health, education, and welfare systems.

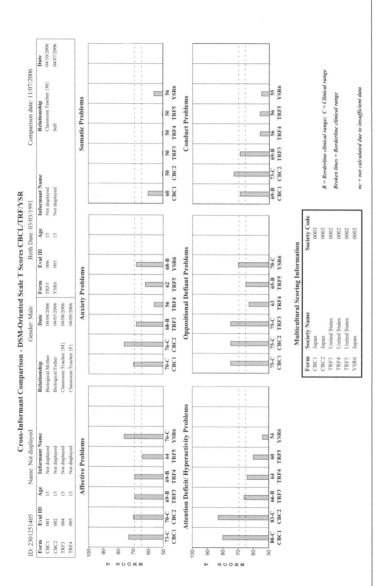

FIGURE 2–5.   Cross-informant comparisons of DSM-oriented scale scores in relation to Child Behavior Checklist (CBCL) norms for low-scoring societies and Teacher's Report Form (TRF) and Youth Self-Report (YSR) norms for medium-scoring societies.

Source.   Reprinted from Achenbach TM, Rescorla LA: *Multicultural Supplement to the Manual for the ASEBA School-Age Forms and Profiles.* Burlington, University of Vermont Research Center for Children, Youth, and Families, 2007. Used with permission.

FUTURE DIRECTIONS

This chapter has focused largely on school-age children and youth. However, the same assessment model has been used for preschoolers, adults, and the elderly (Achenbach and Rescorla 2000, 2003; Achenbach et al. 2004). Consequently, similar multicultural applications can eventually be made to these additional developmental periods. As the developmental study of psychopathology advances, it can illuminate continuities and discontinuities in phenotypic psychopathology and in underlying etiologic factors across the life span. The empirically based syndromes described in this chapter were derived from data for ages 6–18, but similar methods have been used to derive syndromes for ages 1½–5, 18–59, and 60 to over 90 years. Some syndromal patterns are quite similar across multiple developmental periods. Other patterns vary in some respects from one period to another, whereas still others are limited to particular developmental periods.

Just as there may be similarities, variations, and dissimilarities in psychopathology across the lifespan, there may also be similarities, variations, and dissimilarities in psychopathology across different cultural groups. The extension of the developmental study of psychopathology across the lifespan and across more societies can greatly enrich our understanding of the relations between normal and abnormal development.

CONCLUSIONS

Nearly everything about humans is related to genes, to the environment, and to developmental interplays between them. Although the "environment" includes myriad variables, cultural aspects of human environments are becoming increasingly important to consider. To build a generalizable science of psychopathology, we must broaden our database beyond a handful of Western societies. We must also overcome tendencies to view cultures as categorically different from one another. Multicultural research requires that assessment instruments be tested in different societies. If the instruments function well for members of different societies, they can provide a multicultural basis for research, training, and treatment. They can also be used by the mental health, education, and welfare systems of host societies to evaluate the needs of millions of immigrants from other societies.

No assessment instrument can be expected to include everything that is important about psychopathology in all societies. Nevertheless, it is important to apply the same methods to different cultural groups in order to identify both similarities and differences on a common core set of attributes. This chapter summarized applications of the same standardized assessment instruments to tens of thousands of children and youth in many societies.

Syndromes of co-occurring problems were found to be similar across all the societies in parent ratings, teacher ratings, and self-ratings. Although there were statistically significant variations in problem scores across societies, the scores for most societies were close to the omnicultural mean (the arithmetical average of the mean scores from all societies).

To take account of differences between societies with relatively low versus medium versus high scores, researchers have constructed three sets of multicultural norms. Individuals' scores on syndromes, DSM-oriented scales, Internalizing, Externalizing, and Total Problems can be displayed in relation to norms for low-scoring, medium-scoring, and high-scoring societies. Comparisons between ratings by different informants can also be displayed in relation to the low, middle, and high norms.

Despite differences in mean problem scores among societies, the distributions of scores from each society overlap the distributions from all the other societies. Statistical analyses showed that individual differences in scores accounted for far more variance than differences between societies. Studies in several societies have found significant correlates of the individual differences in scores, including psychiatric diagnoses, referral for mental health services, genetic factors, SES, developmental course, and outcomes. The applicability of the same standardized assessment instruments to different cultural groups has enabled comparisons of psychopathology among immigrants to psychopathology among the immigrants' peers who remained in their home society and to psychopathology among members of the host society.

The same standardized instruments can be applied to clinical assessment, to research, and to documentation of needs and outcomes for people served by mental health, education, and welfare systems. Although most of the multicultural findings to date are for school-age children and youth, the availability of similar standardized assessment instruments for preschoolers, adults, and the elderly make it possible to extend the multicultural developmental study of psychopathology across the lifespan.

REFERENCES

Achenbach TM: A factor-analytic study of juvenile psychiatric symptoms. Paper presented at Society for Research in Child Development, Minneapolis, MN, March 1965

Achenbach TM: The classification of children's psychiatric symptoms: a factor-analytic study. Psychol Monogr 80:1–37, 1966

Achenbach TM: Developmental Psychopathology. New York, Wiley, 1974

Achenbach TM: Developmental Psychopathology, 2nd Edition. New York, Wiley, 1982

Achenbach TM, Rescorla LA: Manual for the ASEBA Preschool Forms and Profiles. Burlington, University of Vermont, Research Center for Children, Youth, and Families, 2000

Achenbach TM, Rescorla LA: Manual for the ASEBA School-Age Forms and Profiles. Burlington, University of Vermont, Research Center for Children, Youth, and Families, 2001

Achenbach TM, Rescorla LA: Manual for the ASEBA Adult Forms and Profiles. Burlington, University of Vermont, Research Center for Children, Youth, and Families, 2003

Achenbach TM, Rescorla LA: Multicultural Supplement to the Manual for the ASEBA School-Age Forms and Profiles. Burlington, University of Vermont Research Center for Children, Youth, and Families, 2007a

Achenbach TM, Rescorla LA: Multicultural Understanding of Child and Adolescent Psychopathology: Implications for Mental Health Assessment. New York, Guilford, 2007b

Achenbach TM, McConaughy SH, Howell CT: Child/adolescent behavioral and emotional problems: Implications of cross-informant correlations for situational specificity. Psychol Bull 101:213–232, 1987

Achenbach TM, Newhouse PA, Rescorla LA: Manual for the ASEBA Older Adult Forms and Profiles. Burlington, VT, University of Vermont, Research Center for Children, Youth, and Families, 2004

Achenbach TM, Krukowski RA, Dumenci L, et al: Assessment of adult psychopathology: meta-analyses and implications of cross-informant correlations. Psychol Bull 131:361–382, 2005

American Psychiatric Association: Diagnostic and Statistical Manual: Mental Disorders. Washington, DC, American Psychiatric Association, 1952

American Psychiatric Association: Diagnostic and Statistical Manual of Mental Disorders, 4th Edition, Text Revision. Washington, DC, American Psychiatric Association, 2000

Bengi-Arslan L, Verhulst FC, van der Ende J, et al: Understanding childhood (problem) behavior from a cultural perspective: comparison of problem behaviors and competencies in Turkish immigrant, Turkish and Dutch children. Soc Psychiatry Psychiatr Epidemiol 32:477–484, 1997

Bérubé RL, Achenbach TM: Bibliography of Published Studies Using the Achenbach System of Empirically Based Assessment (ASEBA): 2008 Edition. Burlington, VT, University of Vermont, Research Center for Children, Youth, and Families, 2008

Cicchetti D, Cohen DJ (eds): Developmental Psychopathology. New York, Wiley, 1995

Cicchetti D, Cohen DJ (eds): Developmental Psychopathology, 2nd Edition. Hoboken, NJ, Wiley, 2006

Cohen J: Statistical Power Analysis for the Behavioral Sciences, 2nd Edition. New York, Academic Press, 1988

Crijnen AAM, Bengi-Arslan L, Verhulst FC: Teacher-reported problem behaviour in Turkish immigrant and Dutch children: A cross-cultural comparison. Acta Psychiatr Scand 102:439–444, 2000

Gove PB (ed): Webster's Third New International Dictionary of the English Language. Springfield, MA, Merriam, 1971

Hermans HJM, Kempen HJG: Moving cultures: the perilous problems of cultural dichotomies in a globalizing society. Am Psychol 53:1111–1120, 1998

Hermans HJM, Kempen HJG: Categorical thinking is the target. Am Psychol 54:840–841, 1999

Ivanova MY, Achenbach TM, Rescorla LA, et al: The generalizability of the Youth Self-Report syndrome structure in 23 societies. J Consult Clin Psychol 75:729–738, 2007a

Ivanova MY, Achenbach TM, Dumenci L, et al: Testing the eight-syndrome structure of the Child Behavior Checklist in 30 societies. J Clin Child Adolesc Psychol 36:405–417, 2007b

Ivanova MY, Achenbach TM, Rescorla LA, et al: Testing the Teacher's Report Form syndromes in 20 societies. Sch Psychol Rev 36:468–483, 2007c

McConaughy SH, Achenbach TM: Manual for the Semistructured Clinical Interview for Children and Adolescents, 2nd Edition. Burlington, VT, University of Vermont, Research Center for Children, Youth, and Families, 2001

McConaughy SH, Achenbach TM: Manual for the Test Observation Form for Ages 2–18. Burlington, VT, University of Vermont, Research Center for Children, Youth, and Families, 2004

Meyer GJ, Finn SE, Eyde LD, et al: Psychological testing and psychological assessment: a review of evidence and issues. Am Psychol 56:128–165, 2001

Murad SD, Joung IM, van Lenthe FJ, et al: Predictors of self-reported problem behaviours in Turkish immigrant and Dutch adolescents in the Netherlands. J Child Psychol Psychiatry 44:412–423, 2003

Rescorla LA, Achenbach TM, Ginzburg, S, et al: Consistency of teacher-reported problems for students in 21 countries. Sch Psychol Rev 36:91–110, 2007a

Rescorla LA, Achenbach TM, Ivanova MY, et al: Behavioral and emotional problems reported by parents of children ages 6 to 16 in 31 societies. J Emot Behav Disord 15:130–142, 2007b

Rescorla LA, Achenbach TM, Ivanova MY, et al: Epidemiological comparisons of problems and positive qualities reported by adolescents in 24 countries. J Consult Clin Psychol 75:351–358, 2007c

Roza SJ, Hofstra MB, van der Ende J, et al: Stable prediction of mood and anxiety disorders based on behavioral and emotional problems in childhood: a 14-year follow-up during childhood, adolescence and young adulthood. Am J Psychiatry 160:2116–2121, 2003

Rutter M: Genes and Behavior: Nature-Nurture Interplay Explained. Malden, MA, Blackwell Publishing, 2006

Rutter M, Garmezy N: Developmental psychopathology, in Handbook of Child Psychology, 4th Edition, Vol 4: Socialization, Personality, and Social Development. Edited by Mussen PH (series ed), Hetherington EM (volume ed). New York, Wiley, 1983, pp 775–911

Sowa H, Crijnen AA, Bengi-Arslan L, et al: Factors associated with problem behaviors in Turkish immigrant children in the Netherlands. Soc Psychiatry Psychiatr Epidemiol 35:177–184, 2000

Stanger C, MacDonald VV, McConaughy SH, et al: Predictors of cross-informant syndromes among children and youths referred for mental health services. J Abnorm Child Psychol 24:597–614, 1996

Visser JH, van der Ende J, Koot HM, et al: Predicting change in psychopathology in youth referred to mental health services in childhood or adolescence. J Child Psychol Psychiatry 44:509–519, 2003

Wadsworth ME, Achenbach TM: Explaining the link between low socioeconomic status and psychopathology: testing two mechanisms of the social causation hypothesis. J Consult Clin Psychol 73:1146–1153, 2005

Chapter 3

SOCIAL CONTEXT AND DEVELOPMENTAL PSYCHOPATHOLOGY

Dana March, M.P.H.
Ezra Susser, M.D., Dr.P.H.

The developmental psychopathology perspective grew in the 1970s in response to the conceptual limitations of its seeding disciplines, psychiatry and developmental psychology. At its core is a concern with the factors, which tend to be specific to the developmental context, that influence cognitive, affective, and behavioral outcomes (Achenbach 1974; Buka et al. 2001; Costello et al. 1991, 1996, 1997, 2006; Rutter and Sroufe 2000; Rutter et al. 1976). In other words, at different stages in development, different factors may play important roles or the same factors may have different effects. Concerned explicitly with the origins and course of individual patterns of behavioral maladaption over the life course, developmental psychopathology seeks to illuminate the processes underlying both continuity and change in those patterns (Rutter and Sroufe 2000; Sroufe and Rutter 1984).

Over several decades, this perspective has provided a crucial framework for investigating the causes, course, and variable manifestations of mental disorders. It has gained further currency by its integration with the study of genetic susceptibility. Some of the key findings on genetic determinants of mental disorders have, in fact, derived from studies that accord with this perspective. The Dunedin study, for example, traced the course of psychopathology from birth up to adulthood and examined genetic and environmental exposures in tandem (Caspi et al. 2003a, 2003b; Kim-Cohen et al. 2003; Silva and Stanton 1996).

We propose that developmental psychopathology can be similarly enhanced by integration with the study of social context. The effect of exposures associated with psychopathology also varies according to social context. Indeed, social context may shape the *meaning* of exposures for individuals. Most investigators in this field would readily agree that social factors are important, demonstrated by the approaches put forward and the landmark studies conducted over the past 50 years (e.g., Costello et al. 1996, 2003; Leighton 1959; Rutter et al. 1976). Nonetheless, social context has not been the main focus of developmental psychopathology and presents a unique set of conceptual and methodological challenges (Boyce et al. 1998; Rutter 1988; Sullivan 1998). Embracing these challenges would naturally extend the perspective of developmental psychopathology and enrich our understanding of the etiology of psychopathology.

As reflected by research in developmental psychopathology, the characteristics, continuities, and discontinuities of the social context within which the developing individual is situated are less well characterized than either individuals or developmental processes themselves. One of the challenges in the study of social context is the conceptualization and measurement of exposures at different levels of social organization. In this chapter, therefore, we discuss the concept of levels of organization and describe how it could be applied to investigate the social context in developmental psychopathology by using an example from schizophrenia research. Another challenge in the study of social context is to understand how its importance varies over the life course. Thus, in this chapter, we also address the need to advance etiologic research that encompasses both the developmental and the social context.

LEVELS OF ORGANIZATION

In *Uses of Epidemiology*, first published in 1957, J.N. Morris advanced notions that populations have unique properties representing more than just the amalgamation of their constituents' properties and that population health differs from individual health. *Uses of Epidemiology* was followed by *Causal Thinking in the Health Sciences*, in which Mervyn Susser sought "to develop causal models in a manner that will foster understanding of the relationships between states of health and the environment" (M. Susser 1973, p. viii). He formally introduced levels of organization into epidemiology, building on Morris's notion that populations differ from their constituent individuals, and extended the understanding that each level has unique properties and dynamics. These ideas only recently have been taken up quantitatively in the mainstream of epidemiology (Diez Roux 1998).

The fundamental idea behind levels of organization is that phenomena can be arranged in a hierarchy of increasing complexity. Each level of organization is a more complex whole consisting of less complex parts. In relation to its parts, each whole is one level of organization higher and provides the context in which its constituent parts are situated. A whole on one level of organization is a part on a higher level of organization. Conversely, a part on one level of organization is a whole on a lower level of organization. This general concept is applied widely, although here we concern ourselves with its usefulness for studying social context and its influence on health (Schwartz et al. 2006).

Suppose we wish to study how variations in the social context within a large metropolitan area influence the health of people in that area. The metropolitan area comprises towns that organize their own municipal services, such as garbage collection, schools, transportation, and parks. The towns consist of neighborhoods that have distinctive ethnic and socioeconomic profiles. Each neighborhood includes thousands of individuals. In this schema, a neighborhood is a whole consisting of individuals—they are the neighborhood's constituent parts. At the same time a neighborhood is part of a town, which consists of many neighborhoods. Thus, a neighborhood is both a part and a whole. The neighborhood provides the context in which individuals are situated, whereas the town provides the context in which both individuals and neighborhoods are situated.

Each whole has characteristics or properties that are unique from those of its constituent parts. In our hypothetical example, the range and quality of municipal services would be best understood as reflecting a property of the town. Municipal services could vary a great deal across towns, and this variation might explain part of the variation in health across towns. Nonetheless, municipal services could be the same for neighborhoods within a town and for individuals within a neighborhood. Variation in municipal services may not explain any of the variation in health among individuals within a town.

Likewise, neighborhoods have properties that individuals do not. For example, some neighborhoods are ethnically homogeneous; others are ethnically diverse. This characteristic of ethnic diversity varies across neighborhoods, and the ethnic diversity of a given neighborhood certainly contributes to the unique lived experience of all individuals residing therein.

Most often, research in developmental psychopathology focuses on explaining variation in disease risk among individuals within a given population. Yet as our hypothetical example shows, the factors that cause variation in the rates of disorder across populations—or social groups at a specific level of organization—may differ from the factors that cause variation in disease risk among the individuals within a population (Rose 1985; Schwartz and Diez-Roux 2001; E. Susser et al. 2006). If we limit ourselves to the study designs suitable for detecting the factors that cause interindividual variation, we are unlikely to detect the impact of factors at other levels. It follows that focusing exclusively on the individual, although instructive, is also restrictive. Explaining variation in rates of disorder at other levels of social organization is essential to uncovering the full range and sequence of causes of disorder.

In theory, the number of levels of social organization is infinite, beginning with the entire population of the globe and descending through levels such as societies, regions, towns, neighborhoods, families, and, ultimately, individuals. Our first task, then, in any particular investigation of social context, is to select the levels we believe to be most important to the question at hand. In our example, it would be reasonable to limit our investigation to towns, neighborhoods, and individuals. There would be, however, other meaningful levels of organization. For example, the family is a social unit that lies in between the neighborhood and the individual. We cannot possibly encompass all levels in a single study; being cognizant of this limitation helps to prevent misleading or overly narrow interpretations of our results.

The Ecologic Fallacy

Many researchers are familiar with the *ecologic fallacy*. This refers to the circumstance in which an investigator makes a comparison across populations and then mistakenly infers causation at the individual level (Robinson 1950; Schwartz 1994; E. Susser et al. 2006; M. Susser 1973). For example, a study might find that wealthier populations have higher rates of cardiovascular disease. This does not mean that within these populations the wealthier individuals have a higher risk of cardiovascular disease.

Fewer are familiar with the equally important converse fallacy, sometimes referred to as the *atomistic fallacy* (Riley 1963; M. Susser 1973). Suppose we find that within populations the individuals with lower incomes have a higher risk of cardiovascular disease. This does not mean that populations with lower incomes will have higher rates of cardiovascular disease. We cannot reliably infer from an observation of interindividual variation the causes of variation across populations.

Caution about the ecologic fallacy in group-level studies is appropriate, although caution about the atomistic fallacy in individual-level studies is equally appropriate. The key point is that when we study variation at one level of organization, we have to guard against mistakenly inferring causation at another level.

Measurement and Analysis

The most rigorous studies of social context measure it directly at the relevant levels of organization and compare rates of disorder across varying contexts. Such studies, however, are the exception. It is more common to add measures thought to indirectly reflect social context to our studies of individuals. We may, for example, ask people about the municipal services in their town rather than actually measuring them at the level of the town. In addition, we infrequently design our studies so as to ensure sufficient variation at higher levels of organization such as the town in this example.

With the advent of multilevel modeling, analytic approaches do not compel the investigator to prejudice the individual over the contextual variables (Diez Roux 1998). Given the requisite data, it is possible to analyze group-level as well as individual-level variation within the same study. Still, it must be acknowledged that study designs and statistical methods are much better developed for studying variation across individuals than across contexts. For this very reason, it is important to begin a more systematic appraisal of context in developmental psychopathology.

SOCIAL CONTEXT AND SCHIZOPHRENIA

The perspective of developmental psychopathology has enriched our understanding of schizophrenia by focusing on the developmental origins and early manifestations of the disorder. In turn, studies of the developmental origins of schizophrenia have strengthened developmental psychopathology by demonstrating that it is relevant to adult as well as to childhood disorders. Thus, the example of schizophrenia seems apt for illustrating the import of embracing social context.

We share the prevailing view that schizophrenia is a complex neurodevelopmental disorder that has strong genetic causes and is also influenced by environmental exposures early in development (Murray et al. 2002). Yet, social context has a potentially important role to play at every point in the pathogenesis and course of this brain disorder.

At the time of conception the sociocultural environment exerts influence; paternal age at conception, which is determined in part by sociocultural factors, has been established as a risk factor for schizophrenia (Malaspina et al. 2001). During gestation, the mother, the fetus, and the placenta (which mediates the distribution to the fetus of nutrients and toxins taken in by the mother) function collectively as a system. After birth, the child becomes an individual, and the family becomes one of the most meaningful social groupings. It provides the context most proximal to the individual in which development occurs. Moreover, the family provides a meaningful context for offspring with respect to exposures incurred in broader social environments. It is possible that families retain exposures incurred in one social environment and carry them into another social environment, which affects offspring. For instance, recent research exploring the urban-rural difference in schizophrenia demonstrated that children born in rural areas were at increased risk if their families had lived in an urban area prior to their birth (Pedersen and Mortensen 2006). This highlights the importance of the family social grouping for children during gestation and early development with respect to the etiology of schizophrenia (March and Susser 2006). However, social context influences not only the etiology but also the course of psychopathology. Research comparing the course of schizophrenia in developing countries with that of developed countries indicates that affected individuals in developing countries experience a more favorable course of the disorder despite the relative lack of pharmacological and other treatments in such settings (Bresnahan et al. 2003; Hopper and Wanderling 2000; Jablensky et al. 1992; Leff et al. 1992; World Health Organization 1973).

IMMIGRATION AND SCHIZOPHRENIA

The importance of considering social context in the study of schizophrenia is set into relief by a number of examples. Perhaps the most salient example, however, exists in the relationship between immigration and schizophrenia. Immigration itself is defined by the movement from one particular social context to another; thus, it is a phenomenon that cannot be understood without consideration of the characteristics of the social context itself and other potentially operative social factors. Furthermore, the timing of immigration during development may be important for the etiology of schizophrenia. However, as illustrated below, research regarding the association between immigration and schizophrenia is itself at a certain stage of development and requires some encouragement and attention if our understanding is to grow.

Associations between social factors and schizophrenia—or at least insanity—have been observed since the nineteenth century. In a classic study, Edward Jarvis (Jarvis 1855/1971) of Massachusetts identified two social factors associated with insanity: being of low socioeconomic status and being an immigrant (from Ireland). The association with low socioeconomic status was confirmed in numerous studies of schizophrenia and well established by the mid-twentieth century. Then, over a long period, researchers sought to determine the direction of the causal relationship underlying the association: whether low socioeconomic status was a cause or a consequence of schizophrenia. The results overall suggest that it is largely the latter. In studies that measure socioeconomic status antecedent to the disorder—for example, in the family of origin—there is not a consistent association between low socioeconomic status and risk of schizophrenia; when an association is detected, it is generally modest (e.g., Byrne et al. 2004; Wicks et al. 2005).

Jarvis's observation of increased insanity among Irish immigrants was not confirmed; a reanalysis of Jarvis's data suggests the association was probably a result of confounding by low socioeconomic status (Vander Stoep and Link 1998). Later, a classic study conducted by Ödegaard (1932) in the 1930s found immigrants from Norway to the United States to have an increased risk of schizophrenia. Ultimately, Ödegaard concluded that this association was an artifact of selective migration. In the decades following, many studies addressing immigration and schizophrenia lacked a certain standard of rigor and were often regarded with skepticism.

Recently, however, interest in the association between immigration and schizophrenia has been rejuvenated. One of the most remarkable and consistent findings on schizophrenia is the elevated rate of the disorder among some immigrant groups in Western Europe (Jones and Fung 2006; Kirkbride et al. 2006; Veling et al. 2006). In a recent meta-analysis, Cantor-Graae and Selten (2005) examined 18 population-based incidence studies and found that for first-generation immigrants the mean weighted relative risk for developing schizophrenia was 2.7 (95% confidence interval [CI]= 2.3–3.2), whereas that for second-generation immigrants was 4.5 (95% CI=1.5–13.1). These findings on immigrants are not explained by diagnostic bias, selective migration, or higher incidence in countries of origin, nor are they explained by variation in suspected risk factors such as obstetric complications and cannabis use. Because the increased risk is at least as high in the second generation—the offspring of immigrants—the causal factor cannot reside in the experience of immigration per se.

It seems likely that the high rates among immigrants offer a clue to some still unknown major cause of schizophrenia. Increasingly, researchers are turning to the social experience of immigrants for the explanation. The challenge is to determine whether certain social contexts contribute to the development of schizophrenia in members of immigrant groups situated therein. Our first task, therefore, is to conceptualize the relevant social experiences at different levels of organization and consider the research designs that could be used to study them. For immigrants, this task is not as straightforward as in the hypothetical example provided earlier.

The Level of the Immigrant Group

Between Groups

We can start by considering the level of organization of the immigrant group. The experience of being an immigrant, whether first- or second-generation, differs by group with respect to the experience within the same host country. These differences include the variation in reception of the different immigrant groups upon arrival as well as variation in the ongoing lived experience in the host country. Stigma and discrimination experienced by an immigrant group in the host country would be an example of a factor at this level. It may infuse the attitudes of nonimmigrants toward all members of a given immigrant group. The individual members of the immigrant group may vary, however, in their awareness of it and in their perception of its impact on their encounters with nonimmigrants. Thus, the group-level factor and the individual measures are not synonymous. For some research questions it is the group-level factor that will be most relevant.

In studying causes at this level of organization, it is most strategic to employ a between-group approach. For instance, we can compare the rates of schizophrenia in first- and second-generation immigrants, grouped by country of origin, within a particular destination country. We may postulate that a group-level factor, such as discrimination, is important. Then we can examine how it varies among immigrant groups and whether this explains variation in rates of schizophrenia across these groups.

There is, indeed, evidence of substantial variation in rates of schizophrenia across immigrant groups, which requires explanation. In the United Kingdom, for example, Afro-Caribbean immigrants have higher rates of schizophrenia than South Asian immigrants (Jones and Fung 2006; Kirkbride et al. 2006). Moreover, in the Netherlands, Moroccan immigrants have higher incidence rates of schizophrenia than all other immigrants (Veling et al. 2006). It is intriguing that in both the United Kingdom and the Netherlands, the immigrant groups that experience the most discrimination have the highest rates of schizophrenia.

Also, it has been noted that in several European countries the immigrants from countries with a black majority—who presumably suffer the most stigma and discrimination in host countries with a white majority population— have the highest rates of schizophrenia (Cantor-Graae and Selten 2005). As yet, published reports have not explicitly articulated and tested this hypothesis—or other causal hypotheses—at the immigrant group level. To do so requires a good measure of stigma and discrimination or other group-level factors of interest for different immigrant groups as well as a measure of the incidence of schizophrenia in these groups. Some studies of this kind, however, are presently under way (Veling et al. 2007).

The Level of the Neighborhood

Within Groups

Once we have detected variation between different immigrant groups within the broad social context of a given host country, we can adopt a within-group approach to examine the contribution of the local, more proximal social context. One such social context is the *neighborhood*. Most immigrants to Western Europe are ethnic minorities, and the social experience of being an ethnic minority might differ according to the neighborhood context. One important characteristic of the neighborhood context is *ethnic density*— that is, the proportion of people living in the neighborhood who belong to a given ethnic group.

Increasingly, neighborhood characteristics are being investigated with respect to a host of health outcomes, and ethnic density seems to capture some important characteristics of the neighborhood context. Among them is *social cohesion*, or the degree to which a community is bound together by social ties. This and other characteristics of immigrant enclaves appear to have a direct relationship with many physical and mental health outcomes; the more socially cohesive the neighborhood, the better the health of the neighborhood (see, e.g., Landale et al. 2000).

As with the relationship between immigration and schizophrenia, the relevance of neighborhood characteristics, and ethnic density in particular, to schizophrenia has long been considered. In their classic 1939 study *Mental Disorders in Urban Areas*, Faris and Dunham set out to study the relationship between mental health and social organization. For them, one aspect of social organization was ethnic density. They observed that the rates of schizophrenia and other psychoses for the foreign born in Chicago were significantly lower in areas primarily populated by their own members. This also held for African Americans and the native born (Faris and Dunham 1939). Nearly three decades later, Mintz and Schwartz (1964) reported a similar finding among Italians living in 27 Boston communities.

In the first study in the current era to examine this hypothesis, in the United Kingdom, Boydell et al. (2001) compared rates of schizophrenia for ethnic minorities living in low- versus high-density neighborhoods. Those living in higher-density neighborhoods had lower rates of schizophrenia. Because members of ethnic minority groups in the United Kingdom are mainly first- or second-generation immigrants, this result suggests that, as anticipated by the work of Faris and Dunham, the ethnic mix of the local social context modifies the relationship between immigration and schizophrenia. Boydell and colleagues did not differentiate specific immigrant groups in their study of ethnic density; however, another group in the Netherlands is currently examining the relationship between ethnic density, specific immigrant groups, and schizophrenia (Veling et al., in press). In future studies, our charge will be to investigate the specific aspects of ethnic density that contribute to the observed relationship with schizophrenia because the proportion of ethnic minorities in a given set of neighborhoods alone is insufficient to understand causal mechanisms. We will have to ask what it is about higher-ethnic density neighborhoods that seems to be protective. Is it, for example, social cohesion or social support that is operative? If so, we must meaningfully measure and examine these phenomena at the neighborhood level and determine at what points in development these phenomena are important and how they operate.

The Individual Level

We have emphasized that the factors that cause variation in the rate of disorder between groups need not be the same as the factors that cause variation in risk among individuals within a group. In some instances, however, they will be the same. Suppose separation from parents during childhood increases the risk of developing schizophrenia. Suppose also that people with a history of immigration—either first- or second-generation immigrants—are more likely than natives to be separated from parents during childhood. Then this exposure, which is measured in individuals and can be considered a characteristic of individuals, would explain part of the increased risk in immigrant groups. To detect this cause, we do not need to study any level of organization beyond the individual. Ordinary cohort and case–control designs comparing the disease risk among individuals with different histories of immigration and of childhood separation from parents are appropriate for this purpose. Preliminary evidence supporting this explanation has in fact been found in a case–control study in the United Kingdom (Morgan et al. 2006).

Interaction Between Levels

Often the interaction between causes at different levels of organization turns out to be of primary interest. A history of immigration may place an individual at risk in some but not other social contexts; the social context may modify the effect of or "interact with" the individual's history of immigration. It may also interact with factors at higher levels of organization. Suppose that only some immigrant groups have an increased risk of schizophrenia when living in low–ethnic density neighborhoods. This could indicate an interaction between a characteristic of the immigrant group (e.g., experience of stigma and discrimination), a characteristic of the neighborhood (e.g., ethnic density), and a characteristic of the individual (e.g., history of immigration).

Other Relationships

With the introduction of too many levels of causation, and interactions among them, the study of multilevel causation quickly becomes unwieldy. It should be noted, however, that in any particular study, some more complex relationships will need to be considered. For example, some immigrant groups may have been minorities in their country of origin and experienced more discrimination in their country of origin than in the host country, or an immigrant group from the same country of origin may be sharply divided by religion or other factors. A finer distinction then may be needed to define a meaningful group.

Our discussion has also assumed that a history of immigration is a necessary condition for the increased risk observed among immigrant groups. It is also possible, however, that it is an antecedent of some other social experience that can be brought about in other ways. For example, groups that suffer discrimination in the absence of any recent history of cross-national migration might also have an increased risk of schizophrenia, such as African Americans in the United States. Some evidence supports this as a plausible hypothesis (Bresnahan et al. 2007).

A DEVELOPMENTAL PERSPECTIVE ON SOCIAL CONTEXT

Developmental psychopathology has much to gain by considering the social context in a more systematic way. Social context shapes the meaning of individual experience, and we need to better characterize social context in order to uncover important causal mechanisms. The example of schizophrenia underscores this point. The large magnitude of the immigrant effect indicates that, to quote J.N. Morris, one of the first epidemiologists to articulate the significance of social context for health, "gold awaits the imaginative traveler" (Morris 1957).

To study social context, however, calls for a shift in the perspective and the practice of developmental psychopathology. We will need to focus on designing studies so as to detect the effects of levels of social organization beyond the individual. Equally important, the perspective of developmental psychopathology can greatly inform the study of social context. Just as there is a need to measure various individual phenomena over the life course, as developmental psychopathology has done, there is a need to measure social context over the life course so that the interaction between individuals and their environments might be better understood. Often, even in what we consider the most comprehensive longitudinal studies, social context is measured with less frequency and less vigilance than the individual him- or herself. Sometimes, characterization of social context occurs at birth and then at a given end point such as the development of a disease or disorder. Fewer questions are asked about the continuities and discontinuities of the social context than about the individual despite the fact that the two are critically linked.

This does not always require initiation of entirely new studies. We can, for example, capitalize on the information available in extant birth cohorts. For schizophrenia, this can be illustrated with the Prenatal Determinants of Schizophrenia (PDS) study birth cohort (E. Susser et al. 2000). A recent study suggests that African Americans in this cohort born between 1959 and 1967 were three times more likely to develop schizophrenia than their white counterparts (Bresnahan et al. 2007). As previously discussed, we can explore this between-groups finding by examining within-group variation, and, importantly, over the course of development. One strategy is investigating characteristics of the social context that might differ over time within groups. Researchers are beginning to examine the within-group differences by examining the role of the local (e.g., neighborhood) context by conducting both qualitative and quantitative research to determine the relevant aspects of that context and linking them to the developmental stage of cohort members. Quantitative measures of relevant aspects of the local social context over the course of development would capture underlying constructs thought to be meaningful with respect to schizophrenia; these constructs include social cohesion, social support, and social organization, which may well account for the decades-old ethnic density findings in the United States and the more current findings in Western Europe. These measures, which might vary across contexts and historical periods, could assume the form of a quantum of community involvement—for example, the number, membership, and activities of community groups and organizations, among others. There is much latitude for creativity in marrying relevant social theory and knowledge about developmental processes and applying them to this area of investigation.

CONCLUSIONS

There is a need to integrate the strengths of the developmental psychopathology perspective with an understanding of social context. Just as it has been necessary to elucidate the relationship between developmental processes and psychopathology, it is necessary to understand the relationship between social context and development. It is equally necessary to remain tethered to the biology and genetics of such illnesses. In essence, to fully understand the etiology of psychopathology, we must integrate macrolevel phenomena (i.e., those occurring at levels of organization higher than the individual) with microlevel phenomena (i.e., those occurring at levels of organization lower than the individual) over the individual life course and across historical time. An integrative, multilevel approach advocated by eco-epidemiology and other similar frameworks is necessary for such endeavors (March and Susser 2006; E. Susser 2004; E. Susser et al. 2006; M. Susser and Susser 1996). Indeed, a broader lens encompassing developmental psychopathology, biology, and the historical and social context is necessary to further develop our perspective and thereby our understanding of mental disorders.

REFERENCES

Achenbach T: Developmental Psychopathology. New York, Wiley, 1974

Boyce WT, Frank E, Jensen PS, et al: Social context in developmental psychopathology: recommendations for future research from the MacArthur Network on Psychopathology and Development. The MacArthur Foundation Research Network on Psychopathology and Development. Dev Psychopathol 10:143–164, 1998

Boydell J, Van Os J, McKenzie K, et al: Incidence of schizophrenia in ethnic minorities in London: ecological study into interactions with environment. BMJ 323:1336–1338, 2001

Bresnahan M, Menezes P, Varma VK, et al: Geographical variation in incidence, course and outcome of schizophrenia: a comparison of developing and developed countries, in The Epidemiology of Schizophrenia. Edited by Murray R, Jones P, Susser E, et al. Cambridge, UK, Cambridge University Press, 2003

Bresnahan M, Begg MD, Brown A, et al: Race and risk of schizophrenia in a U.S. birth cohort: another example of health disparity? Int J Epidemiol 36:751–758, 2007

Buka S, Tsuang M, Torrey E, et al: Maternal infections and subsequent psychosis among offspring. Arch Gen Psychiatry 58:1032–1037, 2001

Byrne M, Agerbo E, Eaton W, et al: Parental socioeconomic status and risk of schizophrenia: a Danish national register based study. Soc Psychiatry Psychiatr Epidemiol 39:87–96, 2004

Cantor-Graae E, Selten JP: Schizophrenia and migration: a meta-analysis and review. Am J Psychiatry 162:12–24, 2005

Caspi A, Harrington H, Milne BJ, et al: Children's behavioral styles at age 3 are linked to their adult personality traits at age 26. J Pers 71:495–513, 2003a

Caspi A, Sugden K, Moffitt TE, et al: Influence of life stress on depression: moderation by a polymorphism in the 5-HTT gene. Science 301:386–389, 2003b

Costello EJ, Angold A, Cicchetti D, et al: Developmental epidemiology, in Rochester Symposium on Developmental Psychopathology, Vol 3: Models and Integrations. Edited by Cicchetti D, Cohen D. Hillsdale, NJ, Erlbaum, 1991, pp 23–56

Costello EJ, Angold A, Burns BJ, et al: The Great Smoky Mountains Study of Youth: goals, design, methods, the prevalence of DSM-III-R disorders. Arch Gen Psychiatry 53:1129–1136, 1996

Costello E, Farmer E, Angold A, et al: Psychiatric disorders among American Indian and white youth in Appalachia: the Great Smoky Mountains Study. Am J Public Health 87:827–832, 1997

Costello EJ, Compton SN, Keeler G, et al: Relationships between poverty and psychopathology: a natural experiment. JAMA 290:2023–2029, 2003

Costello E, Foley D, Angold A: 10-year research update review: the epidemiology of child and adolescent psychiatric disorders: II. Developmental epidemiology. J Am Acad Child Adolesc Psychiatry 45:8–25, 2006

Diez Roux AV: Bringing context back into epidemiology: variables and fallacies in multilevel analyses. Am J Public Health 88:216–222, 1998

Faris R, Dunham H: Mental Disorders in Urban Areas: An Ecological Study of Schizophrenia and Other Psychoses. Chicago, IL, University of Chicago Press, 1939

Hopper K, Wanderling J: Revisiting the developed versus developing country distinction in course and outcome in schizophrenia: results from ISoS, the WHO collaborative follow-up project. International Study of Schizophrenia. Schizophr Bull 26:835–846, 2000

Jablensky A, Sartorius N, Ernberg G, et al: Schizophrenia: manifestations, incidence and course in different cultures: a World Health Organization ten-country study. Psychol Med 20:1–97, 1992

Jarvis E: Insanity and Idiocy in Massachusetts: Report of the Commission on Lunacy (1855). Cambridge, MA, Harvard University Press, 1971

Jones P, Fung W: Ethnicity and mental health: the example of schizophrenia in the African-Caribbean population in Europe, in Ethnicity and Causal Mechanisms. Edited by Rutter M, Tienda M. New York, Cambridge University Press, 2006, pp 227–261

Kim-Cohen J, Caspi A, Moffitt TE, et al: Prior juvenile diagnoses in adults with mental disorder: developmental follow-back of a prospective-longitudinal cohort. Arch Gen Psychiatry 60:709–717, 2003

Kirkbride J, Fearon P, Morgan C, et al: Heterogeneity in incidence rates of schizophrenia and other psychotic syndromes: findings from the 3-center AeSOP study. Arch Gen Psychiatry 63:250–258, 2006

Landale N, Oropresa R, Gorman B: Migration and infant death: assimilation or selective migration among Puerto Ricans? Am Sociol Rev 65:888–909, 2000

Leff J, Sartorius N, Jablensky A, et al: The international pilot study of schizophrenia: five-year follow-up findings. Psychol Med 22:131–145, 1992

Leighton AH: My Name is Legion: Foundations for a Theory of Man in Relation to Culture, Vol 1: The Stirling County Study of Psychiatric Disorder and Sociocultural Environment. New York, Basic Books, 1959

Malaspina D, Harlap S, Fennig S, et al: Advancing paternal age and the risk of schizophrenia. Arch Gen Psychiatry 58:361–367, 2001

March D, Susser E: Invited commentary: taking the search for causes of schizophrenia to a different level. Am J Epidemiol 163:979–981, 2006

Mintz M, Schwartz D: Urban ecology and psychosis: community factors in the incidence of schizophrenia and manic-depression among Italians in Greater Boston. Int J Soc Psychiatry 10:101–118, 1964

Morgan C, Kirkbride J, Leff J, et al: Parental separation, loss, and psychosis in different ethnic groups: a case-control study. Psychol Med 37:495–503, 2006

Morris JN: Uses of Epidemiology. Edinburgh, Scotland, Livingstone, 1957

Murray RM, Jones PB, Susser E, et al (eds) : The Epidemiology of Schizophrenia. New York, Cambridge University Press, 2002

Ödegaard Ö: Emigration and insanity. Acta Psychiatr Neurol Scand Suppl 4:1–206, 1932

Pedersen CB, Mortensen PB: Are the cause(s) responsible for urban-rural differences in schizophrenia risk rooted in families or in individuals? Am J Epidemiol 163:971–978, 2006

Riley MW: Commentary: special problems of sociological analysis, in Sociological Research. Edited by Merton R. New York, Harcourt, Brace & World, 1963, pp 700–738

Robinson WS: Ecological correlations and the behavior of individuals. Am Sociol Rev 15:351–357, 1950

Rose G: Sick individuals and sick populations. Int J Epidemiol 14:32–38, 1985

Rutter M: Epidemiological approaches to developmental psychopathology. Arch Gen Psychiatry 45:486–495, 1988

Rutter M, Sroufe L: Developmental psychopathology: concepts and challenges. Dev Psychopathol 12:265–296, 2000

Rutter M, Tizard J, Yule W, et al: Research report: Isle of Wight Studies, 1964–1974. Psychol Med 6:313–332, 1976

Schwartz S: The fallacy of the ecological fallacy: the potential misuse of a concept and the consequences. Am J Public Health 84:819–824, 1994

Schwartz S, Diez-Roux AV: Commentary: causes of incidence and causes of cases: a Durkheimian perspective on Rose. Int J Epidemiol 30:435–439, 2001

Schwartz S, Diez Roux AV, Susser E: Causal explanation outside the black box, in Psychiatric Epidemiology: Searching for the Causes of Mental Disorders. Edited by Susser E, Schwartz S, Morabia A, et al. New York, Oxford University Press, 2006, pp 441–460

Silva P, Stanton WR (eds): From Child to Adult: The Dunedin Multidisciplinary Health and Development Study. New York, Oxford University Press, 1996

Sroufe L, Rutter M: The domain of developmental psychopathology. Child Dev 55:17–29, 1984

Sullivan ML: Integrating qualitative and quantitative methods in the study of developmental psychopathology. Dev Psychopathol 10:377–393, 1998

Susser E: Eco-epidemiology: thinking outside the black box. Epidemiology 15:519–520, 2004

Susser E, Schaefer CA, Brown A, et al: The design of the prenatal determinants of schizophrenia study. Schizophr Bull 26:257–273, 2000

Susser E, Schwartz S, Morabia A, et al: Psychiatric Epidemiology: Searching for the Causes of Mental Disorders. New York, Oxford University Press, 2006

Susser M: Causal Thinking in the Health Sciences. New York, Oxford University Press, 1973

Susser M, Susser E: Choosing a future for epidemiology: II. From black box to Chinese boxes and eco-epidemiology. Am J Public Health 86:674–677, 1996

Vander Stoep A, Link B: Social class, ethnicity, and mental illness: the importance of being more than earnest. Am J Public Health 88:1396–1402, 1998

Veling W, Selten J-P, Veen N, et al: Incidence of schizophrenia among ethnic minorities in the Netherlands: a four-year first-contact study. Schizophr Res 86:189–193, 2006

Veling W, Selten J-P, Susser E, et al: Discrimination and the incidence of psychotic disorders among ethnic minorities in The Netherlands. Int J Epidemiol 36(4):761–768, 2007

Veling W, Susser E, van Os J, et al: Ethnic density of neighborhoods and incidence of psychotic disorders among immigrants. Am J Psychiatry (in press)

Wicks S, Hjern A, Gunnell D, et al: Social adversity in childhood and the risk of developing psychosis: a national cohort study. Am J Psychiatry 162:1652–1657, 2005

World Health Organization: The International Pilot Study of Schizophrenia. Geneva, Switzerland, World Health Organization, 1973

Part 2

GENERAL CONCEPTS OF GENE–ENVIRONMENT INTERACTION ON CHILD DEVELOPMENT

Chapter 4

TEMPERAMENT AND CHILD PSYCHOPATHOLOGY

Beyond Associations

David C. Rettew, M.D.

Our understanding of the relations between temperament and psychopathology has come full circle over the past 2,000 years. The ancient Greeks, most notably Galen, originally hypothesized that varying concentrations of four humors in the body contributed to both personality style and psychiatric symptoms alike (Kagan 1994). In the era of psychoanalysis, Freud similarly viewed the processes underlying personality development and psychopathology to be one and the same. Perhaps in an effort to legitimatize psychiatric disorders, psychopathology began to be more "medicalized," and studies of personality and temperament began to drift apart from the study of psychiatric disorders. In so doing, psychiatric symptoms were explained in language similar to that used for other medical syndromes. One is afflicted by major depression, for example, in a similar way that one gets the flu or diabetes and through a process that has very little to do with someone's basic tendencies.

The seminal work of Thomas and Chess in the 1970s brought these worlds together again with their findings of strong links between temperament and later psychopathology (Thomas and Chess 1984). Interestingly, their argument was not to work against the increasing evidence for biological substrates of psychiatric disorders but rather to highlight the intrinsic nature of temperament and its adaptability to particular environments.

Mercifully, the field has finally begun to make substantial moves away from the anachronistic nature-versus-nurture debates, first with the acknowledgment that the distinction between biological and psychological processes are and must be artificial and, more recently, with investigations into the precise mechanisms through which genetic and environmental events interact. No longer is the environment seen either as an epiphenomon of genetic destiny or as an overwhelmingly powerful and independent force. Genetic influences not only interact with environmental events, they cause certain environmental events to be more likely (Rutter et al. 1997). Similarly, the influence of environmental events depends on an individual's genetic makeup and vice versa (Caspi et al. 2003).

Thus, it is into these waters where the temperament and psychopathology research must go. Since Thomas and Chess's work, an increasing body of research has been devoted to demonstrating extensive links between temperament, personality, and virtually all types of psychopathology (Rettew and McKee 2005). These findings have been critical to justify the next generation of research now beginning to take place. The question no longer is *if* temperament and psychopathology are related but *how* and *how much* temperament and psychopathology are related.

In this chapter, I first briefly define the construct of temperament and personality as it relates to psychopathology and provide a concise summary of the association studies that have been conducted. The rest of the text will then be devoted to efforts that potentially could expand and sharpen our understanding of the complex interplay between these once-parallel domains. This chapter is not meant to be an exhaustive review of the relevant literature but rather a guide, using illustrative examples, to issues and techniques that could potentially advance this fascinating area of study even further.

DEFINITIONS

The precise definition of temperament has remained elusive. Although debate is likely to continue, most experts agree that *temperament* refers to individual differences in emotional reactivity and perhaps to regulations that appear early in life, are at least moderately stable, and are genetically influenced (Goldsmith et al. 1987). Some theorists frame temperament more in terms of variation in behavioral approach, avoidance, and maintenance (Cloninger et al. 1993), although these frameworks are not mutually exclusive.

The degree of overlap between *temperament* and *personality* is murkier still and beyond the scope of this chapter. Interested readers are advised to consult more in-depth discussions on this topic (McCrae et al. 2000; Rothbart et al. 2000). In general, it is probably fair to say that most researchers see temperament as an early-appearing determinant of personality that in turn incorporates more sophisticated cognitive functions and cultural influences. Nevertheless, there does appear to be a movement toward increasing conceptual overlap between these constructs, and for the purposes of this chapter, we will use the two terms somewhat interchangeably.

Given these conceptual difficulties, it should come as no surprise that a major factor that makes synthesis of temperament and personality literature difficult is the existence of multiple conceptual frameworks of temperament and personality dimensions with different names and partially overlapping definitions. Despite this confusion, however, some consensus has emerged as to the primary higher-order temperament traits. Most theorists include a dimension related to behavioral approach and characterized by an individual's tendency to seek out and enjoy novel-situation and high-stimulation activities. This dimension has been variably named *novelty seeking*, *surgency*, and, especially when a social component is included, *extraversion* (Costa and McCrae 1992; Luby et al. 1999; Rothbart et al. 2001). Another dimension usually considered refers to a person's proclivity to experience negative emotions such as sadness, fear, and anger with regard to threshold, amplitude, frequency, and duration of response. In the temperament literature, this trait has been called *negative affectivity*, whereas in personality frameworks the somewhat arcane term *neuroticism* has often been preserved (Eysenck and Eysenck 1975). Dimensions of sociability and activity level are sometimes but not always described as higher-order traits (Buss and Plomin 1984), whereas in other models they are subsumed under dimensions such as novelty seeking and extraversion. Finally, a dimension that encompasses an ability to regulate emotions and persevere in the face of obstacles is often included under labels such as *effortful control* or *persistence*.

ASSOCIATION STUDIES

As mentioned, there has been a surge of interest in the links between temperament and psychopathology. By far the most common methodology employed so far is to measure both temperament and psychopathology (either at one point in time or longitudinally) and statistically test an association. In most cases, temperament is examined as a continuous trait, whereas psychopathology is measured categorically (meeting criteria or not for a psychiatric disorder) so that mean temperament scores are compared between subjects who do and do not meet criteria for a particular diagnosis. When psychopathology is measured quantitatively, such as with scores on the Child Behavior Checklist (CBCL; Achenbach and Rescorla 2001) or other instruments, or when temperament is measured categorically, such as with the trait of behavioral inhibition (Kagan et al. 1988), methods such as correlations, regression, and χ^2 statistics have been employed.

By use of these approaches, significant links between many temperament and personality dimensions and a host of psychiatric diagnoses have been discovered (Shiner and Caspi 2003). Indeed, it is difficult to think of any type of psychopathology in which this link has not been established through one method or another. As psychiatry increasingly begins to consider quantitative and dimensional models of psychopathology, the magnitude of these associations can only be expected to increase (Krueger et al. 2005).

High levels of negative affectivity, harm avoidance, or neuroticism has been associated with multiple types of psychopathology, most notably affective and anxiety disorders but also disruptive behavior disorders, personality disorders, eating disorders, and substance use (Austin and Chorpita 2004; Goodyer et al. 1993; Nigg et al. 2002; Ongur et al. 2005). High levels of novelty seeking has been linked to disruptive behavior disorders and attention-deficit/hyperactivity disorder (ADHD), mania, and some substance abuse, whereas low levels appear to be associated with anxiety and depressive disorders (Schmeck and Poustka 2001; Tillman et al. 2003). Dimensions related to emotion regulation and effortful control have been hypothesized to be a common factor to a wide spectrum of psychopathology, including substance abuse and externalizing disorders (Oldehinkel et al. 2004; Rettew et al. 2004a; Wills and Dishion 2004). Low sociability, reward dependence, and agreeableness have been linked to conduct, antisocial, and autism spectrum disorders, whereas high activity level, not surprisingly, is strongly related to ADHD (Nigg et al. 2002).

One difficulty that inevitably surfaces with this research is the content overlap between criteria items that load onto a temperament dimension and criteria items for psychopathology assessed both categorically and dimensionally (Frick 2004). This traditionally has been represented as a methodological problem, although it is also a theoretical problem when nearly identical language is used to describe and define both a temperamental trait and a psychiatric diagnosis. Table 4–1 shows items used to assess temperament in addition to psychopathology assessed both categorically and quantitatively. Typically, studies tend to acknowledge this difficulty rather than actively confront it through statistical methods or study design. Some researchers have tried to remove overlapping items and then examine the associations (Lemery et al. 2002). Although this procedure can remove some

TABLE 4–1. Content overlap between temperamental items and psychopathology

Temperament[a]	Quantitative psychopathology[b]	Categorical psychopathology[c]
"…loses temper more easily than other children" (NS)	"Temper tantrums or hot temper" (AG)	"Often loses temper" (ODD)
"…seems to be shy with new people" (HA)	"Too shy or timid" (W/D)	"Marked or persistent fear of one or more social situations" (SP)
"…wouldn't bother my child to be alone all the time" (RD-r)	"Withdrawn, doesn't get involved with others" (W/D)	"Neither desires nor enjoys close relationships" (SPD)

Note. Comparison of criteria items for temperamental dimensions and psychopathology. Parentheses indicate diagnosis or subscale on which item loads.

AG=aggression; HA=harm avoidance; NS=novelty seeking; ODD=oppositional defiant disorder; RD-r=reward dependence–reversed; SP=social phobia; SPD=schizoid personality disorder; W/D=withdrawn/depressed.

[a]From Junior Temperament and Character Inventory (Luby et al. 1999).
[b]From Child Behavior Checklist (Achenbach and Rescorla 2001).
[c]From DSM-IV (American Psychiatric Association 1994).

of the methodological concerns, it raises others when analyzing links between two constructs each of whose integrity has been compromised.

STRATEGIES TO DISENTANGLE THE TEMPERAMENT/PSYCHOPATHOLOGY ASSOCIATIONS

Longitudinal Studies

One of the most common and potentially valuable approaches to this dilemma is to design a prospective study that is able to assess temperament before the onset of psychopathology. This has been the principal method employed by Kagan, Snideman, and Hirshfeld-Becker in their prospective studies of children who are assessed around age 2 years for behavioral inhibition, a hypothesized temperament trait that reflects reticence and restraint in novel situations as assessed through a laboratory protocol (Kagan 1994). This research has demonstrated important links between behavioral inhibition and later psychopathology assessed many years later, particularly anxiety disorders. For example, as adolescents, 44% of previously inhibited girls had current impairing social anxiety in comparison with 6% of previously uninhibited girls (Schwartz et al. 1999).

The well-known Dunedin study assessed over a thousand individuals from age into adulthood (Caspi 2000). Temperament was assessed observationally at age 3 years, and children were divided into three groups designated "well adjusted," "under controlled," and "inhibited." At age 21 years, these categories were associated with various psychiatric diagnoses. Depression was more prevalent among children classified as inhibited, while under-controlled children were more likely to be diagnosed with antisocial personality disorder and alcohol dependence as adults. Not surprisingly, there was significant continuity found between temperament at age 3 years and adult personality.

Unfortunately, longitudinal studies do not necessarily satisfy critics who maintain that temperament scales actually measure subthreshold psychopathology, particularly when a study does not assess and control for psychopathology at time 1 under the assumption that it is too soon to see it. A provision to make yes/no psychiatric diagnoses at the time temperament is assessed is unlikely to solve this problem because the thresholds are too high to pick up milder symptoms. One strategy for addressing this issue would be to assess both temperament and psychopathology at time 1 (preferably using quantitative measures) and then statistically control for the covariance using multiple regression or structural equation modeling. A related strategy is to assess personality after an acute illness phase has passed, although similar concerns remain. In individuals with eating disorders, for example, high harm avoidance and low self-directedness were found to persist in those with a history of eating disorders who are not currently ill (Klump et al. 2004).

Quantifying the Association

Perhaps the first step beyond the yes/no decision of whether the temperament/psychopathology association is statistically significant is to begin quantifying this association. In our own lab, we have used multiple regression to determine that over 50% of the variance in disruptive behavior disorder diagnoses can be explained from temperament as measured by the Junior Temperament and Character Inventory (JTCI) in a school-age sample (Rettew et al. 2004a). In addition, we have attempted to use receiver operating characteristic analysis to quantify the degree of temperament/psychopathology overlap (Rettew et al. 2006a). Using the Harm Avoidance scale of the Temperament and Character Inventory (TCI) and the JTCI to predict a DSM-IV-TR (American Psychiatric Association 2000) diagnosis of generalized anxiety disorder (GAD), we found large area-under-the-curve values of 0.82 and 0.79 for children and adults, respectively. Inspection of the distribution of Harm Avoidance scores by GAD status revealed some interesting trends. Many individuals with very high Harm Avoidance scores do not meet the criteria for GAD, a minority of persons with intermediate Harm Avoidance scores meet the criteria for GAD, and almost no one with low Harm Avoidance scores meets the criteria for GAD. Putting this together, harm avoidance appears to be much more necessary than sufficient in the diagnosis of GAD, yet many extremely worried and anxious people do not meet GAD criteria.

What separates two individuals with the same level of harm avoidance such that one person meets criteria for GAD and another one does not? One possibility may have to do with other temperament dimensions such as those relating to emotion regulation and effortful control. This hypothesis, in turn, speaks to the use of another potentially useful strategy in the temperament/psychopathology investigation.

Profiles Rather Than Pairs

Answering the question posed above compels us to leave behind analyses of one trait and one disorder and to examine the potential moderating influence of other factors, including other temperament and personality dimensions. Externalizing disorders and ADHD, for example, were found to be associated with the *combination* of low constraint and high negative emotionality (Cukrowicz et al. 2006). A similar finding was reported using a different temperament nomenclature. In this study, the dimensions of frustration and effortful control were linked with both internalizing and externalizing problems, whereas dimensions such as shyness and high-intensity pleasure were more related to the direction of psychopathology (Oldehinkel et al. 2004). Even before these studies, Cloninger and colleagues proposed that personality disorders in particular can be visualized as a point in three-dimensional space, with each axis being a particular dimension of temperament or character (Cloninger and Carmen 1999). Each axis alone is insufficient in adequately describing the disorder.

From our own work, we have been investigating the hypothesis that particular diagnoses are principally related not to a single temperament dimension but to multiple dimensions that can potentially modify each other's effect. In children with ADHD without comorbid conditions, a particular combination of high novelty seeking and low harm avoidance was found, whereas these two dimensions were more independent in control subjects (Rettew et al. 2004a). This study also suggested the possibility that some dimensions, such as self-directedness and persistence, were associated with psychopathology in general, whereas other dimensions, such as novelty seeking and harm avoidance, were more related to the specific type of diagnosis.

In examining the qualitative differences between definitions of temperament dimensions and definitions of psychopathology (especially according to DSM standards), one immediate distinction that emerges is that diagnoses require the presence of impairment and temperamental traits do not. Two children potentially can have the same levels of motor activity, yet for one child this behavior leads to substantial difficulties in multiple settings, and for the other child there are minimal problems if any. When thinking about children, impairment can be a function not only of other factors within the individual but of factors across individuals (i.e., parents and caretakers). This hypothesis harkens back to Thomas and Chess's description of "goodness of fit" (Thomas and Chess 1984). Surprisingly, this cornerstone of developmental psychopathology teaching has received little empirical investigation since it was originally proposed. We recently tested this hypothesis within a sample of approximately 200 families and found evidence to support this theory, although not in total (Rettew et al. 2006b). High levels of maternal novelty seeking, for example, were related to child attention problems in high novelty-seeking children but had no effect among low novelty-seeking children. Evidence was also found, however, for main effect associations between child temperament and child behavior problems controlling for parent temperament, socioeconomic status, and other types of psychopathology.

One weakness of the profile or interaction approach is the assumption that there is only one temperament profile that is related to each disorder. If, instead, there are many, this effect easily could be diluted when looking at group means, even using a profile-based analysis. To test this, a different approach is needed—one that takes the focus off of the variable in question and returns it to the individual.

Person-Centered Rather Than Variable-Centered Analyses

Temperament assessment is most commonly done using questionnaires that yield a score on one of the dimensions mentioned previously. For most of the commonly used instruments, these particular dimensions have been developed or at least supported by means of empirical strategies such as exploratory or confirmatory factor analysis. The unit of division for these procedures is the instrument itself, not the individual, although obviously there should be substantial overlap. In other words, these statistical procedures help establish how the instrument should be divided into *subscales* and not how the participants who completed the instrument should be divided into *subgroups*. In turn, when these scales are used in research, the typical method of analysis is to compare scores on particular dimensions between previously defined groups such as girls versus boys or ADHD versus no ADHD. Although this strategy has led to many important findings, it assumes that our subject groupings have captured meaningful differences. As previously mentioned, these analyses also work best if there is basically one profile that underlies a particular type of psychopathology rather than many. If these assumptions are not correct, it is possible that additional information can be gained by analyses that empirically create subject groups as the main division for study rather than the temperament dimensions themselves. These types of analyses have the further advantage of being able to identify the existence and prevalence of empirically based clusters of individuals who tend to resemble each other along a number of important variables. This, in turn, can suggest how these different variables may or may not interact.

As a hypothetical example, let us assume a simplified model of temperament similar to Gray's model of separate behavioral activating and inhibiting systems (Gray 1987) or, as a metaphor, the brake and accelerator of a car. Supposing, then, that these systems underlie ADHD, one could imagine that some individuals are "going too fast" because their overactive accelerator is overriding a normally functioning brake. Another group going the same speed, however, could be due to a deficient brake trying to control a normal accelerator. If both groups are found in an ADHD sample in equal proportions, then measuring the accelerator and brake levels compared with control subjects may not yield significant group differences because of a dilution effect from the two ADHD subgroups. A clustering procedure focusing on the individual, however, could succeed in distinguishing the high accelerator/low brake group from the low accelerator/high brake group in addition to other subgroups. These naturally occurring groups could then potentially be better phenotypic targets for other studies such as neuroimaging or molecular genetic investigations.

One particular example of this type of analysis is *latent class analysis* (LCA), which can be used to identify clusters of individuals who have similar responses to a series of yes/no questions (McCutcheon 1987). By use of individual DSM-IV-TR diagnostic criteria, this technique has been employed to propose different subtypes of eating and bipolar disorders and ADHD. For example, Rasmussen and colleagues examined the clustering of empirically defined subtypes of ADHD within a genetically informative sample to support the hypothesis that these groups may represent more meaningful distinctions than the current DSM-based subtypes (Rasmussen et al. 2004). These analyses have also been applied to responses on the Anxiety/Depression, Aggression, and Attention Problems scales of the CBCL. In one study, LCA identified one group with high scores on all three scales that may represent children now diagnosed with pediatric bipolar disorder (Althoff et al. 2006). In addition, however, the procedure identified other groups with elevations of two of the three scales and at different levels of severity. Should these classes truly represent clusters of children, one can easily understand why so many clinicians debate the pediatric bipolar disorder diagnosis.

In temperament research, we applied LCA to eight yes/no items of the JTCI Harm Avoidance scale that describe Kagan's temperament of behavioral inhibition in a family study of 184 children (Rettew et al. 2004b). As the current definition of behavioral inhibition includes a fear of novelty in both social and nonsocial domains, our goal was to see if the procedure would find two groups of individuals approximating children with or without behavioral inhibition or alternatively might describe additional groups. Interestingly, the LCA identified four groups: those who responded no to most or all questions (uninhibited group), those who responded yes to most all questions (inhibited groups), and two additional groups of individuals who tended to respond yes only to the social or nonsocial items, respectively. Although this example is illustrative of the procedure, there remain limitations to this particular study because the analysis used questionnaire data that may be subject to bias and whose yes/no format may not be able to represent the degree of severity captured in a full behavioral inhibition assessment. Nevertheless, person-centered analyses such as LCA represent an underutilized approach to phenotypic refinement in both temperament and psychopathology.

Behavior and Molecular Genetic Studies

In many areas of medicine, a particular illness or phenotype is described first and researchers then go about looking at the relative genetic and environmental contributions through behavior and molecular genetic studies. In psychiatry, however, this direction of reasoning has been applied in the opposite direction: that is, using results of genetic analyses to help us refine our definition of the phenotype.

Perhaps the two most investigated temperamental traits with regard to genetic studies are novelty seeking and negative affectivity/neuroticism. As previously discussed, novelty seeking describes the degree to which individuals approach and enjoy new experiences and higher stimulation activities. The dimension has also been shown to be related to potentially less desirable attributes such as impulsivity and extravagance. Possible associations between novelty seeking and genes related to dopamine transmission, particularly with the number of 48–base pair (bp) repeats in the dopamine D_4 receptor gene (*DRD4*), have received a great deal of attention (see Plomin and Caspi 1999 for a review).

Interestingly, many of these studies have demonstrated that the amount of genetic influence for novelty seeking and other traits may be less than originally assumed. These findings challenge the model that temperament is an innate risk factor that interacts with environmental factors to promote development toward or away from psychopathology. Rather, as with psychiatric disorders themselves, the expression of certain traits is moderated by particular environmental variables. One study on the expression of novelty seeking, for example, found that a more hostile child-rearing environment was required in those with genetic vulnerabilities for the expression of high novelty seeking (Keltikangas-Jarvinen et al. 2004), working through a gene–environment interaction similar to some widely studied findings in depression and stressful events (Caspi et al. 2003).

Traits related to the tendency toward experiencing negative emotions have been linked to many genes involved with serotonergic transmission (Schinka et al. 2004). A recent compelling study by Pezawas and coworkers demonstrated that the short allele of the promoter region in the gene for the serotonin transporter was related to reduced coupling in the feedback loop between the amygdala and the anterior cingulate cortex (Pezawas et al. 2005). This level of functional connectivity was strongly related to the temperament trait of harm avoidance. This same gene, and indeed the same brain regions, have been implicated in a number of psychiatric disorders, most notably depressive and anxiety disorders (Nemeroff and Owens 2002).

Unfortunately, behavioral and genetic investigations of temperament and psychopathology have tended to proceed in parallel, with both not typically assessed in the same study. It is perhaps, then, even more persuasive that candidate genes for psychiatric disorders and temperament or personality traits have converged on some of the same targets. Recently, however, researchers have begun to look at the amount of shared genetic and environmental influences between a psychiatric disorder and its temperamental counterparts as a way to delineate the boundaries between the two constructs. Behavior genetic studies have similarly begun to quantify the amount of common genetic and environmental factors between temperament and psychopathology using sophisticated genetic analyses. A study of Dutch twins found significant genetic overlap between neuroticism and levels of anxiety/depression measured quantitatively (Boomsma et al. 2000). Hettema et al. (2004) measured both the trait of neuroticism and the diagnosis of GAD in a group of adult twins. The authors found evidence for substantial overlap of the genetic factors related to both neuroticism and GAD and substantial differences in the environmental influences of the two entities. This "same genes, different environments" hypothesis is intriguing and now needs to be followed by more in-depth investigation into the issue of *which* genes and *which* environmental factors are related to these continuities and discontinuities. Obviously, the implications of these results hold importance not only in terms of phenotypic refinement but also in terms of clinical intervention.

Despite these promising findings, molecular studies of temperament and personality have been quite inconsistent and even contradictory (Van Gestel and Van Broeckhoven 2003). One recent strategy used to improve the yield of molecular genetic association studies is to test associations with temperament and *combinations* of alleles at multiple loci. For example, Lee et al. (2003) found no significant associations between novelty seeking and either the number of 48-bp repeats in exon 3 of the dopamine D_4 receptor or the C/T single-nucleotide polymorphism (SNP) at position –521 of the promoter region of the same gene. A finding was observed for the 48-bp variable number of tandem repeats (VNTR), however, among subjects with at least one C allele at the –521 SNP. Similarly, Lakatos et al. (2003) found infant activity and novelty seeking related to a combined effect of both the 48-bp VNTR on *DRD4* and a polymorphism in the serotonin transporter gene. A multivariate study of 59 candidate genes spanning multiple transmitter systems found evidence suggesting that the links between ratios of related groups of genes were stronger with personality traits than direct one-to-one association between a particular SNP and a single personality dimension (Comings et al. 2000). As our field leaves behind the notion of "one gene, one disorder," additional strategies are needed to incorporate the effects of large numbers of relevant genes and polymorphisms.

Neuroimaging Studies

Some of the early behavioral inhibition cohorts are now adults and continue to be followed. Schwartz et al. (2003) conducted a functional magnetic resonance imaging study in a small subsample of 13 subjects who at age 2 years were labeled as having behavioral inhibition versus 9 subjects who were designated as uninhibited. Adult subjects categorized as inhibited in the second year of life showed increased activation of both the left and right amygdala when shown pictures of novel faces compared with the uninhibited group. No group differences were found when participants were shown pictures of familiar faces. The finding held even after current anxiety disorder diagnosis was controlled for, as two previously subjects with behavioral inhibition met the criteria for GAD at the time of the study. The authors concluded that their amygdala findings might represent a temperamental predisposition for a disorder rather than being a marker for psychopathology itself. This conclusion implies a clear qualitative distinction between temperament and psychopathology, according to what might be called a "dry paint" model when considered developmentally. In other words, specific brain activity underlies a temperamental trait that in early childhood can be readily observed as a phenotype. Over time, however, the phenotype of many individuals changes in that they appear less overtly inhibited. Nevertheless, this underlying brain activity persists and can be seen by scraping off the layers using, in this case, functional neuroimaging. This model stands in contrast to a "wet paint" model in which developmental changes continue to mix and alter brain physiology to the point that there exist no older or underlying patterns to observe, just as a mixing wet red on top of wet blue paint yields purple with no red paint remaining underneath. Although the former is an intriguing hypothesis, it would be bolstered by measuring current temperament and perhaps a quantitative measurement of psychopathology. Returning to our discussion of somewhat distinct but interacting temperamental dimensions, a compromise hypothesis might be that many adults who previously were observed as inhibited are no longer so not because that original brain activity is no longer there but because its output is moderated by other circuits emerging later in development, such as improved emotion regulation. This specific hypothesis could be tested by identifying increased activity in cortical regions of the brain in those previously inhibited individuals.

The previously mentioned study by Pezewas et al. (2005) illustrates this point. In this study of healthy adults with no history of psychiatric illness, the authors studied a feedback circuit between the amygdala and regions of the cingulate gyrus that is involved in extinguishing a fear response. The authors demonstrated that subjects with the short allele of the serotonin transporter showed less coupling of these brain regions than subjects with the long allele and that this uncoupling was associated with the temperamental trait of harm avoidance (measured currently, not in childhood). Because these subjects are described as being at risk for depression, a particularly compelling design would be to reimage those who later become depressed to search for quantitative (greater differences in the same process compared with baseline) or qualitative differences (new abnormalities in different brain circuits). Obviously, a study like this would require a very large sample in order to have sufficient power.

Improving Temperament Assessment

As in all clinical research, if we are unable to characterize and measure the phenotypes of interest in an accurate and valid manner, any results downstream from this point are going to suffer. Previously, the issue of improving our ability to describe naturally occurring phenotypes was discussed in terms of applying new statistical techniques to existing instruments. Although this remains a very valuable approach potentially, it does assume that the data used for these techniques capture in a valid manner the true temperamental differences between measured. By far the most widely used assessment method in temperament research is the questionnaire either by self-report or, in younger children, by parent report (Saudino et al. 2001). These methods have been criticized by some as vulnerable to many sources of bias in the argument to use more observational protocols. In turn, these observational methods may be subject to their own, albeit different, concerns in assessing one point in time in an unusual setting. Inasmuch as criticism for both approaches appears legitimate, more deliberate efforts to capture the benefits from different techniques and different informants could go far toward improving results that depend on valid assessments. Similar developments could also be applied to the measurement of many of the potential mediating and moderating factors presumed to be involved in the temperament/psychopathology interplay.

CONCLUSIONS

Temperamental traits that reflect differences in emotional reactivity and control have been found to be closely linked to nearly every type of psychopathology. Research is beginning to move away from straightforward association studies between a single temperamental trait and a single psychiatric disorder toward designs that can begin to elucidate the complex mechanisms of their interactions. Building upon improvements in temperament assessment that incorporate multiple informants and methods, quantification of the cross-sectional overlap between temperament and psychopathology can serve as a starting point from which to further understand the mechanisms and development of these interactions in prospective studies. Identifying clusters of individuals who differ in their profiles across many temperamental traits may allow researchers to describe how particular dimensions work together in propelling children toward or away from more pathological trajectories. Genetic and neuroimaging studies that include measurement of both temperament and psychopathology can then anchor these findings to specific brain regions and activity. These developments currently taking place stand poised to provide us with much more specific knowledge regarding the precise interface of temperament and psychopathology over time. This knowledge, in turn, can be used to identify targets for interventions to turn previously identified genetic–environmental correlations into genetic–environmental interactions.

REFERENCES

Achenbach TM, Rescorla LA: Manual for the ASEBA School-Age Forms and Profiles. Burlington, University of Vermont, Research Center for Children, Youth, and Families 2001

Althoff RR, Rettew DC, Faraone SV, et al: Latent class analysis shows strong heritability of the Child Behavior Checklist—Juvenile Bipolar Phenotype. Biol Psychiatry 60:903–911, 2006

American Psychiatric Association: Diagnostic and Statistical Manual of Mental Disorders, 4th Edition. Washington, DC, American Psychiatric Association, 1994

American Psychiatric Association: Diagnostic and Statistical Manual of Mental Disorders, 4th Edition, Text Revision. Washington, DC, American Psychiatric Association, 2000

Austin AA, Chorpita BF: Temperament, anxiety, and depression: comparisons across five ethnic groups of children. J Clin Child Adolesc Psychol 33:216–226, 2004

Boomsma DI, Beem AL, van den Berg M, et al: Netherlands twin family study of anxious depression (NETSAD). Twin Res 3:323–334, 2000

Buss AH, Plomin R: Temperament: Early Developing Personality Traits. Hillsdale, NJ, Erlbaum, 1984

Caspi A: The child is father of the man: personality continuities from childhood to adulthood. J Pers Soc Psychol 78:158–172, 2000

Caspi A, Sugden K, Moffitt TE, et al: Influence of life stress on depression: moderation by a polymorphism in the 5-HTT gene. Science 301:386–389, 2003

Cloninger CR, Carmen B: Measurement of psychopathology as variants in personality, in Personality and Psychopathology. Edited by Cloninger CR. Washington, DC, American Psychiatric Press, 1999, pp 33–65

Cloninger CR, Svrakic DM, Przybeck TR: A psychobiological model of temperament and character. Arch Gen Psychiatry 50:975–990, 1993

Comings DE, Gade-Andavolu R, Gonzalez N, et al: A multivariate analysis of 59 candidate genes in personality traits: the temperament and character inventory. Clin Genet 58:375–385, 2000

Costa PT, McCrae RR: Revised NEO Personality Inventory and NEO Five-Factor Inventory: Professional Manual. Odessa, FL, Psychological Assessment Resources, 1992

Cukrowicz KC, Taylor J, Schatschneider C, et al: Personality differences in children and adolescents with attention-deficit/hyperactivity disorder, conduct disorder, and controls. J Child Psychol Psychiatry 47:151–159, 2006

Eysenck HJ, Eysenck SBG: Manual for the Eysenck Personality Inventory (Adult and Junior). San Diego, CA, DIGITS, 1975

Frick PJ: Integrating research on temperament and childhood psychopathology: its pitfalls and promise. J Clin Child Adolesc Psychol 33:2–7, 2004

Goldsmith HH, Buss AH, Plomin R, et al: Roundtable: What is temperament? Four approaches. Child Dev 58:505–529, 1987

Goodyer IM, Ashby L, Altham PM, et al: Temperament and major depression in 11 to 16 year olds. J Child Psychol Psychiatry 34:1409–1423, 1993

Gray JA: The Psychology of Fear and Stress. New York, Cambridge University Press, 1987

Hettema JM, Prescott CA, Kendler KS: Genetic and environmental sources of covariation between generalized anxiety disorder and neuroticism. Am J Psychiatry 161:1581–1587, 2004

Kagan J: Galen's Prophecy. Boulder, CO, Westview Press, 1994

Kagan J, Reznick JS, Snidman N: Biological bases of childhood shyness. Science 240:167–171, 1988

Keltikangas-Jarvinen L, Raikkonen K, Ekelund J, et al: Nature and nurture in novelty seeking. Mol Psychiatry 9:308–311, 2004

Klump KL, Strober M, Bulik et al: Personality characteristics of women before and after recovery from an eating disorder. Psychol Med 34:1407–1418, 2004

Krueger RF, Markon KE, Patrick CJ, et al: Externalizing psychopathology in adulthood: a dimensional-spectrum conceptualization and its implications for DSM-V. J Abnorm Psychol 114:537–550, 2005

Lakatos K, Nemoda Z, Birkas E, et al: Association of D4 dopamine receptor gene and serotonin transporter promoter polymorphisms with infants' response to novelty. Mol Psychiatry 8:90–97, 2003

Lee HJ, Lee HS, Kim YK, et al: Allelic variants interaction of dopamine receptor D4 polymorphism correlate with personality traits in young Korean female population. Am J Med Genet B Neuropsychiatr Genet 118:76–80, 2003

Lemery KS, Essex MJ, Smider NA: Revealing the relation between temperament and behavior problem symptoms by eliminating measurement confounding: expert ratings and factor analyses. Child Dev 73:867–882, 2002

Luby JL, Svrakic DM, McCallum K, et al: The Junior Temperament and Character Inventory: preliminary validation of a child self-report measure. Psychol Rep 84 (part 2):1127–1138, 1999

McCrae RR, Costa PT Jr, Ostendorf F, et al: Nature over nurture: temperament, personality, and life span development. J Pers Soc Psychol 78:173–186, 2000

McCutcheon AL: Latent Class Analysis. Newbury Park, CA, Sage, 1987

Nemeroff CB, Owens MJ: Treatment of mood disorders. Nat Neurosci (suppl 5):1068–1070, 2002

Nigg JT, John OP, Blaskey LG, et al: Big five dimensions and ADHD symptoms: links between personality traits and clinical symptoms. J Pers Soc Psychol 83:451–469, 2002

Oldehinkel AJ, Hartman CA, De Winter AF, et al: Temperament profiles associated with internalizing and externalizing problems in preadolescence. Dev Psychopathol 16:421–440, 2004

Ongur D, Farabaugh A, Iosifescu DV, et al: Tridimensional personality questionnaire factors in major depressive disorder: relationship to anxiety disorder comorbidity and age of onset. Psychother Psychosom 74:173–178, 2005

Pezawas L, Meyer-Lindenberg A, Drabant EM, et al: 5-HTTLPR polymorphism impacts human cingulate-amygdala interactions: a genetic susceptibility mechanism for depression. Nat Neurosci 8:828–834, 2005

Plomin R, Caspi A: Behavioral genetics and personality, in Handbook of Personality: Theory and Research, 2nd Edition. Edited by Pervin LA, John OP. New York, Guilford, 1999, pp 251–276

Rasmussen ER., Neuman RJ, Heath AC, et al: Familial clustering of latent class and DSM-IV defined attention-deficit/hyperactivity disorder (ADHD) subtypes. J Child Psychol Psychiatry 45:589–598, 2004

Rettew DC, McKee L: Temperament and its role in developmental psychopathology. Harv Rev Psychiatry 13:14–27, 2005

Rettew DC, Copeland W, Stanger C, et al: Associations between temperament and DSM-IV externalizing disorders in children and adolescents. J Dev Behav Pediatr 25:383–391, 2004a

Rettew DC, Doyle A, Althoff RR, et al: Does fear of novelty in social and nonsocial domains exist together or apart? A latent class approach. Poster presented at the 51st Annual Conference of the American Academy of Child and Adolescent Psychiatry, Washington, DC, October 2004b

Rettew DC, Doyle AC, Kwan M, et al: Exploring the boundary between temperament and generalized anxiety disorder: a receiver operating characteristic analysis. J Anxiety Disorders 20:931–945, 2006a

Rettew DC, Stanger C, McKee L, et al: Interactions between child and parent temperament and child behavior problems. Compr Psychiatry 47:412–420, 2006b

Rothbart MK, Ahadi SA, Evans DE: Temperament and personality: Origins and outcomes. J Pers Soc Psychol 78:122–135, 2000

Rothbart MK, Ahadi SA, Hershey K, et al: Investigations of temperament at three to seven years: The children's behavior questionnaire. Child Dev 72:1394–1408, 2001

Rutter M, Dunn J, Plomin R, et al: Integrating nature and nurture: Implications of person-environment correlations and interactions for developmental psychopathology. Dev Psychopathol 9:335–364, 1997

Saudino KJ, Cherny SS, Emde RN, et al: Sources of continuity and change in observed temperament, in Infancy to Early Childhood: Genetic and Environmental Influences on Developmental Change. Edited by Emde RN, Kewitt JK. New York, Oxford University Press, 2001, pp 89–110

Schinka JA, Busch RM, Robichaux-Keene N: A meta-analysis of the association between the serotonin transporter gene polymorphism (5-HTTLPR) and trait anxiety. Mol Psychiatry 9:197–202, 2004

Schmeck K, Poustka F: Temperament and disruptive behavior disorders. Psychopathology 34:159–163, 2001

Schwartz CE, Snidman N, Kagan J: Adolescent social anxiety as an outcome of inhibited temperament in childhood. J Am Acad Child Adolesc Psychiatry 38:1008–1015, 1999

Schwartz CE, Wright CI, Shin LM, et al: Inhibited and uninhibited infants "grown up": adult amygdalar response to novelty. Science 300:1952–1953, 2003

Shiner R, Caspi A: Personality differences in childhood and adolescence: measurement, development, and consequences. J Child Psychol Psychiatry 44:2–32, 2003

Thomas A, Chess S: Genesis and evolution of behavioral disorders: from infancy to early adult life. Am J Psychiatry 141:1–9, 1984

Tillman R, Geller B, Craney JL, et al: Temperament and character factors in a prepubertal and early adolescent bipolar disorder phenotype compared to attention deficit hyperactive and normal controls. J Child Adolesc Psychopharmacol 13:531–543, 2003

Van Gestel S, Van Broeckhoven C: Genetics of personality: are we making progress? Mol Psychiatry 8:840–852, 2003

Wills TA, Dishion TJ: Temperament and adolescent substance use: a transactional analysis of emerging self-control. J Clin Child Adolesc Psychol 33:69–81, 2004

Chapter 5

GENETICS OF PERSONALITY AND COGNITION IN ADOLESCENTS

Margaret J. Wright, Ph.D.

Nathan A. Gillespie, Ph.D.

Michelle Luciano, Ph.D.

Gu Zhu, M.P.H., M.D.

Nicholas G. Martin, Ph.D.

Disturbances in normal personality and cognitive development underlie much childhood and adolescent psychopathology. It is therefore of value to study these aspects of human behavior in normal adolescents and to try and

We thank the twins and their family members for their continued support, generosity of time, and interest in this research. We also are greatly appreciative of the assistance of research nurses Ann Eldridge and Marlene Grace as well as many other research assistants and support staff in the genetic epidemiology unit at QIMR. Phenotyping has been supported from multiple sources: National Health and Medical Research Council (NHMRC) (901061, 950998, 241944), Queensland Cancer Fund, Australian Research Council (A79600334, A79801419, A79906588, DP0212016, DP0343921), Human Frontiers Science Program (RG0154/1998-B), Beyond Blue, and The Eysenck Memorial Fund. Genotyping has been supported by the Australian NHMRC's Program in Medical Genomics (219178) and the Center for Inherited Disease Research (CIDR; Director, Dr. Jerry Roberts) at The Johns Hopkins University. CIDR is fully funded through a federal contract from the National Institutes of Health to The Johns Hopkins University (Contract Number N01-HG-65403).

unravel the genetic and environmental factors that contribute to individual differences. Since 1992 we have been conducting a longitudinal study of adolescent twins and their nontwin siblings to estimate the importance of genes and environment in personality and cognition. More recently, we have been using gene mapping techniques to pinpoint the particular genes responsible for variation. In this chapter we describe the study and the methods we are using and present some of the results across the domains of personality and cognition.

METHODOLOGY

Twin Sample

A large sample of adolescent and young adult twins (3,408 individuals) and their nontwin singleton siblings (1,572), constituting 1,703 families, is a common resource for several key studies at the Queensland Institute of Medical Research (QIMR) in Australia (Wright and Martin 2004). The twins were recruited from primary and secondary schools in the greater Brisbane area, by media appeals, and by word of mouth. The sample includes both monozygotic (MZ) and dizygotic (DZ) twin pairs, including opposite-sex twin pairs, the singleton siblings of twins, and the twins' parents. The twins and siblings attend QIMR for testing as close as possible to their 12th, 14th, and 16th birthdays and are measured on a range of phenotypes, with personality being measured at 12, 14, and 16 years and cognition at 16 years. In addition, blood is collected for DNA and various hematological and immunological measures. Where possible, any singleton siblings of the twins who are within 5 years of age of the twins are also recruited and tested on an identical protocol. The benefits of a twin and sibling design include increased statistical power to detect genetic and shared environmental influences on a measured variable and the testing of several assumptions of the classical twin design. Thus, the design provides important information on whether estimates based on twin samples can be generalized to a nontwin population (Posthuma and Boomsma 2000). Also, by adding a sibling, MZ pairs become informative for linkage and within-pair association analysis. (By themselves they are not.) Families of DZ twins also become more informative (Dolan et al. 1999). Parents of twins are not phenotyped, but their DNA is used in error detection of marker genotypes and contributed to identity by descent (IBD; see below) estimation as well as haplotype determination.

For all same-sex twin pairs, zygosity is established by DNA polymorphisms using a commercial kit (AmpFlSTR Profiler Plus PCR Amplification Kit, Applied Biosystems, Foster City, CA) and cross-checked with blood group results (ABO, MNS, and Rh) and/or phenotypic data such as hair, skin, and eye color, giving an overall probability of correct zygosity assignment of greater than 99.99%. For DZ pairs this is subsequently confirmed by genome-wide genotyping for linkage scans. All participants give written, informed consent before participating in the study.

Phenotyping of Personality and Cognition

The personality questionnaire we are using in our adolescent studies is the full 81-item Junior Eysenck Personality Questionnaire (JEPQ) (Eaves et al. 1989; H.J. Eysenck and Eysenck 1975; S.B.G. Eysenck 1972), which assesses the three major dimensions of personality: Psychoticism (17 items), Extraversion (24 items), and Neuroticism (20 items). In addition, the questionnaire contains the 20-item Lie scale, which is a measure of social desirability. The JEPQ is scored on a 3-point scale (yes, don't know, and no), with "don't know" responses recorded as missing.

A broad array of cognitive data is being collected, and the measures have been described in detail elsewhere (Wright and Martin 2004; Wright et al. 2001a). Briefly, psychometric IQ is assessed using the Multidimensional Aptitude Battery and the Digit Symbol Substitution subtest from the Wechsler Adult Intelligence Scale—Revised, which provides a Full Scale IQ score, Verbal and Performance IQ scores, and scores for several specific cognitive abilities (Information, Arithmetic, Vocabulary, Spatial, Object Assembly, Digit Symbol). Processing speed is assessed at multiple levels: inspection time assesses early perception; choice reaction time (2-, 4-, and 8-choice reaction time [RT]) assesses information/response processing; and an event-related brain potential (ERP) measure, P300 latency, assesses stimulus evaluation. Similarly, working memory is assessed by performance accuracy and speed measures on a delayed response task, and ERP P300 amplitude and slow-wave amplitude assess attention and visuospatial processing, respectively. Resting electroencephalogram (EEG) measures— (individual) alpha frequency, EEG power (delta, theta, alpha, beta), and EEG coherence—provide psychophysiological measures of brain processing. In addition, two measures of reading ability, the Cambridge Contextual Reading Test (CCRT) and the Schonell Graded Word Fluency Test (SGWFT), are included. The CCRT is a contextualized adaptation of the National Adult Reading Test, which is widely used as a measure of premorbid IQ (Franzen et al. 1997) because of the correlation of word reading ability with IQ and the greater resilience of word reading performance to neurological insult compared with other cognitive measures. Lastly, the battery includes a measure of academic achievement, the Queensland Core Skills Test (QCST), which the majority of grade 12 Queensland students take in their final year at secondary school (i.e., a Queensland equivalent of the SAT).

Genome Scan for the Purpose of Linkage Analysis

Two separate genome-wide marker scans have been completed on a subset of these families (525 families, 2,123 individuals), one by the Australian Genome Research Facility, Melbourne, and a second by the Center for Inherited Disease Research, Bethesda, Maryland (supported by the National Institutes of Health). Combining the two scans results in 795 microsatellite markers (each of the separate but intercollating scans had approximately 400 markers), including 761 markers on the autosomes and 34 markers on the X chromosome, with an average heterozygosity of 79% and an average intermarker distance of 4.8 centimorgans (cM).

Locations of markers were determined from the sex-averaged deCODE genetic map (Kong et al. 2002; Leal 2003). For twins/siblings the number of markers ranged from 211 to 790, with an average of 601 (±192) total markers. Extensive crosschecking and data cleaning included pedigree error checking, genotype error checking via Mendelian error detection, and detection of spurious double recombination events (see Zhu et al. 2004 for a detailed description). Genotype data from approximately 80% of parents also assisted with error detection.

THE PERSONALITY STUDY

Numerous reports based on adult twin data have examined the heritability of personality, in particular for the domains of neuroticism and extraversion. Heritability estimates in the vicinity of 50% have been reported (Eaves and Eysenck 1975; Eaves et al. 1998; Heath et al. 1997; Jinks and Fulker 1970; Kendler et al. 1993; Martin et al. 1979). Given this strong empirical support for genetic contributions to personality, more recently several studies have attempted to locate quantitative trait loci (QTLs) for personality traits (Abkevich et al. 2003; Boomsma et al. 2000; Fullerton et al. 2003; Kirk et al. 2000; Thorgeirsson et al. 2003; Zubenko et al. 2003). These linkage studies have focused on neuroticism, neuroticism-like traits, and genetically related measures of mood and anxiety, and as yet there have been no genome scans for extraversion or psychoticism.

In the next section we summarize our findings of the magnitude of genetic and environmental effects on the multidimensional structure of personality across time (i.e., at ages 12, 14, and 16 years) using genetic simplex modeling (reported in full in Gillespie et al. 2004). We also report our linkage findings for the four domains of personality as assessed by the JEPQ in a subsample of these adolescent twins (see Gillespie et al., in press, for an in depth report).

Genetic Simplex Modeling of Personality in Adolescence

The sample included 670 twin pairs (253 MZ, 417 DZ) at age 12, 578 (216 MZ, 362 DZ) at age 14, and 545 (249 MZ, 296 DZ), at age 16 years. Personality scores were analyzed in the Mx statistical package (Neale et al. 2003) with genetic simplex modeling that explicitly took into account the longitudinal nature of the data. Genetic correlations between personality scores measured at 12, 14, and 16 years were moderate to high (0.61–1.00). Consistent with previous research findings for personality, familial aggregation for each dimension was significant and explained approximately 30%–50% of the total variance at each age. With the exception of the Lie dimension, model-fitting results revealed that familial aggregation was entirely explained by additive genetic effects, accounting for approximately 30%–50% of the total variance at each age, and that large proportions of the additive genetic variance observed at ages 14 and 16 years could be explained by genetic effects present at age 12 years. However, there was evidence for smaller but significant genetic innovations at ages 14 and 16 years for Neuroticism in boys and girls, at 14 years for male Extraversion, at 14 and 16 years for female Psychoticism, and at 14 years for male Psychoticism. These smaller genetic innovations not only suggest that genetic variation is not completely determined by age 12 years but potentially hint at age-specific genetic effects related to developmental or hormonal changes during puberty and psychosexual development.

Genome-Wide Linkage Scan for the Four Dimensions of Personality

Methods

Linkage analysis, using a variance components approach, was based on a subsample of 493 families (1,280 twins and sibs) for whom both genotyping and phenotypic data were available and included only the first twin of a MZ pair. Univariate variance components linkage analysis, parameterized as a function of the variance due to a major QTL, a polygenic component, and unique environment, was performed in Mx, with age and sex specified as a covariate on the means. Estimation of the QTL effect requires the calculation of multipoint IBD probabilities using the software program MERLIN (Abecasis et al. 2002). The covariance of a pair of siblings is modeled according to the extent to which they share alleles IBD at a typed polymorphic marker locus (maximum likelihood, multipoint IBD probabilities: P[IBD=0,1,2]). QTL linkage is present if omission of the QTL from the model causes a significant worsening of fit as evidenced by the χ^2 change. This produces a logarithm of odds (LOD=χ^2/4.6) score that is compatible with the parametric linkage analysis index. Linkage was considered significant if LOD scores exceeded 3.6 and suggestive if LOD scores exceeded 2.2 (Lander and Kruglyak 1995).

In addition, to increase the power to detect linkage for each of the personality dimensions, we tested, by means of a multivariate model that included measures at ages 12, 14, and 16 years, with age and sex as a covariate, whether a QTL is responsible for the same amount of phenotypic variation at each age by equating the three QTL factor loadings. From this reduced model, we then tested for linkage by examining whether the (equated) QTL could be set to zero (for a detailed description, see Evans et al. 2004).

Results

Genome-wide linkage results for the four personality dimensions are shown in Figure 5–1, with the cumulative map position (cM) plotted on the x-axis and LOD score on the y-axis. Univariate analyses at 12, 14, and 16 years are superimposed so that it is possible to compare the consistency of results across each measurement occasion, and displayed immediately below in the figure is the multivariate scan where the QTL factor loadings across the three waves are equated ($df=1$). LOD scores greater than 1.5 are presented in Table 5–1. Suggestive linkage, defined as the a priori criterion of a LOD score greater than 2.2, was found for Neuroticism on chromosome 16, Extraversion on chromosomes 2 and 3, and Psychoticism on chromosomes 1, 7, 10, and 13, but no significant linkage peaks (LOD>3.6) were evident. The linkage signal on chromosome 16 was for Neuroticism measured at age 16 years, with no coincident peaks for Neuroticism measured at 12 or 14 years, or for the multivariate analysis. Similarly, the linkage signal on chromosome 2 for Extraversion was specific to age 16 years, as was the signal on chromosomes 10 and 13 for Psychoticism specific to age 12 years. However, there was reasonable consistency for the linkage signal for Extraversion on chromosome 3, with a suggestive LOD score of 2.38 found in the multivariate analysis and overlapping peaks with LODs > 1.5 found for Extraversion measured at 12 and 16 years, with a peak close by at age 14 years. Also, the linkage signals for Psychoticism on chromosomes 1 and 7 were found for more than one measure: on chromosome 1 overlapping peaks were found in the multivariate analysis and at age 12 years, and on chromosome 7 overlapping peaks were found at ages 12 and 14 years, as well as in the multivariate analysis.

Discussion

This is the first genome-wide scan for adolescent Neuroticism and the first in both adolescents and adults for the dimensions of Extraversion, Psychoti-

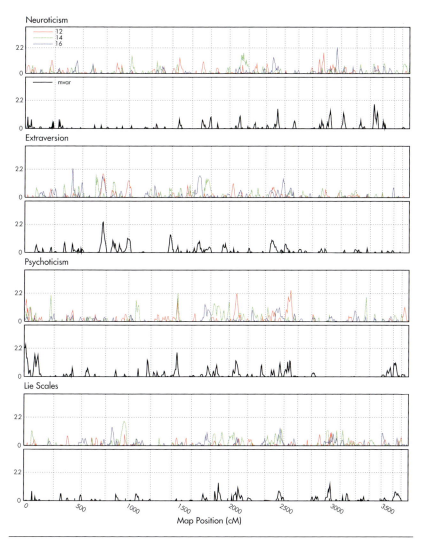

FIGURE 5–1.   Genome screen for personality in the Brisbane adolescent twin sample.

Note.   Linkage plots displaying the significance (LOD [logarithm of odds] scores [y-axis]) of Neuroticism, Extraversion, Psychoticism, and Lie to regions on chromosomes 1 to 22 (distance in centimorgans [cM] along the x-axis) for the univariate analyses at each of the three time points (ages 12 [red], 14 [green], 16 [blue]) and for the multivariate (mvar [black]) analysis. Suggestive linkage is indicated by a LOD> 2.2 (indicated by the horizontal dotted line).

TABLE 5–1.   Regions of suggestive linkage (LOD > 2.2; shown in bold) and LODs greater than 1.50 for personality measures

Chromosome	Measure	Position (cM)	Marker	Peak LOD
1	Psychoticism_12	25.713	D1S450	1.77
	Psychoticism_mvar	25.713	D1S450	**2.46**
	Psychoticism_mvar	116.42	D1S551	1.70
	Psychoticism_14	266.206	D1S2785	2.08
2	Extraversion_16	174.226	D2S2330	**2.29**
3	Extraversion_12	198.435	D3S1262	1.86
	Extraversion_14	126.31	D3S2460	1.81
	Extraversion_16	198.435	D3S1262	1.73
	Extraversion_mvar	203.567	D3S1580	**2.38**
4	Lie_14	181.735	D4S2417	1.92
5	Neuroticism_14	15.873	D5S2505	1.51
	Psychoticism_14	64.933	D5S1457	1.71
7	Psychoticism_12	50.565	D7S817	1.81
	Psychoticism_14	54.925	D7S484	**2.26**
	Psychoticism_mvar	50.565	D7S817	1.88
8	Extraversion_16	69.471	D8S1110	1.73
9	Psychoticism_14	160.92	D9S158	1.58
10	Psychoticism_12	69.072	D10S196	**2.20**
	Neuroticism_14	126.019	D10S597	1.79
12	Neuroticism_mvar	111.14	D12S393	1.56
13	Psychoticism_12	54.01	D13S788	**2.45**
15	Neuroticism_12	106.632	D15S130	1.80
16	Neuroticism_16	113.279	D16S516	**2.29**
18	Psychoticism_14	90.349	D18S68	1.92
19	Neuroticism_mvar	38.55	D19S588	1.90

Note.   mvar=multivariate analysis; 12=at age 12 years; 14=at age 14 years; 16=at age 16 years.

cism, and Lie. Although we found no regions that reached the significance criterion of 3.6, several linkage peaks met the suggestive criterion, identifying a number of regions that may contain genes playing a role in the normal variation of personality in adolescence. For some of these linkage peaks there was good congruency across the three ages, in line with our findings of significant additive genetic continuity across the age bands (Gillespie et al. 2004).

The most consistent evidence for linkage was for Extraversion on chromosome 3, with a maximum LOD score of 2.38 near the marker D3S1580 in the multivariate analysis and LOD scores greater than 1.5 in the same region at ages 12 and 14 years and in an overlapping region at age 14 years. However, note that linkage peaks span chromosomal regions of around 20 cM and many hundreds of genes, making it difficult to identify a gene or nucleotide variant that is responsible for the QTL effect. Other regions that emerged for Extraversion were regions on chromosomes 2 and 8, both for age 16 years. The linkage signal on chromosome 2 is interesting given that it is coincident with our linkage peak on chromosome 2 for general cognitive ability that is described below (see also Luciano et al. 2006; Posthuma et al. 2005; Wainwright et al. 2006), with the present sample being a subsample of that used in the cognition study. There has been recent interest in the relationship between intelligence and personality, with extraversion in particular suggested to influence IQ test performance (Wolf and Ackerman 2005).

The next strongest linkage signals were for Psychoticism on the short arm of chromosome 1, with a reasonably strong signal found in the multivariate analysis and a coincident peak at age 12 years. Indeed a number of areas of interest for this dimension of personality were evident, with a linkage peak on chromosome 7 also reaching the suggestive level with a coincident peak at another time point and in the multivariate analysis. Further single peaks at one time point were evident on chromosomes 10 and 13. As this is the first complete genome scan for Psychoticism, there are no studies with which to compare the location of these peaks. However the linkage peak on chromosome 13 is in the vicinity of the *HTR2A* gene located at 13q14.21, which has been implicated in schizophrenia, psychosis, and impulsivity (e.g., Abdolmaleky et al. 2004; Walitza et al. 2002; Williams et al. 1996).

In contrast to the dimensions of Extraversion and Psychoticism, for Neuroticism only one linkage signal on chromosome 16, at age 16 years, met the suggestive threshold. Evidence for linkage to social phobia for a region nearby on chromosome 16 has been identified previously (Gelernter et al. 2004). There was no evidence for linkage on chromosome 1, which has been the most consistently reported linkage region for Neuroticism in adult studies (e.g., see Fullerton 2006; Fullerton et al. 2003; Nash et al. 2004; B.M. Neale et al. 2005).

The findings of this study represent a first step but should be interpreted cautiously given the modest sample size and the fact that linkage signals were only suggestive. Replication in an independent sample will be required in order to assess the potential role of the chromosomal regions identified.

THE COGNITION STUDY

The Search for Genes Influencing Cognition

Individual differences in cognitive functioning, as measured by IQ tests, are to a large extent caused by differences at a genetic level (Bouchard and McGue 1981; Plomin et al. 1994b). Heritability estimates for various other measures of cognitive functioning (including endophenotypes—quantifiable intermediate constructs that index a behavioral trait) also range from moderate (e.g., 0.38 for perceptual speed) to very high (e.g., 0.83 for EEG power), as shown by us (see below) and others (e.g., Rijsdijk et al. 1998). Despite this evidence for "genes for cognition," the actual identification of genes has not been easy and progress has been slow because genetic influences on cognitive ability, much as with other heritable quantitatively distributed traits, are caused by the combined action of many genes of small effect (QTLs), a perspective that recently has been reaffirmed (Hill 2005).

Initial efforts to identify genetic variants influencing IQ (the IQ-QTL Project [Daniels et al. 1998; Plomin et al. 1995; Plomin et al. 1994a]) provided some evidence for associations of cognitive ability with various genetic polymorphisms (e.g., insulin-like growth factor 2 receptor marker) (Chorney et al. 1998), none of which were replicated in a genome-wide association analysis technique (using 1,842 genetic markers) applied to groups of average and extremely high IQ participants (Plomin et al. 2001). Most recently, a 10K microarray typed on the pooled DNA of cases with mild mental impairment and control subject, then on low-versus-high IQ samples showed association of four single nucleotide polymorphisms (SNPs) with general cognitive ability at 7 years; this was confirmed by individual genotyping in 6,154 children (Butcher et al. 2005b). These four SNPs, coupled with a fifth SNP identified in a study of 432 functional nonsynonymous SNPs expressed in the brain (Butcher et al. 2005a), form a SNP set that has been found to account for 0.86% of variance in g at age 7 years and also predicts variance in general cognitive ability (g) as early as age 2 years (Harlaar et al. 2005).

Another approach comes from targeted candidate gene studies, with findings of polymorphisms in genes coding for brain-derived neurotrophic factor, prion protein, and succinate-semialdehyde dehydrogenase to be associated with normal variation in IQ (Plomin et al. 2004; Rujescu et al. 2003; Tsai et al. 2004). Allelic associations with tasks measuring the specific cognitive processes of cued discrimination, memory, and attention have also been reported for apolipoprotein E and catechol-*O*-methyltransferase Val158Met polymorphisms (Egan et al. 2001; Flory et al. 2000). Other associations include that for the α_{2C}-adrenergic receptor gene (*ADRA2C*), which has been implicated in learning disability (Comings et al. 1999), and the forkhead box P2 gene (*FOXP2*) on chromosome 7, which is related to severe disruption of speech and language (Lai et al. 2001).

Our study for genes for cognition in adolescent twins includes a range of behavioral and neurophysiological indices of cognitive function in addition to indices of general cognitive ability (IQ) and is part of a collaborative effort with the Netherlands and Japan (Wright et al. 2001a). It was specifically designed to sample cognitive tasks (e.g., information processing speed, working memory, reading ability, academic achievement) that have shown consistent significant correlations with IQ. The rationale for this approach is that cognitive endophenotypes measuring more discrete components of cognition are more upstream and are likely to be influenced by a smaller number of genes. We summarize in the next section our quantitative analyses of IQ and other cognitive phenotypes, including our genome-wide linkage scan of IQ, and report our most recent linkage findings for our information processing and working memory measures.

Genetic Analyses of IQ and Cognitive Endophenotypes

To date we have tested 681 twin pairs and 207 of their nontwin siblings, with a mean age of 16 years, on our cognitive test battery. This is a subsample of the twin sample described previously. As shown in Figure 5–2 we have found pervasive genetic influence on both elementary and higher-order cognitive tasks; high heritability was not just found for the broadest index of cognition (IQ) but also for specific cognitive processes and endophenotypes of cognitive ability. These range from a high of 0.80 for EEG power to a low of 0.40 for inspection time (IT) and slow wave.

In a series of multivariate analyses we have tested whether correlations between the various cognitive phenotypes stem from shared (pleiotropic) genes (pleiotropy occurs when a single gene influences multiple phenotypic traits). We have shown that common genes influence a range of processing speed and working memory indices, and IQ, and established the extent to which genetic (and environmental) sources of covariation explain the phenotypic association between more specific indices of cognitive ability and IQ (Luciano et al. 2001a, 2001b, 2002, 2003, 2004a, 2004b, 2005; Wainwright et al. 2004, 2005a, 2005b; Wright et al. 2000, 2001b, 2002). For ex-

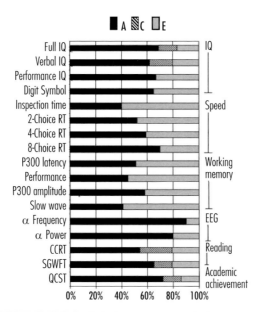

FIGURE 5–2.   Heritability of cognitive measures in the Brisbane adolescent twin sample.

Note.   A=additive genetic; C=common environment; E=unique environment; CCRT=Cambridge Contextual Reading Test; RT=reaction time; SGWFT= Schonell Graded Word Fluency Test; QCST=Queensland Core Skills Test; EEG = electroencephalogram.

ample, we used direction of causation modeling to show that covariation between IT, which taps perceptual speed, and IQ is best explained by pleiotropic genes that influence individual variation in both IT and IQ (Luciano et al. 2005). However, although we found that a common genetic influence primarily explains the relationship between measures, we also found that "group" genetic factors were important. These may exist because of the mutual reliance of some cognitive measures on processes that are mediated by a different set of genes than general cognitive ability. For example, analysis of the covariance among IT, CRT, and IQ subtests showed that three genetic group factors (verbal, visuospatial, broad speediness) were important, in addition to a single genetic factor influencing all measures (Luciano et al. 2004a). These findings are in agreement with findings from other studies (Martin and Eaves 1977; Petrill et al. 1996; Rijsdijk et al. 1998; Wainwright et al. 2004) and suggest that it is likely that QTLs exist for these group factors.

Genome-Wide Linkage Scan for IQ

As was reported elsewhere (Luciano et al. 2006), our first whole genome-wide linkage scan on 361 families (2–5 siblings per family) was performed on the scaled Verbal, Performance, and Full Scale IQ scores, three verbal (information, vocabulary, arithmetic) and three performance (Spatial, Object Assembly, and Wechsler Adult Intelligence Scale—Revised [WAIS-R] Digit Symbol) IQ subtests, and two measures of premorbid IQ (CCRT and SGWFT reading tests). We found converging linkage peaks on chromosome 2 for performance IQ and the CCRT, with respective LOD scores of 3.7 and 4.15. (Empirical LOD scores were estimated [with correction for multiple testing], with performance IQ just falling short of the significance criterion of 3.8 and the CCRT just exceeding the significance criterion of 4.14.) Smaller linkage peaks in this same region were found for the performance IQ subtests, Spatial and Object Assembly, and the SGWFT, and also for academic achievement as measured by the QCST in a subsample of twins (Wainwright et al. 2006). Importantly this linkage peak was found in an independent sample from the Netherlands as well as for the combined Australian and Dutch data (Posthuma et al. 2005). Figure 5–3 shows the linkage plots for the cognitive variables showing converging linkage regions on chromosome 2. Our findings suggest that genes in this region influence a breadth of indicators of general cognitive ability. Specific genes potentially implicated include *GAD1*, *NOSTRIN*, *KCNH7*, *TBR1*, *DLX1*, and *DLX2*, with several of these genes involved in glutamanergic neural transmission, and have been discussed in detail by Posthuma et al. (2005) and Luciano et al. (2006).

We have also identified suggestive linkage peaks (LOD > 2.2) on other chromosomes, including a strong peak on the short arm of chromosome 6 for the verbal subtest Arithmetic (LOD=3.05) as well as Full Scale IQ (LOD= 2.24) (Figure 5–3). This region was identified in the Dutch twin pairs, in the combined linkage analysis of the Australian and Dutch data (Posthuma et al. 2005), and most recently in a linkage analysis of IQ in the collaborative study on the genetics of alcoholism sample (Dick et al. 2006). This region has also been implicated in linkage studies of development dyslexia (Kaplan et al. 2002; Marlow et al. 2003). In addition, a further linkage peak was identified on 6q, with convergence of peaks for verbal test measures (SGWFT, Information, Verbal IQ).

Genome-Wide Linkage for Information Processing and Working Memory

We report here genome-wide linkage findings for information processing measures, including 2-, 4-, and 8-choice RT and inspection time, and for

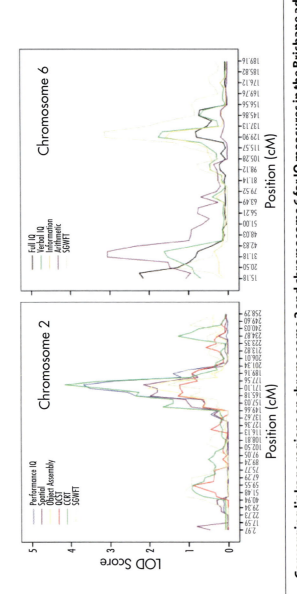

FIGURE 5–3.   Converging linkage regions on chromosome 2 and chromosome 6 for IQ measures in the Brisbane adolescent twin sample.

Left.   Significant linkage (indicated by a logarithm of odds [LOD] of 3.6) for Performance IQ and the Cambridge Contextual Reading Test (CCRT) on chromosome 2. Overlapping linkage peaks were also evident for the IQ subtests Spatial and Object Assembly, the Schonell Graded Word Fluency Test (SGWFT), and the Queensland Core Skills Test (QCST). Both IQ and reading measures peak in the same region on 2q, suggesting a general cognitive ability gene.

Right.   Suggestive linkage on chromosome 6p for the IQ subtest arithmetic with overlapping peaks for full IQ and verbal IQ, and on 6q convergence of peaks for verbal test measures (SGWFT, information, verbal IQ). The x axis indicates position of markers in centimorgans (cM).

Source.   Adapted from Luciano et al. 2006.

working-memory behavioral measures during a delayed response (DR) task, including a measure of accuracy, DR spatial (sensory) precision; a speed measure, DR initiation time; and an omnibus measure of working memory performance (including both accuracy and speed), DR performance.

Methods

The sample included all individuals for whom we had both phenotypic and genotypic data available (378 families [2–5 siblings per family] for information processing; 285 families for delayed-response working memory) and was very similar to the sample used in the linkage analyses on IQ reported previously in this chapter. Univariate, multipoint, variance components linkage analysis was performed in the MERLIN software program. As for the linkage analysis of personality traits, the QTL is estimated using the probabilities that siblings share genes IBD, with the QTL effect evaluated by the difference in log10 likelihood of a model that includes the QTL and a model that fixes it to zero. This produces a LOD score that is compatible with the parametric linkage analysis index. Lander and Kruglyak's (1995) criteria for suggestive and significance linkage were adopted but were not corrected for multiple testing because of the exploratory nature of these analyses.

Results

Genome-wide linkage results are shown in Figure 5–4. Suggestive linkage, using the a priori criterion of LOD greater than 2.2, was indicated on the long arm of chromosome 1 for 8-choice RT, with smaller but coincident peaks for both 2- and 4-choice RT (LODs=1.86 and 1.89, respectively). There was also suggestive linkage for 8-choice RT on chromosome 11, for 4-choice RT on chromosomes 8 and 22, and for working memory measures on chromosomes 7 (DR accuracy) and 14 (DR initiation time). Table 5–2 lists the suggestive linkage regions as well as those regions with LODs greater than 1.5 that did not meet the suggestive criteria. These include regions on chromosomes 12 and 18 for inspection time and on chromosome 22 for 4-choice RT, and for working memory measures, a region on chromosome 2 for DR accuracy, and on chromosome 22 for DR initiation time.

Discussion

These new analyses do not corroborate our linkage findings on chromosomes 2 and 6 for general cognitive ability (IQ) described above. They suggest other chromosomal regions that may be involved in more specific cognitive abilities associated with information processing and working memory. Genetic covariance studies of IQ subtests all find a general genetic factor that explains a significant proportion of cognitive measure variability,

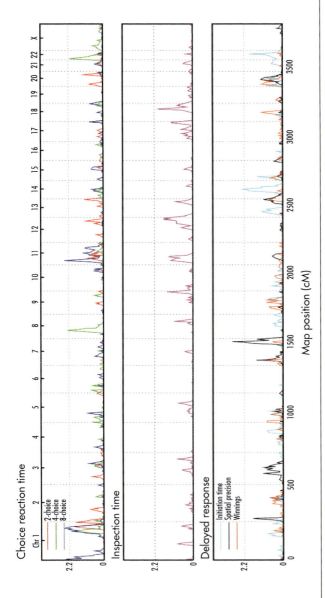

FIGURE 5–4.   Genome screen for information processing and working memory measures in the Brisbane adolescent twin sample.

Note.   Linkage plots displaying the significance (LOD [logarithm of odds] scores [y axis]) of 2-, 4-, and 8-choice reaction time (red, green, and blue, respectively), inspection time, and delayed response measures (initiation time [aqua], spatial precision [black], winnings [brown]) to regions on chromosomes 1–23 (distance in centimorgans [cM] along the x axis) are displayed. Suggestive linkage was defined by a LOD>2.2 and indicated by the horizontal dotted line.

TABLE 5–2. Regions of suggestive linkage (LOD > 2; shown in bold) and LODs greater than 1.50 for the elementary cognitive measures

Chromo-some	Measure	Position[a]	1 LOD Drop	Peak LOD
1	2-choice RT	242.13	228.26–244.40	1.86
	4-choice RT	207.07	199.74–219.23	1.89
	8-choice RT	228.26	194.98–244.40	**2.50**
2	DR spatial precision	19.64	7.60–22.73	1.70
7	DR spatial precision	165.57	159.33–195.13	**2.90**
8	4-choice RT	54.23	52.74–65.47	**2.26**
11	8-choice RT	25.69	17.05–42.49	**2.50**
12	Inspection time	169.54	131.83–169.54	1.67
14	DR initiation time	63.5	36.71–81.46	**2.28**
18	Inspection time	85.12	77.59–92.54	1.97
22	4-choice RT	2.96	2.96–14.68	2.12
	DR initiation time	37.03	32.92–42.26	1.89

Note. DR = delayed response; RT = reaction time.
[a]Comings et al. 1999.

but it is apparent that there is also a large proportion of genetic variability accounted for by genetic group and specific factors (Martin and Eaves 1977; Petrill et al. 1996; Rijsdijk et al. 1998; Wainwright et al. 2004).

The strongest linkage signal was on chromosome 1, in which the linkage peaks for all three levels of the CRT task overlapped. The evidence for linkage was greatest for the 8-choice RT, possibly because this measure had the highest heritability and is the most reliable, as shown by test-retest reliability. As can be seen in Figure 5–4, linkage to this region, albeit nonsignificant, is also observed for IT, and previously we found a small linkage peak (LOD >1) for the IQ subtest Vocabulary and the IQ subtest Digit Symbol (Luciano et al. 2006). Moreover, we found that the CRT tasks share information processing variance with the IQ subtest Digit Symbol that is greater than that shared with other IQ subtests through a genetic general cognitive ability factor, and that IT is also related to choice RT and Digit Symbol through this genetic information processing factor (Luciano et al. 2004a). Thus, it may be that genes in this region on chromosome 1 influence variation in measures that involve information processing efficiency. Independent support for this notion is the finding of small linkage signals in this region for a number of neuropsychological tests, including Digit Symbol, Block Design, and Trails B of the Trail Making Test, which involve an information processing component, in the Collaborative Study on Genetics of Alcoholism Sample (Buyske et al. 2006).

All other regions of "suggestive" linkage (defined as LOD >2.2) were for a single measure. The linkage signal on chromosomes 8 and 22 for 4-choice RT was specific to this measure, and these regions were not implicated in our previous analyses of IQ (Luciano et al. 2006) or academic achievement (Wainwright et al. 2006). Similarly, the peak on chromosome 11 for 8-choice RT also appears to be specific, although we note a weak coincident linkage signal for IT and a small peak for 2-choice RT that is overlapping with this region. However, for the DR working memory measures, the peaks on chromosome 7 for DR accuracy and on chromosome 14 for DR initiation time are coincident with suggestive linkage peaks identified on chromosome 7 for verbal IQ, and on chromosome 14 for both the IQ subtest Arithmetic and the SGWFT (Luciano et al. 2006). The region on chromosome 14 is particularly interesting given the finding of suggestive linkage to this region for the WAIS-R Digit Symbol subtest in the Collaborative Study on the Genetics of Alcoholism Sample (Buyske et al. 2006).

Although the results of this study are not sufficiently strong of themselves to firmly implicate any of the regions identified in cognition, they are of interest in that they possibly identify other chromosomal regions, in addition to those on 2 and 6, that may harbor genes for cognition, and are beginning to reveal patterns of genes that have an impact on related cognitive phenotypes.

CONCLUSIONS

In this ongoing work, a long-term aim has been to provide a powerful resource of brain phenotypes and genotypes to test hypotheses of how putative genetic mechanisms influence variation in normal brain function, in particular with respect to personality and cognition. It is hoped that in time this will dovetail with information being gathered from various clinical studies of neurological and psychiatric disorders and will allow for the piecing together of disjointed parts of the literature in powerful and novel ways.

With the award of a medical genomics grant from the National Health and Medical Research Council of Australia for high-density SNP mapping, we will have available over a period of 4 years a genome-wide association scan using the Affymetrix 500K chip with more than 500,000 SNPs for most of the twins and siblings in our adolescent sample. This will provide us with a unique opportunity to examine the association of genetic polymorphisms, spread across the entire genome, with the personality and cognition phenotypes.

REFERENCES

Abdolmaleky HM, Farone SV, Glatt SJ, et al: Meta-analysis of association between the T102C polymorphism of the 5HT2a receptor gene and schizophrenia. Schizophrenia Res 67:53–62, 2004

Abecasis GR, Cherny SS, Cookson WO, et al: Merlin—rapid analysis of dense genetic maps using sparse gene flow trees. Nat Genet 30:97–101, 2002

Abkevich V, Camp NJ, Hensel CH, et al: Predisposition locus for major depression at chromosome 12q22–12q23.2. Am J Hum Genet 73:1271–1281, 2003

Boomsma DI, Beem AL, van den Berg M, et al: Netherlands twin family study of anxious depression (NETSAD). Twin Res 3:323–334, 2000

Bouchard TJ Jr, McGue M: Familial studies of intelligence: a review. Science 212:1055–1059, 1981

Butcher LM, Meaburn E, Dale PS, et al: Association analysis of mild mental impairment using DNA pooling to screen 432 brain-expressed single-nucleotide polymorphisms. Mol Psychiatry 10:384–92, 2005a

Butcher LM, Meaburn E, Knight J, et al: SNPs, microarrays and pooled DNA: identification of four loci associated with mild mental impairment in a sample of 6000 children. Hum Mol Genet 14:1315–1325, 2005b

Buyske S, Bates ME, Gharani N, et al: Cognitive traits link to human chromosomal regions. Behav Genet 36:65–76, 2006

Chorney MJ, Chorney K, Seese N, et al: A quantitative trait locus associated with cognitive ability in children. Psychol Sci 9:159–166, 1998

Comings DE, Gade-Andavolu R, Gonzalez N, et al: Additive effect of three noradrenergic genes (ADRA2a, ADRA2C, DBH) on attention-deficit hyperactivity disorder and learning disabilities in Tourette syndrome subjects. Clin Genet 55:160–172, 1999

Daniels J, Holmans P, Williams N, et al: A simple method for analyzing microsatellite allele image patterns generated from DNA pools and its application to allelic association studies. Am J Hum Genet 62:1189–1197, 1998

Dick DM, Aliev F, Bierut L, et al: Linkage analyses of IQ in the collaborative study on the genetics of alcoholism (COGA) sample. Behav Genet 36:77–86, 2006

Dolan CV, Boomsma DI, Neale MC: A note on the power provided by sibships of sizes 2, 3, and 4 in genetic covariance modeling of a codominant QTL. Behav Genet 29:163–170, 1999

Eaves L, Eysenck HJ: The nature of extraversion: a genetical analysis. J Pers Soc Psychol 32:102–112, 1975

Eaves L, Eysenck HJ, Martin NG: Genes, Culture, and Personality: An Empirical Approach. London, Academic Press, 1989

Eaves LJ, Heath AC, Neale MC, et al: Sex differences and non-additivity in the effects of genes on personality. Twin Res 1:131–137, 1998

Egan MF, Goldberg TE, Kolachana BS, et al: Effect of COMT Val108/158 Met genotype on frontal lobe function and risk for schizophrenia. Proc Natl Acad Sci U S A 98:6917–6922, 2001

Evans DM, Zhu G, Duffy DL, et al: Multivariate QTL linkage analysis suggests a QTL for platelet count on chromosome 19q. Eur J Hum Genet 12:835–842, 2004

Eysenck HJ, Eysenck SBG: Manual for the Eysenck Personality Questionnaire (Adult and Junior). San Diego, CA, Digits, 1975

Eysenck SBG: Junior Eysenck Personality Inventory. EdITS/Educational and Industrial Testing Service, P.O. Box 7234, San Diego, CA 92167, 1972

Flory JD, Manuck SB, Ferrell RE, et al: Memory performance and the apolipoprotein E polymorphism in a community sample of middle-aged adults. Am J Med Genet 96:707–711, 2000

Franzen MD, Burgess EJ, Smith-Seemiller L: Methods of estimating premorbid functioning. Arch Clin Neuropsychol 12:711–738, 1997

Fullerton J: New approaches to the genetic analysis of neuroticism and anxiety. Behav Genet 36:147–61, 2006

Fullerton J, Cubin M, Tiwari H, et al: Linkage analysis of extremely discordant and concordant sibling pairs identifies quantitative-trait loci that influence variation in the human personality trait neuroticism. Am J Hum Genet 72:879–890, 2003

Gelernter J, Page GP, Stein MB, et al: Genome-wide linkage scan for loci predisposing to social phobia: evidence for a chromosome 16 risk locus. Am J Psychiatry 161:59–66, 2004

Gillespie NA, Evans D, Wright MJ, et al: Genetic simplex modeling of Eysenck's dimensions of personality in a sample of young Australian twins. Twin Res 7:637–648, 2004

Gillespie NA, Zhu G, Evans DM, et al: A genomewide scan for the Eysenckian personality dimensions in adolescent twin sibships: Psychoticism, Extraversion, Neuroticism, and Lie. J Personality (in press)

Harlaar N, Butcher LM, Meaburn E, et al: A behavioural genomic analysis of DNA markers associated with general cognitive ability in 7-year-olds. J Child Psychol Psychiatry 46:1097–1107, 2005

Heath AC, Bucholz KK, Madden PA, et al: Genetic and environmental contributions to alcohol dependence risk in a national twin sample: consistency of findings in women and men. Psychol Med 27:1381–1396, 1997

Hill WG: Genetics: a century of corn selection. Science 307:683–684, 2005

Jinks JL, Fulker DW: Comparison of the biometrical genetical, MAVA, and classical approaches to the analysis of human behavior. Psychol Bull 73:311–349, 1970

Kaplan DE, Gayan J, Ahn J, et al: Evidence for linkage and association with reading disability on 6p21.3–22. Am J Hum Genet 70:1287–1298, 2002

Kendler KS, Neale MC, Kessler RC, et al: A longitudinal twin study of personality and major depression in women. Arch Gen Psychiatry 50:853–862, 1993

Kirk KM, Birley AJ, Statham DJ, et al: Anxiety and depression in twin and sib pairs extremely discordant and concordant for neuroticism: prodromus to a linkage study. Twin Res 3:299–309, 2000

Kong A, Gudbjartsson DF, Sainz J, et al: A high-resolution recombination map of the human genome. Nat Genet 31:241–247, 2002

Lai CS, Fisher SE, Hurst JA, et al: A forkhead-domain gene is mutated in a severe speech and language disorder. Nature 413:519–523, 2001

Lander E, Kruglyak L: Genetic dissection of complex traits: guidelines for interpreting and reporting linkage results. Nat Genet 11:241–247, 1995

Leal SM: Genetic maps of microsatellite and single-nucleotide polymorphism markers: are the distances accurate? Genet Epidemiol 24:243–252, 2003

Luciano M, Smith GA, Wright MJ, et al: On the heritability of inspection time and its covariance with IQ: a twin study. Intelligence 29:443–457, 2001a

Luciano M, Wright M, Smith GA, et al: Genetic covariance among measures of information processing speed, working memory, and IQ. Behav Genet 31:581–592, 2001b

Luciano M, Wright MJ, Smith GA, et al: Genetic covariance between processing speed and IQ, in Behavioral Genetics in the Postgenomic Era. Edited by Plomin R, DeFries JC, Craig IW, et al. Washington, DC, American Psychological Association, 2002, pp 163–182

Luciano M, Wright MJ, Geffen GM, et al: A genetic two-factor model of the covariation among a subset of Multidimensional Aptitude Battery and Wechsler Adult Intelligence Scale—Revised subtests. Intelligence 31:589–605, 2003

Luciano M, Wright MJ, Geffen GM, et al: A genetic investigation of the covariation among inspection time, choice reaction time, and IQ subtest scores. Behav Genet 34:41–50, 2004a

Luciano M, Wright MJ, Geffen GM, et al: A multivariate genetic analysis of cognitive abilities in an adolescent twin sample. Aust J Psychol 56:79–88, 2004b

Luciano M, Posthuma D, Wright MJ, et al: Perceptual speed does not cause intelligence, and intelligence does not cause perceptual speed. Biol Psychol 70:1–8, 2005

Luciano M, Wright MJ, Duffy DL, et al: Genome-wide scan of IQ finds significant linkage to a quantitative trait locus on 2q. Behav Genet 36:45–55, 2006

Marlow AJ, Fisher SE, Francks C, et al: Use of multivariate linkage analysis for dissection of a complex cognitive trait. Am J Hum Genet 72:561–570, 2003

Martin NG, Eaves LJ: The genetical analysis of covariance structure. Heredity 38:79–95, 1977

Martin NG, Eaves LJ, Fulker DW: The genetical relationship of impulsiveness and sensation seeking to Eysenck's personality dimensions. Acta Genet Med Gemellol (Roma) 28:197–210, 1979

Nash MW, Huezo-Diaz P, Williamson RJ, et al: Genome-wide linkage analysis of a composite index of neuroticism and mood-related scales in extreme selected sibships. Hum Mol Genet 13:2173–2182, 2004

Neale BM, Sullivan PF, Kendler KS: A genome scan of neuroticism in nicotine dependent smokers. Am J Med Genet B Neuropsychiatr Genet 132:65–69, 2005

Neale MC, Boker SM, Xie G, et al: Mx; Statistical Modeling, 6th Edition. Richmond, VA, Department of Psychiatry, Virginia Commonwealth University, 2003

Petrill SA, Luo D, Thompson LA, et al: The independent prediction of general intelligence by elementary cognitive tasks: genetic and environmental influences. Behav Genet 26:135–147, 1996

Plomin R, McClearn GE, Smith DL, et al: DNA markers associated with high versus low IQ: the IQ Quantitative Trait Loci (QTL) Project. Behav Genet 24:107–118, 1994a

Plomin R, Pedersen NL, Lichtenstein P, et al: Variability and stability in cognitive abilities are largely genetic later in life. Behav Genet 24:207–215, 1994b

Plomin R, McClearn GE, Smith DL, et al: Allelic associations between 100 DNA markers and high versus low IQ. Intelligence 21:31–48, 1995

Plomin R, Hill L, Craig IW, et al: A genome-wide scan of 1842 DNA markers for allelic associations with general cognitive ability: a five-stage design using DNA pooling and extreme selected groups. Behav Genet 31:497–509, 2001

Plomin R, Turic DM, Hill L, et al: A functional polymorphism in the succinate-semialdehyde dehydrogenase (aldehyde dehydrogenase 5 family, member A1) gene is associated with cognitive ability. Mol Psychiatry 9:582–586, 2004

Posthuma D, Boomsma DI: A note on the statistical power in extended twin designs. Behav Genet 30:147–158, 2000

Posthuma D, Luciano M, de Geus EJ, et al: A genomewide scan for intelligence identifies quantitative trait Loci on 2q and 6p. Am J Hum Genet 77:318–326, 2005

Rijsdijk FV, Vernon PA, Boomsma DI: The genetic basis of the relation between speed-of-information-processing and IQ. Behav Brain Res 95:77–84, 1998

Rujescu D, Hartmann AM, Gonnermann C, et al: M129V variation in the prion protein may influence cognitive performance. Mol Psychiatry 8:937–941, 2003

Thorgeirsson TE, Oskarsson H, Desnica N, et al: Anxiety with panic disorder linked to chromosome 9q in Iceland. Am J Hum Genet 72:1221–1230, 2003

Tsai SJ, Hong CJ, Yu YW, et al: Association study of a brain-derived neurotrophic factor (BDNF) Val66Met polymorphism and personality trait and intelligence in healthy young females. Neuropsychobiology 49:13–16, 2004

Wainwright MA, Wright MJ, Geffen GM, et al: Genetic and environmental sources of covariance between reading tests used in neuropsychological assessment and IQ subtests. Behav Genet 34:365–376, 2004

Wainwright MA, Wright MJ, Geffen GM, et al: The genetic basis of academic achievement on the Queensland Core Skills Test and its shared genetic variance with IQ. Behav Genet 35:133–415, 2005a

Wainwright MA, Wright MJ, Luciano M, et al: Multivariate genetic analyses of academic skills of the Queensland core skills test and IQ highlight the importance of genetic g. Twin Res Hum Genet 8:602–608, 2005b

Wainwright MA, Wright MJ, Luciano M, et al: A linkage study of academic skills defined by the Queensland Core Skills Test. Behav Genet 36:56–64, 2006

Walitza S, Wewetzer C, Warnke A, et al: 5-HT2A promoter polymorphism -1438G/A in children and adolescents with obsessive-compulsive disorders. Mol Psychiatry 7:1054–1057, 2002

Williams J, Spurlock G, McGuffin P, et al: Association between schizophrenia and T102C polymorphism of the 5-hydroxytryptamine type 2a-receptor gene. European Multicentre Association Study of Schizophrenia (EMASS) Group. Lancet 347:1294–1296, 1996

Wolf MB, Ackerman PL: Extraversion and intelligence: a meta-analytic investigation. Pers Individ Diff 39:531–542, 2005

Wright MJ, Martin NG: The Brisbane Adolescent Twin Study: outline of study methods and research projects. Aust J Psychol 56:65–78, 2004

Wright MJ, Smith GA, Geffen GM, et al: Genetic influence on the variance in co-incidence timing and its covariance with IQ: a twin study. Intelligence 28:239–250, 2000

Wright MJ, De Geus E, Ando J, et al: Genetics of cognition: outline of a collaborative twin study. Twin Res 4:48–56, 2001a

Wright MJ, Hansell NK, Geffen GM, et al: Genetic influence on the variance in P3 amplitude and latency. Behav Genet 31:555–65, 2001b

Wright MJ, Luciano M, Hansell NK, et al: Genetic sources of covariation among P3(00) and online performance variables in a delayed-response working memory task. Biol Psychol 61:183–202, 2002

Zhu G, Evans DM, Duffy DL, et al: A genome scan for eye color in 502 twin families: most variation is due to a QTL on chromosome 15q. Twin Res 7:197–210, 2004

Zubenko GS, Maher B, Hughes HB, 3rd, et al: Genome-wide linkage survey for genetic loci that influence the development of depressive disorders in families with recurrent, early onset, major depression. Am J Med Genet B Neuropsychiatr Genet 123:1–18, 2003

Chapter 6

SEX AND DEVELOPMENTAL PSYCHOPATHOLOGY

Adrian Angold, M.R.C.Psych.

This chapter is motivated by two forms of dissatisfaction with the literature on the impact of sex or gender on psychopathology. The first is a response to attempts to separate "biological" from "social" effects of sex and gender on psychopathology in the face of clear evidence that no such separation is appropriate. The second concerns the tendency to treat sex/gender as an invariant feature of the human condition, when, in fact, sex is a *developmental process*, not a fixed condition of the individual at all. I shall spend only a little time in dealing with the first problem because others have made this argument before. The second issue has received rather less attention in relation to psychopathology and so will be the main focus of my discussion. Throughout the chapter I focus on what I regard as being a particularly illuminating example of the need to take a developmental approach to sex if we are to understand sex differences in psychopathology—that of unipolar depression. In conclusion, I shall draw some lessons from this particular example that have wider relevance to the issue of sex differences in psychopathology as a whole. I begin, however, by laying out the bones of the question of sex differences in depression from the perspective of population prevalence research.

PREVALENCE OF DEPRESSION BROKEN DOWN BY AGE AND SEX

Perhaps the best-established fact in psychiatric epidemiology is that major depression is about twice as prevalent in women as it is in men across the reproductive lifespan (Andrade et al. 2003; Bebbington 1996; Bebbington et al. 1981, 1998; Bland et al. 1988a, 1988b; Blazer et al. 1994; Canino et al. 1987; Cheng 1989; Hwu et al. 1989; Jorm 1987; Kessler et al. 1993, 1994; Lee et al. 1987; Weissman and Klerman 1977; Weissman et al. 1993, 1996; Wells et al. 1989; Wittchen et al. 1992). It is also incontestable that depression is *not* more common in girls than in boys before puberty. If anything, depression is more common in immature males than in immature females (Anderson et al. 1987; Angold and Rutter 1992; Angold et al. 1998; Bird et al. 1988; P. Cohen and Brooks 1987; P. Cohen et al. 1993a, 1993b; Costello et al. 1993; Fleming and Offord 1990; Guyer et al. 1989; Hankin et al. 1998; Kashani et al. 1987, 1989; Lewinsohn et al. 1993, 1995; McGee and Williams 1988; McGee et al. 1990, 1992; Nolen-Hoeksema et al. 1991; Reinherz et al. 1993a, 1993b; Rutter et al. 1976; Velez et al. 1989). Although the evidence is very limited for children younger than age 9 years, it seems that the cross-sectional prevalence of DSM-IV-TR unipolar depression (American Psychiatric Association 2000) may not change much between the preschool years and age 13 years. On the other hand, three reasonably large community samples—the Pittsburgh Youth Study (boys only) (Angold et al. 1996), the Virginia Twin Study of Adolescent Behavioral Development, and the Great Smoky Mountains Study (Angold et al. 2002)—have found that self-reported depression scale scores fall in both girls and boys from age 6 to age 11 years, as shown in Figure 6–1. We really do not know how to identify depression, even if it occurs, in children under age 2 years, so we have a complete gap in our understanding of the problem in the earliest years of life.

Both adult studies using retrospective recall and studies of children and adolescents point to adolescence as the period when the prevalence of unipolar depressive disorders rises in girls (Angold et al. 2002). Indeed, we can pinpoint the age period at which the change in prevalence of unipolar depression in girls occurs quite precisely, because all seven epidemiologic studies with sufficient age extension to examine the question place it between ages 13 and 14 years (Angold et al. 1998; Cairney 1998; Hankin et al. 1998; McGee et al. 1992; Velez et al. 1989; Wade et al. 2002). It has also now been shown that a similar pattern of change applies to depression questionnaire scale scores and that there is a shift to the right across the whole range of scores beginning around age 12 years in girls (Angold et al. 2002; Twenge and Nolen-Hoeksema 2002), as shown in Figure 6–1. The period

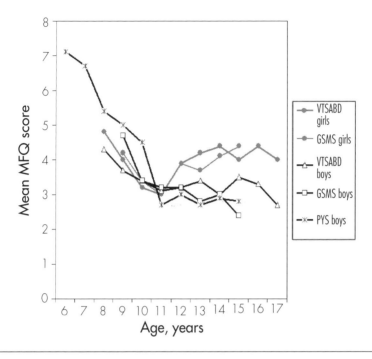

FIGURE 6–1. **Depression scores from ages 6–17 years from three studies.**

GSMS=Great Smoky Mountains Study; MFQ=Mood and Feelings Questionnaire; PYS=Pittsburgh Youth Study; VTSABD=Virginia Twin Study of Adolescent Behavioral Development.

from ages 12 through 14 years, therefore, represents a key transitional period as far as the etiology of depression is concerned, and the key question is why do the rates of depression rise in girls but not boys?

Women continue to have an unambiguously higher prevalence of depression than men up until about age 45 years or so. There are several ways in which higher cross-sectional prevalence could be maintained; if depressive episodes were of longer duration in women, or if they had more frequent episodes, or their episodes were of greater severity than those of men, then their point or short-period prevalences could be higher without a greater proportion of women than men being affected at some point in their lives. However, none of these mechanisms appears to be responsible; rather, the evidence suggests that the higher prevalence in women is generated entirely by an increased *incidence* of new cases of depression beginning in adolescence (Kessler 2000, 2003). Unfortunately, few studies cover the full period of adulthood, but some find that rates of depression actually appear to fall after the age of 45 years or so (Bebbington et al. 2003; Blazer et al. 1994; Butterworth et al. 2006; Henderson et al. 1998; Jorm 2000; Villamil et al. 2006; Wilhelm et al. 2003). On the other hand, it has been argued that standard psychiatric epidemiologic assessments have underestimated the prevalence of depression in late life (Blazer 1994; Lepine and Bouchez 1998; O'Connor 2006) Also, in sharp contrast to the situation in adolescence, in which there is clearly an age effect on rates of depression in females, it is not at all clear whether any change in rates of depression in later life is the result of age, period, or cohort effects (Andrade et al. 2003; Jorm 2000; Wittchen et al. 1994). Although it is generally accepted that depression continues to be more common in women than men in late life (Lepine and Bouchez 1998; Wilhelm et al. 2003), there is evidence that the sex ratio diminishes (Bland et al. 1988b; Robins and Regier 1991), and the British National Survey of Psychiatric Morbidity found that at age 55 years and above men were more often depressed than women (Bebbington et al. 1998).

Figure 6–2 provides a graphical summary of what we know about the prevalence of depression in men and women over a lifespan divided into seven epochs. The darker bars (solid for females, patterned for males) represent solidly established findings, whereas the lighter bars represent areas for which there are few data or the findings are uncertain. The absence of bars indicates the absence of information. The first important point that this figure makes clear is that we have clarity as to the effects of sex on the prevalence of depression for only three of the seven epochs and a complete absence of data on two of them. The second obvious point is that the relationship between sex and depression changes dramatically across the lifespan.

There are two basic ways in which such a relationship change could occur. First, etiologic factors for depression (life events, for example) could be correlated with sex at some epochs but not others; second, sex itself could be changing through life in such a way as to have effects on depression only at certain phases in the development of sex. Of course, both processes may be operative, but here I shall deal with the development of sex because I think that we have not paid sufficient attention to the implications for etiologic research of sex as a *developmental process*.

PROBLEMS WITH TYPICAL CURRENT APPROACHES TO THE ANALYSIS OF SEX AND GENDER EFFECTS

Sex is typically treated analytically as the archetypal *fixed* (i.e., time-invariant) demographic factor in psychiatric research (e.g., Kraemer et al. 1997). It has been pointed out that age is an analytically ambiguous variable be-

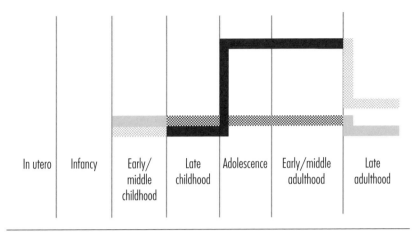

FIGURE 6–2. A graphical summary of what we know about the prevalence of depression in males and females from conception to old age.

cause it averages change over a wide range of developmental domains (Rutter 1989), but at least it incorporates time variation. Sex is even more radically ambiguous because it reduces many complex developmental processes to a lifetime-invariant binomial categorization typically defined by the observation of a single outcome of those processes at a single point in time—these days usually the form of the external genitalia at ultrasound evaluation of the fetus.

Sex Versus Gender: Biological Versus Social

Money's introduction of the concept of gender role (Money 1955) marked the beginning of consistent attempts to differentiate between sex and gender (Haig 2004), with *gender* being used to label sociocultural aspects of differences between men and women, whereas *sex* was limited to biological differences. At first sight such a distinction appears useful, and the apparent divide between *social* and *biological* has often served as a convenient shorthand for consideration of physiological intra-organismic versus extraorganismic factors (e.g., Bebbington et al. 1998; Brooks-Gunn and Warren 1989). However, such usage has become problematic because some authoritative sources seek to maintain a careful separation between sex (biological) and gender (sociocultural) (e.g., Institute of Medicine 2001, Pinn 2003), and I am convinced that this is a serious conceptual and practical mistake. In the first place, the attempt to implement such a terminological distinction has already failed in the scientific (not to mention the lay) literature, as Haig's (2004) analysis of the titles of more than 30 million titles in the scientific literature since the second world war makes clear. *Sex* and *gender* are now functionally synonymous, and gender is now used in both scientific and natural language to index what *sex* has always referred to—any and all of the differences between males and females (Dunnett 2003). It is too late to turn the clock back and attach different meanings to these terms.

Second, there is, in reality, no necessary or even well-demarcated division between human biological and social functions and activities (Rutter et al. 2003). Basic human social functions are substantially hardwired, as the modern literature on autism makes clear (Rutter and O'Connor 2004). But such wiring is not a one-way street, as can be seen from the fact that some seriously psychosocially neglected orphanage-reared Romanian children develop syndromes that look very much like autism phenomenologically (Rutter et al. 1999) but that are partially remediable in a nurturing environment. Therefore the biological/social divide fails to provide a useful scientific distinction.

That is not to say that no useful subsetting of sex/gender differences is possible. Indeed the third problem with the sex/gender division is that quite the contrary is true. As we have learned more about the developmental sociobiology of sex differentiation, it has become clear that many more than two terms are needed to distinguish among the various processes involved, and I shall now go on to distinguish a variety of components of sex that may be relevant to the development of sex differences in psychopathology, following their developmental course. A great deal has been learned about the ontogeny of sex over the last two decades, and my aim here is to show that this new knowledge has many implications for the future of research on the development of sex differences in psychopathology.

DIMENSIONS OF SEX FROM A DEVELOPMENTAL PERSPECTIVE

Sex in Embryogenesis

Chromosomal Sex

Most humans have 46 chromosomes: 22 pairs of autosomes and two sex chromosomes. Typical females have two X chromosomes, and typical males have one X chromosome and one Y chromosome. We are now familiar with the doctrine that the presence of a Y chromosome is required for male development in humans. However, as we shall see, this doctrine is not universally true. Be that as it may, one possible mechanism for the generation of sex differences in psychiatric disorders is the differential dose of X chromosome genes in men and women. The discovery that one X chromosome is randomly inactivated in each female cell seemed to have vitiated this idea for a while, but it turns out that as many as 10%–15% of the inactivated chromosome's genes continue to be expressed (Willard 2000). These genes provide a potential mechanism for inducing male–female differences. The Y chromosome may also have direct effects because the majority of the 78 protein coding genes on the nonrecombinant portion of the Y chromosome (which between them code for 27 discrete proteins) are expressed outside the gonads, including in the brain (Page 2004; Skaletsky et al. 2003).

Genetic Sex

In 1990, a 0.9-kb region, the sex-determining region Y gene (*SRY*), responsible for the masculinization of the fetus, was identified simultaneously by two groups (Berta et al. 1990; Jager et al. 1990). Deletion or dysfunction of *SRY* resulting from mutations (of which several dozen have already been reported; see http://archive.uwcm.ac.uk/uwcm/mg/search/125556.html) results in failure to develop a typical male phenotype in XY individuals (e.g., *SRY* mutations can give rise to XY-apparent females with gonadal dysgenesis), whereas translocation (misplacement during meiosis) of *SRY* onto an X chromosome results in the birth of an XX individual with apparently male genitalia. SRY is a 204–amino acid protein capable of binding to 1) two specific DNA base sequences and 2) sequence-nonspecific DNA four-way junctions. It thereby induces configurational changes in DNA, but how this translates into effects on sexual differentiation is unknown (Jordan and Vilain 2002). However, that is far from the end of genetic sex determination. *SRY* transcription is itself genetically regulated—for instance, by the Wilms tumor gene (*WT1*) on chromosome 11 (Hossain and Saunders 2001; Jordan and Vilain 2002)—and hundreds of genes appear to be involved in sexual differentiation. For instance, in addition to *SRY*, the gene *DMRT1* on chromosome 9 is involved in testicular development (Dewing et al. 2002), and unlike *SRY*, it has to be present in two copies to work properly. XY humans who have lost one copy of the gene fail to develop testes and show gonadal sex reversal, despite having a fully functional *SRY*. We do not know what other functions the cascade of genes involved in differential gonadal development might have, but this cascade represents a second possible source of neuropsychiatric differences between men and women.

Here we need to consider two sorts of effects that parallel the well-known distinction in the steroid hormone literature between early organizational and later activational effects (Romeo 2003). *SRY* is certainly the switch that turns on the organization of male characteristics early in embryogenesis, but then what else does it do? Recent work from Eric Vilain's laboratory has shown that *SRY* is expressed in the substantia nigra of *adult* male rats and that downregulation of that expression is accompanied by reduction in tyrosine hydroxylase levels in the dopaminergic nigrostriatal system, accompanied by behavioral motor deficits (Dewing et al. 2006). So we cannot ignore the possibility that the genes responsible for embryological sex differentiation might also have later direct sex-typed effects on brain function. The key point here is that a particular gene may have quite different effects at different points in development because the organism in which it resides is differently organized at those points. So individual genes might only be associated with risk for depression during certain periods of life or in a certain anatomic-physiological milieu (e.g., mature males or females).

Vilain's group is also responsible for casting serious doubt on another long-standing developmental dogma—that sex differentiation of the brain occurs as a response to testosterone secretion in the male embryo. These investigators found that, even in the absence of testosterone, genetically male and female mice exhibit substantial differences in gene expression in the brain (Dewing et al. 2003). If the same is true of humans, then already in the first few weeks of embryonic development differences in brain function could have implications for sex differences in psychopathology. If this seems at first glance to be an unlikely scenario, consider that there is little sex difference in the anatomy of the anterior chest wall until gonadal release of estrogen kicks in at puberty, at which point rather striking differences emerge.

Gonadal Sex

The sex-determinative genes discussed above initiate the development of ovaries or testes (and their associated structures). So sex may also be defined by the nature of the gonads. Regardless of sex chromosome complement, until the seventh week of gestation the embryonic gonadal region remains undifferentiated, and the precursors of both male and female genital systems (the Wolffian and Müllerian ducts respectively) are present, with the result that human embryos at that point have sexual bipotential (Jordan and Vilain 2002). Testicular differentiation occurs during the eighth and ninth weeks of gestation, but the ovary does not begin to differentiate until about the third month (Vilain 2000).

Genital Sex

It is now also well known that the default anatomical developmental plan for the human embryo is female (Jost 1947). The development of male external genitalia requires the presence of a functional testis (and its hormonal products). Müllerian inhibiting substance produced by Sertoli cells in the seminiferous tubules causes apoptosis of the Müllerian ducts. Testosterone, produced by Leydig cells surrounding the seminiferous tubules, and its derivative, dihydrotestosterone, produced locally in the genital region, are responsible for the development of the male internal and external genitalia (Vilain 2000).

More importantly from our perspective, testosterone production at this stage has also been identified as a key player in the masculinization of the brain and behavior (Vilain 2000), although as we have already noted sex-differentiated brain gene expression is still possible in the absence of testosterone. Differences in hormonal milieu and gene expression could also lead to differential susceptibility to external threats to the fetus, such as nutritional deficiencies, environmental toxins, viral assaults, or placental deficits. The need to take such possibilities seriously has recently been underlined by our finding from the Great Smoky Mountains Study that low birth weight (despite being more common in boys) is associated with increased rates of depression in girls (but not boys) but that this effect does not appear until puberty (see Figure 6–3).

Assigned Sex

Historically at birth, but more recently at ultrasound, the external genitalia of the newborn or fetus are observed, and the child is declared to be either a boy or a girl. However, it is also possible to manipulate the assigned sex of a child, as has been done in genetically and gonadally male children with cloacal exstrophy (who have often had their histologically normal testes removed) or in children who have suffered catastrophic penile damage and been raised as girls (Reiner and Gearhart 2004). The key point here is that the child enters a social world and that the social world treats boys and girls differently. Here we have another potential mechanism for generating psy-

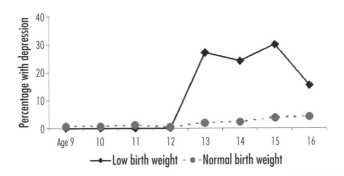

FIGURE 6–3. Low birth weight and depression in girls.

chopathological differences between males and females. However, following the demise of psychoanalytic theory as a scientific guide, a girl's lack of a penis per se is no longer thought to be important in the etiology of depression.

In most people the assignment of sex at or before birth settles the issue from a labeling standpoint. They will remain male or female, at first as a girl or as a boy, growing up to be a woman or a man, and they will die as such. But in considering progress through life it is immediately apparent that the meaning of being male or female changes dramatically across the life span after birth—biologically, socially, and psychologically. Even the words we use to denote males and females are different in childhood and adulthood.

Continuing Sexual Development in Childhood: Adrenarche and the Beginnings of the Emergence of "Secondary" Sexual Characteristics

Although the hypothalamic-pituitary-gonadal (HPG) and hypothalamic-pituitary-adrenal axes show a brief burst of activity in the first months after birth (Skuse 1984), circulating concentrations of gonadotropins and gonadal and adrenal steroids are very low in early to mid-childhood, apparently due to the suppression of luteinizing hormone–releasing hormone (LHRH; also known as gonadotropin-releasing hormone [GnRH]) secretion by γ-aminobutyric acid (GABA)–ergic (and perhaps neuropeptide Y) neural systems (Plant 2001; Terasawa and Fernandez 2001).

An increase in adrenal androgen output (adrenarche) occurs at around 6–8 years in both boys and girls (DePeretti and Forest 1976; Ducharme et al. 1976; Lashansky et al. 1991; Parker et al. 1978; Reiter et al. 1977; Sizonenko and Paunier 1975). Indeed, a substantial proportion of the androgens (including testosterone) secreted by women from then on continues to be contributed by the adrenals, whereas in boys the massive later output of testosterone by the testes far outweighs the adrenal contribution to the masculinization of adult body morphology. However, the adrenal contribution of androgens is sufficient to initiate the early stages of pubic hair development in many cases, with the result that, despite its traditional inclusion in Tanner's stages (Tanner 1962) of puberty for both boys and girls, the initial appearance of pubic hair is not a clean marker of *pubertal* development.

Adrenarche precedes the earliest changes of puberty on the HPG axis by about age 2 years (beginning around ages 6–8 years) and was once thought to act as a trigger for its onset (Collu and Ducharme 1975). We now know that this is not the case (Counts et al. 1987; Korth-Schutz et al. 1976; Wierman et al. 1986), but adrenarche is still suspected to play a facilitative role in the initiation of puberty. Despite the fact that these prepubertal changes in androgen levels are similar in boys and girls, they still have to be considered as possible factors in generating changes in the sex ratios for psychiatric disorders, because they act on already sexually differentiated brains and patterns of behavior. It is also important to bear in mind that levels of the most abundant androgen of all, dehydroepiandrosterone (DHEA), and of its sulfated metabolite, DHEA-S, increase enormously over this period (and continue to do so into the 20s), and that DHEA is a neurosteroid (Baulieu 1998) with reported protective effects against cortisol neurotoxicity (e.g., Gubba et al. 2000; Kaminska et al. 2000; Karishma and Herbert 2002; Kimonides et al. 1998). Adrenal androgen levels also continue to rise throughout the 20s in men but peak about a decade earlier in women.

This serves as a reminder that there may be sex differences in responses to protective factors as well as risk factors. Some tantalizing evidence in this direction is provided by a series of studies by Ian Goodyer and colleagues. In clinically referred children and adolescents with major depressive disorder (MDD), they found that those with MDD had lower morning (8 A.M.) DHEA (but not DHEA-S) levels (Goodyer et al. 1996). A follow-up indicated that those with persistent depression were more likely to have had cortisol/DHEA ratios above the 60th percentile at 8 P.M. and midnight (but not at 8 A.M., 12 P.M., or 4 P.M.) at presentation than were those who were later free of psychiatric disorder or those who manifested only nondepressive disorders (Goodyer et al. 1997). At a 72-week follow-up (Goodyer et al. 2001), there was no continuing significant effect of DHEA or cortisol/DHEA ratio. In a mixed-sex community-based study of initially nondepressed early adolescents, however, DHEA hypersecretion predicted the onset of major depression over the next year (Goodyer et al. 2000). Those whose depression then persisted over the following (i.e., second) year had lower DHEA levels at 8 A.M. and higher morning cortisol/DHEA ratios than those who recovered (Goodyer et al. 2003). Other pubertal hormone levels were not measured in these studies, and they all involved mixed-sex groups of children and adolescents, which is problematic because depression trajectories are so different for boys and girls across this age period (Angold 2003).

Puberty (Hormonal Sex)

Leptin (Clayton and Trueman 2000; Ebling 2005; Gueorguiev et al. 2001) and the happily named kisspeptin (actually named for Hershey's Kisses before its role in puberty was described) (Dhillo et al. 2005; Dungan et al. 2006; Han et al. 2005; Messager 2005; Seminara 2005, 2006) have a necessary permissive role in the onset of puberty, but the ultimate trigger for puberty remains unknown (Terasawa and Fernandez 2001).

Declining GABAergic LHRH suppression results in increases in release of glutamate (and other neurotransmitters), permitting the onset of puberty, manifested initially as closely sleep-entrained nighttime pulses of luteinizing hormone, beginning in late childhood (Beck and Wuttke 1980; Dunkel et al. 1990; Judd et al. 1977; Kulin et al. 1976; Wu et al. 1990). LHRH pulse amplitude and frequency increase across the late prepubertal stage to early and middle stages of puberty (Hale et al. 1988; Landy et al. 1992) and show progressive diminution of diurnal variation in early to middle puberty. Pulse frequency decreases in late puberty as LHRH release becomes more sensitive to negative feedback control from gonadal steroids (Dunger et al. 1991; Marshall et al. 1991; Wennink et al. 1989). A critical sex difference established over the course of puberty is that females develop pulsatile GnRH release along with fluctuating estradiol and progesterone levels (Marshall et al. 1991). Maturation of this pattern extends from before menarche to several months or years beyond in the course of establishing regular ovulation and luteal function (Vihko and Apter 1980; Wennink et al. 1990). These changes are, of course, associated with enormous changes in cognitive, psychological, social, and sexual functioning. All of these have potential for changing the patterns of psychopathology manifested by females and males. It also brings a whole new meaning to the word *sex*—as a libidinous act. As far as psychopathology is concerned, adolescence is a developmental period during which a variety of female-typical psychopathologies arise, the best-documented examples being unipolar depression and eating disorders (Rutter et al. 2003).

Research on the relationship between puberty and depression has typically focused on one of two types of parameter: 1) the timing of puberty, and 2) pubertal level or stage as measured by Tanner stages, multi-item questionnaire, or hormone levels. At any point during the teenage years the timing of puberty and the level of maturity achieved will be related because early maturers will have had more time to advance through the pubertal process. Despite this, few studies have looked at both parameters simultaneously, with the result that it is difficult to know how much apparent timing effects are actually the result of variation in level and vice versa.

Timing Effects of Puberty

The age at which puberty occurs, relative to the norm, has often been suggested to be related to risk of depression. In particular, early puberty *in girls* has been regarded as being a bad thing. There is now very strong evidence that for conduct problems, early puberty is a substantial risk factor, but only in girls (Persson et al. 2004; Stattin and Magnusson 1990; Stattin et al. 2005). The evidence for effects of early puberty on depression in girls has been much more mixed (Angold and Rutter 1992; Brooks-Gunn and Warren 1989;

Cairns and Cairns 1994; Ge et al. 1996; Greif and Ulman 1982; Olweus et al. 1988; Paikoff et al. 1991; Stattin and Magnusson 1990; Susman et al. 1987a; Weichold et al. 2003). More recently, however, stronger evidence has appeared for negative effects of earlier pubertal timing in both boys (Alsaker 1992; Ge et al. 2001b; Huddleston and Ge 2003) and girls (Ge et al. 1996, 2001a). In the case of girls there are also new challenges to the notion that truly early puberty is what matters (as opposed to there being a linear association between pubertal timing and depression), and there have continued to be indications from some studies that late maturation is also a problem for boys (Alsaker 1992; Graber et al. 1997; Nottelmann et al. 1987b).

By far the largest study of this question involved Beck Depression Inventory (BDI) scores collected from more than 30,000 Finnish 14- to 16-year-olds (Kaltiala-Heino et al. 2003). Data from this study on the relationship between depression (BDI score≥8), sex, and pubertal timing are shown graphically in Figure 6–4 (oigarche is age at first ejaculation). There are a number of striking features in these data. Looking first at the girls, there is a linear decrease in risk for depression with increasing age at menarche. The issue seems not to be that early starters are at risk compared with all the rest but that the rates of depression are higher in girls than in boys in this age range. It is worth noting that the design of the study means that the 15+ group also contains 14- to 16-year-olds who had not yet reached menarche/oigarche. If, as we shall argue below, the increase in depression in girls is an effect of relatively advanced puberty, then we would not expect these individuals with late onset of menarche to show much increase in depression because they were not yet sufficiently physiologically mature. In other words, these data are consistent with the idea that puberty is a risk factor for depression in girls whenever it occurs but that the level of risk decreases linearly with the age at which puberty occurs. Failures to find increased risk for "on-time" puberty compared with late puberty in many earlier studies could well result from the fact that no study has had anything close to the power of the Finnish survey to detect such effects. The other notable feature of these data is that the shape of the curve in boys is quite different from that for girls, being U shaped, with early puberty (approximately the earliest 20%) being associated with a substantial increase in risk for depression and late puberty (approximately the latest 10%) indexing a much smaller increase.

A further finding from this study was that higher levels of sexual experience (and particularly sexual intercourse) were associated with depression, even when timing of menarche/oigarche was controlled for. This finding highlights the inappropriateness of attempts to partition sex effects into biological and social components. Is having sexual intercourse a biological or a social phenomenon? Of course, it is both. Libido is related to androgen

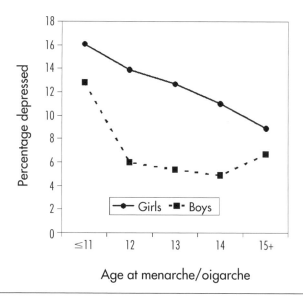

FIGURE 6–4.   Depression and age at puberty in a large Finnish sample.

levels (Davis and Tran 2001; Guay and Jacobson 2002; Travison et al. 2006), and it does not require a doctoral degree to discover that puberty produces an interest in sexual behavior that was absent in childhood, and no one doubts that this change is a result of hormones. However, whether a person has had sexual intercourse by age 14–16 years depends on a lot more than his or her libido. Factors such as religious affiliation, parental supervision, peer group social norms, availability of alcohol, and a host of others all play an obvious part. Understanding of *how* having had sexual intercourse is related to depression demands that we try to understand the interplay among all such possible contributions. Attempts to parse causal pathways of this sort into biological and social components are no help at all.

Level or Stage Effects of Puberty

Body morphological (e.g., Tanner) stage and depression.   Earlier studies of menarche or morphological development (secondary sex characteristics—usually measured by Tanner stages [Tanner 1962]), mostly on the basis of relatively small and nonrepresentative samples, suggested that levels (as opposed to timing) of these pubertal status markers per se were not significantly related to mood or other behavioral disturbances over and above the effects of age or relative pubertal timing (Angold and Rutter 1992; Brooks-Gunn and Warren 1989; Ge et al. 1996; Paikoff et al. 1991; Susman et al.

1987b, 1991). In contrast, in the Great Smoky Mountains Study of 1,420 children followed over three annual waves of data collection, we found a substantial effect of pubertal status on depression in girls. At or after Tanner stage 3, girls were 3.4 times more likely to have a 3-month history of major or minor depression or dysthymia than girls in Tanner stages 1 and 2, regardless of the timing of puberty (Angold et al. 1998). Similarly, Patton et al. (1996) found from a sample of more than 2,500 Australian adolescents that effects of age on depression were explained by time since menarche (which can be seen as a marker of pubertal stage) rather than menarcheal timing. These relatively large studies both used psychiatric diagnostic interviews to assess depression status and provide quite strong evidence that there is a specific association between advancing pubertal status and depression in girls over and above the effect of age in general.

Adrenal androgens, gonadotropins, gonadal steroids, and depression. Several pioneering studies from the mid-1980s onward provided spotty but tantalizing indications that risk for depression in girls could be related specifically to changes in pituitary-gonadal function, as measured by gonadotropins and steroid hormones (Booth et al. 2003; Brooks-Gunn and Warren 1989; Granger et al. 2003; Nottelmann et al. 1987a, 1987b, 1990; Paikoff et al. 1991; Susman et al. 1985, 1987a, 1987b, 1991, 1998).

In contrast to these mixed, small-sized, and unstable effects, data from the first three waves of the Great Smoky Mountains Study identified very substantial independent effects of testosterone and estradiol on depression in girls ages 9–15 years (Angold et al. 1999). Levels of these two hormones explained all of the apparent effects of Tanner stage mentioned earlier. There were also no additional effects of androstenedione, DHEA-S, follicle-stimulating hormone, luteinizing hormone, or age on depression rates once testosterone and estradiol had been accounted for. We also found that adding the molarities of testosterone and estradiol provided a reasonable fit to the data. The logic behind this approach is that one molecule of testosterone can be aromatized to one molecule of estradiol intracellularly, and in some animal models, behavioral effects of testosterone have been found to be mediated at estrogen receptors (Hutchison et al. 1990; Rasmussen et al. 1990). We do not know whether this is the case in humans, but for our purposes here, the combination of estradiol and testosterone, to produce a single sex steroid level (SSL) (Angold et al. 2003), provides an easily digestible summary of our findings as shown in Figure 6–5. The curve appears to have three regions. First there is a somewhat flat portion with low levels of depression corresponding to SSLs up to 1.3 nmol. The second region with rates of depression about five times as high is generated by SSLs between 1.3 nmol and 2.3 nmol. The final region involving a further quadrupling of

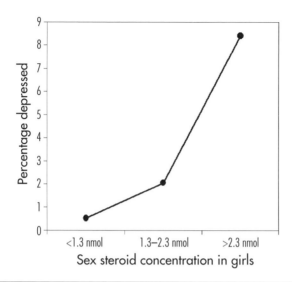

FIGURE 6–5.   **Sex steroid levels and depression in girls ages 9–15 years.**

the rate of depression is associated with SSL levels above 2.3 nmol. We divided the observations into SSL groups on the basis of these three cut points. The differences in rates of depression among them were all significant. It is also notable that it was not until age 13 years that mean SSL rose over 1.3 nmol. This study, therefore, suggests that there is a threshold that must be reached before the sex steroids have any effect on depression and perhaps a further threshold that results in the appearance of adult levels of depression. The argument here is that above a certain sex steroid threshold the risk for depression in girls and women rises to adult levels. In other words, at any level of other risk factors, all women with normal SSLs become at greater risk for depression than men or prepubertal girls with the same level of other risk factors. Another way of putting this is to say that the sex steroids lower the threshold for becoming depressed in women. Once adult levels of sex steroids are reached, however, there is no necessary relationship between SSL and depression, because the vast majority of women remain above the level of sex steroid secretion necessary to maintain this pattern of increased susceptibility.

We (Angold et al. 2003) also found that the higher levels of depression in more mature girls could not be explained either by an increase in the occurrence of life events in more mature girls (there was no such increase) or by increased sensitivity to the occurrence of life events in more mature girls. Depression was equally strongly related to life events in both immature and more mature girls. (In fact, there was a very slight, nonsignificant, decrease in the strength of the association with increasing maturity.)

Despite these findings, we should not dismiss the possibility that external stressors in adolescence do increase in girls during adolescence, because a number of studies have found that girls experience greater levels of stressors resulting from the exigencies of peer relationships, and such stressors are related to the onset of depressive episodes (Compas et al. 1994; Goodyer 1990, 1995; Goodyer and Altham 1991; Goodyer et al. 1986, 1987, 1990, 1993; Jensen et al. 1991; Laitinen-Krispijn et al. 1999; Lewinsohn et al. 1995, 1998; Olsson et al. 1999; Sandberg et al. 2001; Williamson et al. 1998). Therefore apparent pubertal effects could be generated in part by mechanisms that have nothing to do with HPG axis maturation but that are temporally correlated with it. In a situation such as this, we need studies using multiple markers of pubertal status and timing, reflecting multiple levels of the pubertal maturation, if we are to understand the mechanisms by which puberty might affect rates of depression. There have been few such studies, and those that exist have mostly been too small to support the multiple complex tests required to identify key causal factors.

Continuing Sexual Development in Adulthood

The development of sex as a biological phenomenon does not end at puberty. The menstrual cycle, with its enormous monthly swings in neuroactive hormone levels, also presents a challenge to psychological well-being, with many women reporting emotional symptoms perimenstrually and with some meeting the criteria for premenstrual dysphoric disorder (Burt and Stein 2002). It may be that it is the repeated changes in hormonal levels rather than any transition from one average level to another that is the culprit in increasing risk for unipolar depression, for instance. At this point there is no evidence that cycling per se is the key factor in relation to any disorder other than premenstrual dysphoric disorder, but it must be admitted that this is a difficult parameter to separate from the others.

Only women become pregnant, and so only women can suffer postpartum depressions. Only women take contraceptive pills or breastfeed, and women still bear the brunt of child rearing. Therefore sex continues to present newly differentiated challenges to males and females as they age. It appears, however, that the postpartum period is characterized by recurrent episodes or relapses of depression rather than new onsets (Burt and Stein 2002; L.S. Cohen et al. 2006a; Kessler 2003).

There is yet a final stage in sexual development that affects men and women rather differently. In both sexes levels of androgens fall dramatically in later life (Labrie et al. 1997; Young et al. 1999), but women also experience the menopause, with its much more rapid and dramatic hormonal change. But, as I have noted already, the picture here is very uncertain even at the most straightforward level of relative prevalence, and we must set against the possibility that rates of depression fall in women in later life findings from studies suggesting that the menopause is associated with new onsets of depression (L.S. Cohen et al. 2006b). Here we must recognize that both could be true. It is possible that as sex steroids fall below the threshold for generating the depressions characteristic of the female reproductive life span, other depressogenic mechanisms come into play that place previously unaffected individuals at risk. If the physiological, psychological, and social meaning of sex changes in later life, then the ways in which sex might be related to depression and other forms of psychopathology can be expected to change also.

SEX AND DEVELOPMENTAL PSYCHOPATHOLOGY: WHERE DO WE GO FROM HERE?

Depression is one of the better-researched areas as far as its life-course epidemiology is concerned, but, as we have seen, there are still huge gaps in our understanding of even the most basic questions of prevalence at many points in the lifespan. When we consider sex as a developmental process it also becomes obvious that we have hardly begun to study, let alone understand, the nature of sex differences in this strikingly sex-differentiated, prevalent, and disabling disease. When it comes to other disorders, our lack of knowledge is typically even greater. However, treating sex as a developmental phenomenon provides us with a powerful analytic tool, which will only sharpen as our understanding of the process of sex differentiation per se unfolds.

Let us briefly consider two other examples of ways in which sex differences can provide insights into the nature of psychopathology (see Rutter et al. 2003 for further discussion). Overall, male conceptuses appear to be more susceptible to a variety of early developmental hazards, and it is now well established that boys are more likely to have a number of developmental disorders, such as autism, attention-deficit/hyperactivity disorder (ADHD), and antisocial behavior, suggesting that a broad range of neurodevelopmental mechanisms are more prone to be disrupted early in boys than girls (Rutter et al. 2003). However, there is little evidence that boys are more susceptible to psychosocial risk for psychiatric disorders overall (Rutter et al. 2003), so explanations of sex differences in this area have tended to concentrate on fetal and early life neurodevelopmental processes. The key point here is that the timing of the onsets of these disorders predisposes to consideration of certain classes of putative sex-differentiated causes. At different life stages, sex is manifest in different ways, and so different classes of potential causes can be called into play. Therefore, for example, concurrent testosterone level does not offer itself as a good candidate for explaining sex differences in the rates of ADHD because ADHD is prevalent during developmental periods when both boys and girls have very low levels of testosterone.

To take a rather different example, the median age at onset of schizophrenia is later in women (late 20s) than in men (early to mid 20s), and premorbid adjustment and outcomes have been reported to be better in women. These sex differences point to different explanations than do those seen in unipolar depression because they obviously cannot be accounted for by pubertal hormonal changes. On the other hand, they call to mind the same two questions as does depression: What characteristics of the concurrent nature of sex (i.e., the characteristics of sex at the developmental period at which the disease arises) and what characteristics of the ontogeny of sex might explain the observed sex differences? The former question is asked relatively often (but not often enough), but the latter is rarely asked. The purpose of this chapter is to promote the consideration of sex as a developmental phenomenon and to promote the ontogenetic question in psychiatric research.

REFERENCES

Alsaker FD: Pubertal timing, overweight, and psychological adjustment. J Early Adolesc 12: 396–419, 1992

American Psychiatric Association: Diagnostic and Statistical Manual of Mental Disorders, 4th Edition, Text Revision. Washington, DC, American Psychiatric Association, 2000

Anderson JC, Williams S, McGee R, et al: DSM-III disorders in preadolescent children: prevalence in a large sample from the general population. Arch Gen Psychiatry 44:69–77, 1987

Andrade L, Caraveo-Anduaga JJ, Berglund P, et al: The epidemiology of major depressive episodes: results from the International Consortium of Psychiatric Epidemiology (ICPE) Surveys. Int J Methods Psychiatr Res 12:3–21, 2003

Angold A: Adolescent depression, cortisol and DHEA. Psychol Med 33:573–581, 2003

Angold A, Rutter M: The effects of age and pubertal status on depression in a large clinical sample. Dev Psychopathol 4:5–28, 1992

Angold A, Erkanli A, Loeber R, et al: Disappearing depression in a population sample of boys. J Anxiety Disord 4:95–104, 1996

Angold A, Costello EJ, Worthman CM: Puberty and depression: the roles of age, pubertal status, and pubertal timing. Psychol Med 28:51–61, 1998

Angold A, Costello EJ, Worthman CM: Pubertal changes in hormone levels and depression in girls. Psychol Med 29:1043–1053, 1999

Angold A, Erkanli A, Silberg J, et al: Depression scale scores in 8–17-year-olds: effects of age and gender. J Child Psychol Psychiatry 43:1052–1063, 2002

Angold A, Worthman CM, Costello EJ (eds): Puberty and depression, in Gender Differences at Puberty. Edited by Hayward C. New York, Cambridge University Press, 2003, pp 137–164

Baulieu E: Neurosteroids: a novel function of the brain. Psychoneuroendocrinology 23:963–987, 1998

Bebbington P: The origins of sex differences in depressive disorder: bridging the gap. Int Rev Psychiatry 8:295–332, 1996

Bebbington PE, Hurry J, Tennant C, et al: Epidemiology of mental disorders in Camberwell. Psychol Med 11:561–579, 1981

Bebbington PE, Dunn G, Jenkins R, et al: The influence of age and sex on the prevalence of depressive conditions: report from the National Survey of Psychiatric Morbidity. Psychol Med 2:9–10, 1998

Bebbington PE, Dunn G, Jenkins R: The influence of age and sex on the prevalence of depressive conditions: report from the National Survey of Psychiatric Morbidity. Int Rev Psychiatry 15:74–83, 2003

Beck W, Wuttke W: Diurnal variations of plasma luteinizing hormone, follicle-stimulating hormone, and prolactin in boys and girls from birth to puberty. J Clin Endocrinol Metab 50:635–639, 1980

Berta P, Hawkins JR, Sinclair AH: Genetic evidence equating SRY and the testis-determining factor. Nature 348 (suppl 6300):448–450, 1990

Bird HR, Canino G, Rubio-Stipec M, et al: Estimates of the prevalence of childhood maladjustment in a community survey in Puerto Rico: the use of combined measures. Arch Gen Psychiatry 45:1120–1126, 1988

Bland RC, Newman SC, Orn H: Lifetime prevalence of psychiatric disorders in Edmonton. Acta Psychiatr Scand 77 (suppl 338):24–32, 1988a

Bland RC, Newman SC, Orn H: Period prevalence of psychiatric disorders in Edmonton. Acta Psychiatr Scand 77:33–42, 1988b

Blazer DG: Is depression more frequent in late life? An honest look at the evidence. Am J Geriatr Psychiatry 2:193–199, 1994

Blazer DG, Kessler RC, McGonagle KA, et al: The prevalence and distribution of major depression in a national community sample: the National Comorbidity Survey. Am J Psychiatry 151:979–986, 1994

Booth A, Johnson DR, Granger DA, et al: Testosterone and child and adolescent adjustment: the moderating role of parent-child relationships. Dev Psychol 39:85–98, 2003

Brooks-Gunn J, Warren MP: Biological and social contributions to negative affect in young adolescent girls. Child Dev 60:40–55, 1989

Burke KC, Burke JD, Regier DA, et al: Age at onset of selected mental disorders in five community populations. Arch Gen Psychiatry 47:511–518, 1990

Burt VK, Stein K: Epidemiology of depression throughout the female life cycle. J Clin Psychiatry 63:9–15, 2002

Butterworth P, Gill SC, Rodgers B, et al: Retirement and mental health: analysis of the Australian national survey of mental health and well-being. Soc Sci Med 62:1179–1191, 2006

Cairney J: Gender differences in the prevalence of depression among Canadian adolescents. Can J Public Health 89:181–182, 1998

Cairns RB, Cairns BD: Lifelines and Risks: Pathways of Youth in Our Time. New York, Cambridge University Press, 1994

Canino GJ, Bird HR, Shrout PE, et al: The prevalence of specific psychiatric disorders in Puerto Rico. Arch Gen Psychiatry 44:727–735, 1987

Cheng TA: Sex difference in the prevalence of minor psychiatric morbidity: a social epidemiological study in Taiwan. Acta Psychiatr Scand 80:395–407, 1989

Clayton P, Trueman J: Leptin and puberty. Arch Dis Child 83:1–3, 2000

Cohen LS, Altshuler LL, Harlow BL, et al: Relapse of major depression during pregnancy in women who maintain or discontinue antidepressant treatment. JAMA 295:499–507, 2006a

Cohen LS, Soares CN, Vitonis AF, et al: Risk for new onset of depression during the menopausal transition. Arch Gen Psychiatry 63:385–390, 2006b

Cohen P, Brooks JS: Family factors related to the persistence of psychopathology in childhood and adolescence. Psychiatry 50:332–345, 1987

Cohen P, Cohen J, Brook J: An epidemiological study of disorders in late childhood and adolescence: 2. Persistence of disorders. J Child Psychol Psychiatry 34:869–877, 1993a

Cohen P, Cohen J, Kasen S, et al: An epidemiological study of disorders in late childhood and adolescence: 1. Age- and gender-specific prevalence. J Child Psychol Psychiatry 34:851–867, 1993b

Collu R, Ducharme JR: Role of adrenal steroids in the regulation of gonadotropin secretion at puberty. J Steroid Biochem 6:869–872, 1975

Compas BE, Grant KE, Ey S: Psychosocial stress and child and adolescent depression: can we be more specific? in Handbook of Depression in Children and Adolescents. Edited by Reynolds WM, Johnston HF. New York, Plenum, 1994, pp 509–523

Costello EJ, Stouthamer-Loeber M, DeRosier M: Continuity and change in psychopathology from childhood to adolescence. Paper presented at the Annual Meeting of the Society for Research in Child and Adolescent Psychopathology, Santa Fe, NM, February 1993

Counts DR, Pescovitz OH, Barnes KM: Dissociation of adrenarche and gonadarche in precocious puberty and in isolated hypogonadotropic hypogonadism. J Clin Endocrinol Metab 64:1174–1178, 1987

Davis SR, Tran J: Testosterone influences libido and well being in women. Trends Endocrinol Metab 12:33–37, 2001

DePeretti E, Forest MG: Unconjugatyed dehydroepiandrosterone plasma levels in normal subjects from birth to adolescence in human: the use of a sensitive radioimmunoassay. J Clin Endocrinol Metab 43:962–969, 1976

Dewing P, Bernard P, Vilain E: Disorders of gonadal development. Semin Reprod Med 20:189–198, 2002

Dewing P, Shi T, Horvath S, et al: Sexually dimorphic gene expression in mouse brain precedes gonadal differentiation. Brain Res Mol Brain Res 118:82–90, 2003

Dewing P, Chiang CW, Sinchak K, et al: Direct regulation of adult brain function by the male-specific factor SRY. Curr Biol 16:415–420, 2006

Dhillo WS, Chaudhri OB, Patterson M, et al: Kisspeptin-54 stimulates the hypothalamic-pituitary gonadal axis in human males. J Clin Endocrinol Metab 90:6609–6615, 2005

Ducharme JR, Forest MG, DePeretti E, et al: Plasma adrenal and gonadal sex steroids in human pubertal development. J Clin Endocrinol Metab 42:458–467, 1976

Dungan HM, Clifton DK, Steiner RA: Minireview: kisspeptin neurons as central processors in the regulation of gonadotropin-releasing hormone secretion. Endocrinology 147:1154–1158, 2006

Dunger DB, Villa AK, Matthews DR, et al: Pattern of secretion of bioactive and immunoreactive gonadotrophins in normal pubertal children. Clin Endocrinol 35:267–275, 1991

Dunkel L, Alfthan H, Stenman UH, et al: Gonadal control of pulsatile secretion of luteinizing hormone and follicle stimulating hormone in prepubertal boys evaluated by ultrasensitive time-resolved immunofluorometric assay. J Clin Endocrinol Metab 70:107–114, 1990

Dunnett S: Sex and gender in Brain Research Bulletin. Brain Res Bull 60:187–188, 2003

Ebling F: The neuroendocrine timing of puberty. Reproduction 129:675–683, 2005

Fleming JE, Offord DR: Epidemiology of childhood depressive disorders: a critical review. J Am Acad Child Adolesc Psychiatry 29:571–580, 1990

Ge X, Conger RD, Elder GH: Coming of age too early: pubertal influences on girls' vulnerability to psychological distress. Child Dev 67:3386–3400, 1996

Ge X, Conger R, Elder G: Pubertal transition, stressful life events, and the emergence of gender differences in adolescent depressive symptoms. Dev Psychol 37:404–417, 2001a

Ge X, Conger RD, Elder G: The relation between puberty and psychological distress in adolescent boys. J Res Adolesc 11:49–70, 2001b

Goodyer IM: Life Experiences, Development, and Childhood Psychopathology. Chichester, UK, Wiley, 1990

Goodyer I: Life events and difficulties: their nature and effects, in The Depressed Child and Adolescent: Developmental and Clinical Perspectives. Edited by Goodyer IM. New York, Cambridge University Press, 1995, pp 171–193

Goodyer I, Altham P: Lifetime exit events and recent social and family adversities in anxious and depressed school-age children and adolescents—II. J Affect Disord 21:229–238, 1991

Goodyer I, Kolvin I, Gatzanis S: Do age and sex influence the association between recent life events and psychiatric disorders in children and adolescents? A controlled enquiry. J Child Psychol Psychiatry 27:681–687, 1986

Goodyer I, Kolvin I, Gatzanis S: The impact of recent undesirable life events on psychiatric disorders in childhood and adolescence. Br J Psychiatry 151:179–184, 1987

Goodyer I, Wright C, Altham P: The friendships and recent life events of anxious and depressed school-age children. Br J Psychiatry 156:689–698, 1990

Goodyer I, Cooper P, Vize C, et al: Depression in 11–16 year-old girls: the role of past parental psychopathology and exposure to recent life events. J Child Psychol Psychiatry 34:1103–1115, 1993

Goodyer I, Herbert J, Altham P, et al: Adrenal secretion during major depression in 8- to 16-year-olds, I: altered diurnal rhythms in salivary cortisol and dehydroepiandrosterone (DHEA) at presentation. Psychol Med 26:245–256, 1996

Goodyer I, Herbert J, Secher S, et al: Short-term outcome of major depression, I: comorbidity and severity at presentation as predictors of persistent disorder. J Am Acad Child Adolesc Psychiatry 36:179–187, 1997

Goodyer I, Herbert J, Tamplin A, et al: First-episode major depression in adolescents: affective, cognitive and endocrine characteristics of risk status and predictors of onset. Br J Psychiatry 176:142–149, 2000

Goodyer IM, Park RJ, Herbert J: Psychosocial and endocrine features of chronic first-episode major depression in 8–16 year olds. Biol Psychiatry 50:351–357, 2001

Goodyer IM, Herbert J, Tamplin A: Psychoendocrine antecedents of persistent first episode major depression in adolescents: a community based longitudinal inquiry. Psychol Med 33:601–610, 2003

Graber JA, Lewinsohn PM, Seeley JR, et al: Is psychopathology associated with the timing of pubertal development? J Am Acad Child Adolesc Psychiatry 36:1768–1776, 1997

Granger DA, Shirtcliff EA, Zahn-Waxler C, et al: Salivary testosterone diurnal variation and psychopathology in adolescent males and females: individual differences and developmental effects. Dev Psychopathol 15:431–449, 2003

Greif EB, Ulman KJ: The psychological impact of the menarche on early adolescent females: a review of the literature. Child Dev 53:1413–1430, 1982

Guay AT, Jacobson J: Decreased free testosterone and dehydroepiandrosterone-sulfate (DHEA-S) levels in women with decreased libido. J Sex Marital Ther 28:129–142, 2002

Gubba EM, Netherton CM, Herbert J: Endangerment of the brain by glucocorticoids: experimental and clinical evidence. J Neurocytol 29:439–449, 2000

Gueorguiev M, Goth M, Korbonits M: Leptin and puberty: a review. Pituitary 4:79–86, 2001

Guyer B, Lescohier I, Gallagher S, et al: Intentional injuries among children and adolescents in Massachusetts. N Engl J Med 321:1584–1589, 1989

Haig D: The inexorable rise of gender and the decline of sex: social change in academic titles, 1945–2001. Arch Sex Behav 33:87–96, 2004

Hale PM, Khoury S, Foster CM, et al: Increased luteinizing hormone pulse frequency during sleep in early to midpubertal boys. J Clin Endocrinol Metab 66:785–791, 1988

Han SK, Gottsch ML, Lee KJ, et al: Activation of gonadotropin-releasing hormone neurons by kisspeptin as a neuroendocrine switch for the onset of puberty. J Neurosci 25:11349–11356, 2005

Hankin BL, Abramson LY, Moffitt TE, et al: Development of depression from pre-adolescence to young adulthood: emerging gender differences in a 10-year longitudinal study. J Abnorm Psychol 107:128–140, 1998

Henderson AS, Jorm AF, Korten AE, et al: Symptoms of depression and anxiety during adult life: evidence for a decline in prevalence with age. Psychol Med 28:1321–1328, 1998

Hossain A, Saunders GF: The human sex-determining gene SRY is a direct target of WT1. J Biol Chem 276:16817–16823, 2001

Huddleston J, Ge X (eds): Boys at puberty: psychosocial implications, in Gender Differences at Puberty. Edited by Hayward C. New York, Cambridge University Press, 2003, pp 113–136

Hutchison JB, Schumacher M, Steimer T, et al: Are separable aromatase systems involved in hormonal regulation of the male brain? J Neurobiol 21:743–759, 1990

Hwu HG, Yeh EK, Chang LY: Prevalence of psychiatric disorders in Taiwan defined by the Chinese Diagnostic Interview Schedule. Acta Psychiatr Scand 79:136–147, 1989

Institute of Medicine: Exploring the Biological Contributions to Human Health: Does Sex Matter? Washington, DC, National Academy Press, 2001

Jager RJ, Anvret M, Hall K, et al: A human XY female with frame shift mutation in the candidate sex determining gene, SRY. Nature 348:452–454, 1990

Jensen PS, Richters J, Ussery T, et al: Child psychopathology and environmental influences: discrete life events versus ongoing adversity. J Am Acad Child Adolesc Psychiatry 30:303–309, 1991

Jordan B, Vilain E: Sry and the genetics of sex determination. Adv Exp Med Biol 511:1–14, 2002

Jorm AF: Sex and age differences in depression: a quantitative synthesis of published research. Aust N Z J Psychiatry 21:6–53, 1987

Jorm AF: Does old age reduce the risk of anxiety and depression? A review of epidemiological studies across the adult life span. Psychol Med 30:1–22, 2000

Jost A: Recherches sur la differenciation sexuelle de l'embryon de lapin. III. Role des gonades foetales dans la differenciation sexuelle somatique. Arch Anat Microsc Morphol Exp 36:271–315, 1947

Judd HL, Parker DC, Yen SSC: Sleep-wake patterns of LH and testosterone release in prepubertal boys. J Clin Endocrinol Metab 44:965–969, 1977

Kaltiala-Heino R, Kosunen E, Rimpela M: Pubertal timing, sexual behaviour and self-reported depression in middle adolescence. J Adolesc 26:531–545, 2003

Kaminska M, Harris J, Gijsbers K, et al: Dehydroepiandrosterone sulfate (DHEAS) counteracts decremental effects of corticosterone on dentate gyrus LTP: implications for depression. Brain Res Bull 52:229–234, 2000

Karishma KK, Herbert J: Dehydroepiandrosterone (DHEA) stimulates neurogenesis in the hippocampus of the rat, promotes survival of newly formed neurons and prevents corticosterone-induced suppression. Eur J Neurosci 16:445–453, 2002

Kashani JH, Beck NC, Hoeper EW, et al: Psychiatric disorders in a community sample of adolescents. Am J Psychiatry 144:584–589, 1987

Kashani JH, Orvaschel H, Rosenberg MA, et al: Psychopathology in a community sample of children and adolescents: a developmental perspective. J Am Acad Child Adolesc Psychiatry 28:701–706, 1989

Kessler RC: Gender differences in major depression: epidemiological findings, in Gender and Its Effects on Psychopathology. Edited by Frank E. Washington, DC, American Psychiatric Publishing, 2000, pp 61–84

Kessler RC: Epidemiology of women and depression. J Affect Disord 74:5–13, 2003

Kessler RC, McGonagle KA, Swartz MS, et al: Sex and depression in the National Comorbidity Survey: I. Lifetime prevalence, chronicity and recurrence. J Affect Disord 29:85–96, 1993

Kessler RC, McGonagle KA, Nelson CB, et al: Sex and depression in the National Comorbidity Survey: II. Cohort effects. J Affect Disord 30:15–26, 1994

Kimonides VG, Khatibi NH, Svendsen CN, et al: Dehydroepiandrosterone (DHEA) and DHEA-sulfate (DHEAS) protect hippocampal neurons against excitatory amino acid-induced neurotoxicity. Proc Natl Acad Sci U S A 95:1852–1857, 1998

Korth-Schutz S, Levine LS, New MI: Serum androgens in normal prepubertal and pubertal children and in children with precocious adrenarche. J Clin Endocrinol Metab 42:117–124, 1976

Kraemer HC, Kazdin AE, Offord DR, et al: Coming to terms with the terms of risk. Arch Gen Psychiatry 54:337–343, 1997

Kulin HE, Moore RW, Satner SJ: Circadian rhythms in gonadotropin excretion in prepubertal and pubertal children. J Clin Endocrinol Metab 42:770–773, 1976

Labrie F, Belanger A, Cusan L, et al: Marked decline in serum concentrations of adrenal C19 sex steriod precursors and conjugated androgen metabolites during aging. J Clin Endocrinol Metab 82:2396–2402, 1997

Laitinen-Krispijn S, Van der Ende J, Hazebroek-Kampschreur AAJM, et al: Pubertal maturation and the development of behavioural and emotional problems in early adolescence. Acta Psychiatr Scand 99:16–25, 1999

Landy H, Boepple PA, Mansfield MJ, et al: Sleep modulation of neuroendocrine function: Developmental changes in gonadotropin-releasing hormone secretion during sexual maturation. Pediatr Res 213:213–217, 1992

Lashansky G, Saenger P, Fishman K, et al: Normative data for adrenal steroidogenesis in a healthy pediatric population: age and sex-related changes after adrenocorticotropin stimulation. J Clin Endocrinol Metab 73:674–686, 1991

Lee CK, Han JH, Choi JO: The epidemiological study of mental disorders in Korea (IX): alcoholism, anxiety, and depression. Seoul Journal of Psychiatry 12:183–191, 1987

Lepine J, Bouchez S: Epidemiology of depression in the elderly. Int Clin Psychopharmacol 13:S7–S12, 1998

Lewinsohn PM, Hops H, Roberts RE, et al: Adolescent psychopathology: I. Prevalence and incidence of depression and other DSM-III-R disorders in high school students. J Abnorm Psychol 102:133–144, 1993

Lewinsohn PM, Gotlib IH, Seeley JR: Adolescent psychopathology: IV. Specificity of psychosocial risk factors for depression and substance abuse in older adolescents. J Am Acad Child Adolesc Psychiatry 34:1221–1229, 1995

Lewinsohn PM, Rohde P, Seeley JR: Major depressive disorder in older adolescents: prevalence, risk factors, and clinical implications. Clin Psychol Rev 18:765–794, 1998

Marshall JC, Dalkin AC, Haisenieder DJ, et al: Gonadotropin-releasing hormone pulses: regulators of gonadotropin synthesis and ovulatory cycles. Recent Prog Horm Res 47:155–187, 1991

McGee R, Williams S: A longitudinal study of depression in nine-year-old children. J Am Acad Child Adolesc Psychiatry 27:342–348, 1988

McGee R, Feehan M, Williams S, et al: DSM-III disorders in a large sample of adolescents. J Am Acad Child Adolesc Psychiatry 29:611–619, 1990

McGee R, Feehan M, Williams S, et al: DSM-III disorders from age 11 to age 15 years. J Am Acad Child Adolesc Psychiatry 31:51–59, 1992

Messager S: Kisspeptin and its receptor: new gatekeepers of puberty. J Neuroendocrinol 17:687–688, 2005

Money J: Hermaphroditism, gender and precocity in hyperadrenocorticism: psychologic findings. Bull Johns Hopkins Hosp 96:253–264, 1955

Nolen-Hoeksema S, Girgus JS, Seligman MEP: Sex differences in depression and explanatory style in children. J Youth Adolesc 20:233–245, 1991

Nottelmann ED, Susman EF, Dorn LD, et al: Developmental processes in early adolescence: relations among chronological age, pubertal stage, height, weight, and serum levels of gonadotropins, sex steroids, and adrenal androgens. J Adolesc Health Care 8:246–260, 1987a

Nottelmann ED, Susman EJ, Inoff-Germain G, et al: Developmental processes in early adolescence: relationships between adolescent adjustment problems and chronological age, pubertal stage, and puberty-related serum hormone levels. J Pediatr 110:473–480, 1987b

Nottelmann ED, Inoff-Germain G, Susman EJ, et al: Hormones and behavior at puberty, in Adolescence and Puberty. Edited by Bancroft J, Reinisch JM. New York, Oxford University Press, 1990, pp 88–123

O'Connor DW: Do older Australians truly have low rates of anxiety and depression? A critique of the 1997 National Survey of Mental Health and Wellbeing. Aust N Z J Psychiatry 40:623–631, 2006

Olsson GI, Nordström ML, von Knorring HA, et al: Adolescent depression: social network and family climate: a case-control study. J Child Psychol Psychiatry 40:227–237, 1999

Olweus D, Mattsson A, Schalling D, et al: Circulating testosterone levels and aggression in adolescent males: a causal analysis. Psychosom Med 50:261–272, 1988

Page DC: On low expectations exceeded; or, the genomic salvation of the Y chromosome. Am J Hum Genet 74:399–402, 2004

Paikoff RL, Brooks-Gunn J, Warren MP: Effects of girls' hormonal status on depressive and aggressive symptoms over the course of one year. J Youth Adolesc 20:191–215, 1991

Parker LN, Sack J, Fisher DA, et al: The adrenarche: prolactin, gonadotropins, adrenal androgens, and cortisol. J Clin Endocrinol Metab 46:396–404, 1978

Patton GC, Hibbert ME, Carlin J, et al: Menarche and the onset of depression and anxiety in Victoria, Australia. J Epidemiol Community Health 50:661–666, 1996

Persson A, Kerr M, Stattin H: Why a leisure context is linked to normbreaking for some girls and not others: personality characteristics and parent-child relations as explanations. J Adolesc 27:583–598, 2004

Pinn V: Sex and gender factors in medical studies: implications for health and clinical practice. JAMA 289:397–400, 2003

Plant T: Neurobiological bases underlying the control of the onset of puberty in the rhesus monkey: a representative higher primate. Front Neuroendocrinol 22:107–139, 2001

Rasmussen JE, Torres-Aleman I, MacLusky NJ, et al: The effects of estradiol on the growth patterns of estrogen receptor-positive hypothalamic cell lines. Endocrinology 126:235–240, 1990

Reiner W, Gearhart J: Discordant sexual identity in some genetic males with cloacal exstrophy assigned to female sex at birth. N Engl J Med 350:333–341, 2004

Reinherz HZ, Giaconia RM, Lefkowitz ES, et al: Prevalence of psychiatric disorders in a community population of older adolescents. J Am Acad Child Adolesc Psychiatry 32:369–377, 1993a

Reinherz HZ, Giaconia RM, Pakiz B, et al: Psychosocial risks for major depression in late adolescence: a longitudinal community study. J Am Acad Child Adolesc Psychiatry 32:1155–1163, 1993b

Reiter EO, Fuldauer VG, Root AW: Secretion of the adrenal androgen, dehydroepiandrosterone sulfate, during normal infancy, childhood, and adolescence, in sick infants, and in children with endocrinologic abnormalities. J Pediatr 90:766–770, 1977

Robins LN, Regier DA: Psychiatric Disorders in America: The Epidemiologic Catchment Area Study. New York, Free Press, 1991

Romeo R: Puberty: a period of both organizational and activational effects of steroid hormones on neurobehavioural development. J Neuroendocrinol 15:1185–1192, 2003

Rutter M: Age as an ambiguous variable in developmental research: some epidemiological considerations from developmental psychopathology. Int J Behav Dev 12:1–34, 1989

Rutter M, O'Connor TG: Are There biological programming effects for psychological development? Findings from a study of Romanian adoptees. Dev Psychol 40:81–94, 2004

Rutter M, Graham P, Chadwick OFD, et al: Adolescent turmoil: fact or fiction? J Child Psychol Psychiatry 17:35–56, 1976

Rutter M, Andersen-Wood L, Beckett C, et al: Quasi-autistic patterns following severe early global privation. J Child Psychol Psychiatry 40:537–549, 1999

Rutter M, Caspi A, Moffitt T: Using sex differences in psychopathology to study causal mechanisms: Unifying issues and research strategies. J Child Psychol Psychiatry 44:1092–1115, 2003

Sandberg S, Rutter M, Pickles ADM, et al: Do high-threat life events really provoke the onset of psychiatric disorder in children? J Child Psychol Psychiatry 42:523–532, 2001

Seminara SB: We all remember our first kiss: kisspeptin and the male gonadal axis. J Clin Endocrinol Metab 90:6738–6740, 2005

Seminara SB: Mechanisms of disease: the first kiss—a crucial role for kisspeptin-1 and its receptor, G-protein-coupled receptor 54, in puberty and reproduction. Nat Clin Pract Endocrinol Metab 2:328–334, 2006

Sizonenko PC, Paunier L: Hormonal changes in puberty III: correlation of plasma dehydroepiandrosterone, testosterone, FSH, and LH with stages of puberty and bone age in normal boys and girls and in patients with Addison's disease or hypogonadism or with premature or late adrenarche. J Clin Endocrinol Metab 41:894–904, 1975

Skaletsky H, Kuroda-Kawaguchi T, Minx PJ, et al: The male-specific region of the human Y chromosome is a mosaic of discrete sequence classes. Nature 423:825–837, 2003

Skuse D: Extreme deprivation in early childhood. J Child Psychol Psychiatry 25:543–572, 1984

Stattin H, Magnusson D: Paths Through Life, Vol 2: Pubertal Maturation in Female Development. Hillsdale, NJ, Erlbaum, 1990

Stattin H, Kerr M, Mahoney J, et al: Explaining why a leisure context is bad for some girls and not for others, in Organized Activities as Contexts of Development: Extracurricular Activities, After-School and Community Programs. Edited by Mahoney JL, Larson RW, Eccles JS. Mahwah, NJ, Erlbaum, 2005

Susman EJ, Nottelmann ED, Inoff-Germain GE, et al: The relation of relative hormonal levels and physical development and social-emotional behavior in young adolescents. J Youth Adolesc 14:245–264, 1985

Susman EJ, Inoff-Germain G, Nottelmann ED, et al: Hormones, emotional dispositions, and aggressive attributes in young adolescents. Child Dev 58:114–1134, 1987a

Susman EJ, Nottelmann ED, Inoff-Germain G, et al: Hormonal influences on aspects of psychological development during adolescence. J Adolesc Health Care 8:492–504, 1987b

Susman EJ, Dorn LD, Chrousos GP: Negative affect and hormone levels in young adolescents: concurrent and predictive perspective. J Youth Adolesc 20:167–190, 1991

Susman EJ, Finkelstein JW, Chinchilli VM, et al: The effect of sex hormone replacement therapy on behavior problems and moods in adolescents with delayed puberty. J Pediatr 133:521–525, 1998

Tanner JM: Growth at Adolescence, With a General Consideration of the Effects of Hereditary and Environmental Factors Upon Growth and Maturation From Birth to Maturity, 2nd Edition. Oxford, UK, Blackwell Scientific, 1962

Terasawa E, Fernandez D: Neurobiological mechanisms of the onset of puberty in primates. Endocr Rev 22:111–151, 2001

Travison TG, Morley JE, Araujo AB, et al: The relationship between libido and testosterone levels in aging men. J Clin Endocrinol Metab 91:2509–2513, 2006

Twenge JM, Nolen-Hoeksema SK: Age, gender, race, SES, and birth cohort differences on the Children's Depression Inventory. J Abnorm Psychol 111:578–588, 2002

Velez CN, Johnson J, Cohen P: A longitudinal analysis of selected risk factors of childhood psychopathology. J Am Acad Child Adolesc Psychiatry 28:861–864, 1989

Vihko H, Apter D: The role of androgens in adolescent cycles. J Steroid Biochem 12:369–373, 1980

Vilain E: Genetics of sexual development. Annu Rev Sex Res 11:1–25, 2000

Villamil E, Huppert FA, Melzer D: Low prevalence of depression and anxiety is linked to statutory retirement ages rather than personal work exit: a national survey. Psychol Med 36:999–1099, 2006

Wade TJ, Cairney J, Pevalin DJ: Emergence of gender differences in depression during adolescence: national panel results from three countries. J Am Acad Child Adolesc Psychiatry 41:190–198, 2002

Weichold K, Silbereisen R, Schmitt-Rodermund E: Short-term and long-term consequences of early versus late physical maturation in adolescents, in Gender Differences at Puberty. Edited by Hayward C. New York, Cambridge University Press, 2003, pp 241–276

Weissman MM, Klerman GL: Sex differences and the epidemiology of depression. Arch Gen Psychiatry 34:98–111, 1977

Weissman MM, Bland R, Joyce PR, et al: Sex differences in rates of depression: cross-national perspectives. J Affect Disord 29:77–84, 1993

Weissman MM, Bland R, Canino GJ, et al: Cross-national epidemiology of major depression and bipolar disorder. JAMA 276:293–299, 1996

Wells JE, Bushnell JA, Hornblow AR, et al: Christchurch Psychiatric Epidemiology Study, part I: methodology and lifetime prevalence for specific psychiatric disorders. Aust N Z J Psychiatry 23:315–326, 1989

Wennink JMB, Delemarre-van de Waal HA, Schoemaker R, et al: Luteinizing hormone and follicle stimulating hormone secretion patterns in boys throughout puberty measured using highly sensitive immunoradiometric assays. Clin Endocrinol 31:551–564, 1989

Wennink JMB, Delemarre-van de Waal HA, Schoemaker R, et al: Luteinizing hormone and follicle stimulating hormone secretion patterns in girls throughout puberty measured using highly sensitive immunoradiometric assays. Clin Endocrinol 33:333–344, 1990

Wierman ME, Beardsworth DE, Crawford JD, et al: Adrenarche and skeletal maturation during luteinizing hormone releasing hormone analogue suppression of gonadarche. J Clin Invest 77:121–126, 1986

Wilhelm K, Mitchell P, Slade T, et al: Prevalence and correlates of DSM-IV major depression in an Australian national survey. J Affect Disord 75:155–162, 2003

Willard HF: The sex chromosomes and X chromosome inactivation, in The Metabolic and Molecular Bases of Inherited Disease. Edited by Scriver CR, Beaudet AL, Sly WS, et al. New York, McGraw-Hill, 2000

Williamson DE, Birmaher B, Frank E, et al: Nature of life events and difficulties in depressed adolescents. J Am Acad Child Adolesc Psychiatry 37:1049–1057, 1998

Wittchen HU, Essau CA, von Zerssen D, et al: Lifetime and six-month prevalence of mental disorders in the Munich Follow-Up Study. Eur Arch Psychiatry Clin Neurosci 241:247–258, 1992

Wittchen HU, Knauper B, Kessler RC: Lifetime risk of depression. Br J Psychiatry Suppl 26:16–22, 1994

Wu FC, Butler GE, Kelnar CJH, et al: Patterns of pulsatile luteinizing hormone secretion before and during the onset of puberty in boys: a study using an immunoradiometric assay. J Clin Endocrinol Metab 70:629–637, 1990

Young DG, Skibinski G, Mason JI, et al: The influence of age and gender on serum dehydropeiandrosterone sulphate (DHEA-S), IL-6, IL-6 soluble receptor (IL-6 sR) and transforming growth factor beta 1 (TGF-beta1) levels in normal healthy blood donors. Clin Exp Immunol 117:476–481, 1999

DISORDER-BASED EXAMPLES OF THE STUDY OF GENE–ENVIRONMENT INTERACTION

GENETIC AND ENVIRONMENTAL MODIFIERS OF RISK AND RESILIENCY IN MALTREATED CHILDREN

Joan Kaufman, Ph.D.

By all standards of measurement, the problem of child maltreatment is enormous in terms of its cost to the individual and its cost to society (Zigler 1980). Child abuse occurs at epidemic rates, with nearly 1,000,000 substantiated reports of child maltreatment each year (U.S. Department of Health and Human Services, Administration on Children, Youth and Families 2006), many reported cases of actual abuse that are not verified (Drake et al. 2003; Kaufman and Zigler 1996), and countless other cases that never come to the attention of authorities (Wolfner and Gelles 1993). Victims of abuse constitute a significant proportion of all child psychiatric admissions, with lifetime incidence of physical and sexual abuse estimated at 30% among child and adolescent outpatients (Lanktree et al. 1991) and as high as 55% among psychiatric inpatients (McClellan et al. 1995).

Child abuse most often occurs in the context of other risk factors. Domestic violence and family history of psychiatric illness and substance abuse are problems that frequently co-occur in association with child maltreatment. It is estimated that 60% of cases involved with protective services involve histories of severe domestic violence (Connelly et al. 2006), close to 80% of parents who lose custody of their children have a substance use disorder (Besinger et al. 1999), and approximately 70% of mothers of maltreated children have a lifetime history of depression (De Bellis et al. 2001). Most children who are maltreated are multiply traumatized and at high-risk for psychopathology for many reasons, including genetic factors.

Although child abuse is frequently associated with long-term significant psychiatric sequelae, not all abused children develop difficulties (Kendall-Tackett et al. 1993). Emerging findings strongly indicate that the likelihood of a given maltreated child developing problems is influenced by *both* genetic and environmental factors. Moreover, understanding the interplay between these two domains is critical to understanding risk and resiliency in maltreated children and to developing effective prevention and treatment interventions. In this chapter, I review sequelae frequently associated with child maltreatment and then discuss emerging findings of the role of genetics in moderating risk for deleterious outcomes in maltreated children.

PSYCHIATRIC DIAGNOSES IN MALTREATED CHILDREN

Child maltreatment is a nonspecific risk factor for many forms of psychopathology (Kendler et al. 2000; Molnar et al. 2001). Compared with community control subjects, maltreated children have elevated externalizing and internalizing behavior problems according to parent and teacher reports (Kaplan et al. 1999). They also have increased rates of posttraumatic stress disorder (Famularo et al. 1992, 1996; Kilpatrick et al. 2003; Ruggiero et al. 2000), depression (Kaufman 1991; Pelcovitz et al. 2000), reactive attachment disorder (Zeanah et al. 2004), dissociative symptoms (Putnam et al. 1995), self-destructive behavior and borderline traits (Noll et al. 2003; Romans et al. 1995), sexually inappropriate behaviors (Cosentino et al. 1995; Noll et al. 2003), drug and alcohol problems (Molnar et al. 2001; Schuck and Widom 2003; Widom et al. 1995), eating disorders (Ackard and Neumark-Sztainer 2003), oppositional defiant disorder (Garland et al. 2001; Kolko 2002), and conduct disorder (Garland et al. 2001; Kolko 2002).

ROLE OF GENETICS IN PSYCHIATRIC AND SUBSTANCE ABUSE DISORDERS

The results of scores of adoption, twin, and family studies indicate a role for both genetics and environment in the pathophysiology of the major psychiatric diagnoses, including the disorders most frequently associated with a history of child maltreatment (Kendler 2005). Advances in molecular biology, however, have enabled more refined investigation of the role of genes in the etiology of these disorders. Specifically, since the mid 1980s numerous DNA markers, or polymorphisms, have been identified, facilitating the testing of associations between variability in specific genes and the presence of different disorders.

DNA is made up of four nucleotide bases repeated in specified sequences. Genes represent a subset of the total DNA, and the nucleotides that make up individual genes provide a template for the synthesis of proteins critical for development and sustaining life. Some of the proteins most relevant in the etiology of psychiatric disorders include those that act as enzymes in the synthesis and degradation of stress hormones and neurotransmitters, and those used as receptors on cells facilitating communication from one brain region to another.

Since 2000, technical advances have eliminated the need for blood draws to obtain DNA. Adequate DNA for genetic analyses can now readily be obtained from saliva. Despite some remaining public concerns, research with DNA is currently considered minimal risk by most institutional review boards, even when the research involves pediatric participants and the creation of data repositories. The greatest risks imposed by genetics research are loss of confidentiality and privacy violations. A recent survey of 49 psychiatric genetics investigators who collectively recruited approximately 30,000 subjects asked about adverse events involving loss of confidentiality and requests for genetic data from outside parties. Through standard practices employed to protect subjects' confidentiality, there were no reports of individuals outside the research teams gaining access to the genetic data (J.F. Cubells, M.D., Ph.D., "Risks in Genotype-Based Research on Human Behavior," unpublished ms., September 2006). The field appears to have developed appropriate informed consent and privacy protection procedures, so the risks posed by genetics research is indeed balanced by the great promises offered by this methodology.

To date, molecular genetic techniques have been applied to the study of the onset of sociopathy, alcohol use, and depression in maltreated children. There is an important caveat to note before reviewing these exciting findings: the individual genes identified in the studies are just one of the many variables that contribute to the onset of these problems. Multiple genetic and environmental factors in combination increase risk for these behaviors. In addition, just as a history of maltreatment need not be associated with deleterious consequences, high-risk genes do not inevitably lead to bad outcomes. The most appropriate models for the etiology of problems associated with a history of maltreatment appear to be those that take into account gene–environment interactions.

Sociopathy

Caspi, Moffitt, and colleagues (Caspi et al. 2002) were the first to examine the role of genetic factors in moderating the outcome of maltreated children. They studied a large sample of 1,037 males from birth to adulthood. The sample was well characterized on indices of environmental adversity, and between the ages of 3 and 11 years, 8% of the children were severely maltreated, and 28% had experiences rated as "probable maltreatment." Although maltreatment significantly increases the risk for later criminality, most maltreated children do not become delinquents or adult criminals.

Caspi et al. (2002) examined differences in a functional polymorphism in the promoter of the monoamine oxidase A (MAO-A) gene (*MAOA*) to determine why some children who are maltreated grow up to develop antisocial behavior and others do not. MAO-A is an enzyme that participates in the metabolism of neurotransmitters such as serotonin, norepinephrine, and dopamine. Human *MAOA* is located on the X chromosome (Levy et al. 1989), and a polymorphism consisting of a variable number of tandem repeats (VNTR) has been reported in the promoter region of this gene. The repeated sequence consists of a 30–base pair unit, and versions of *MAOA* with three and four repeats of this sequence are most common (Inoue-Murayama et al. 2006). The version of the gene, or the allele, with four copies of this repeated base-pair sequence is associated with higher activity of *MAOA* than the allele with three copies. Given genetic deficiencies in *MAOA* activity have been linked with aggression in mice and humans (Caspi et al. 2002), there was strong rationale for examining this gene in association with sociopathy and violent behavior in maltreated individuals.

Males in the severe, probable, and no maltreatment groups did not differ in terms of *MAOA* allele frequency, suggesting genotype did not influence exposure to maltreatment. The functional polymorphism in *MAOA* gene, however, was found to moderate the relationship between maltreatment and later sociopathy. This relationship is depicted in Figure 7–1. Only maltreated males with the low MAO-A activity gene were at increased risk for antisocial outcomes. Maltreated males with the gene associated with high MAO-A activity were approximately half as likely as maltreated males with the low MAO-A activity gene to be convicted of a violent offense, and were not statistically more likely than nonmaltreated peers with the same genotype to have this history.

Maltreated children with the genotype conferring low levels of *MAOA* expression were more likely to develop antisocial problems across all the indices examined by Caspi and colleagues. They had higher rates of conduct disorder in adolescence, more antisocial personality disorder symptoms in adulthood, a greater propensity toward violence, and higher rates of conviction for violent offenses by age 26 years (Caspi et al. 2002). The role

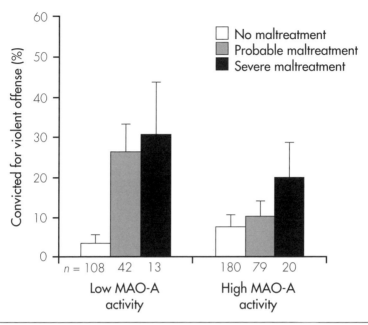

FIGURE 7–1. **Association between childhood maltreatment and subsequent conviction for a violent crime as a function of MAO-A activity.**

Source. Reprinted from Caspi A, McClay J, Moffitt TE, et al.: "Role of Genotype in the Cycle of Violence in Maltreated Children." *Science* 297:851–854, 2002. Used with permission.

of *MAOA* in moderating the development of aggression and sociopathy in maltreated children has now been replicated in several other studies (Kim-Cohen et al. 2006; Widom and Brzustowicz 2006). Understanding additional risk and protective factors associated with variability in aggressive and antisocial behavior is critical for the development of more effective targeted prevention and intervention strategies.

Alcohol Consumption

As noted previously, alcohol dependence is one of the more common sequelae of child abuse (Kendler et al. 2000; Moran et al. 2004). The more severe the child maltreatment (Bulik et al. 2001) and the greater the number of childhood adversities experienced (Dube et al. 2002), the more likely it is that alcohol problems will develop. The importance of both genetic and environmental factors in the etiology of alcoholism has been suggested by findings of preclinical (Caldji et al. 2004), twin (Liu et al. 2004), and adoption (Cutrona et al. 1994) studies.

The serotonin transporter gene (*5-HTTLPR*) is an ideal candidate to examine in gene–environment interaction studies of the development of alcohol problems, because serotonin (5-HT) is a critical modulator of the stress response (Oroszi and Goldman 2004). 5-HT is also one of the main neurotransmitter systems involved in brain reward circuitry (Koob et al. 1997); it is released in response to alcohol (Yoshimoto et al. 1992), and alcohol dependence is associated with serotonergic system dysregulation (Koob 2003). Although prior research investigations reported inconsistent findings in the association between *5-HTTLPR* and alcohol dependence, results of a recent meta-analysis of 17 studies suggest that *5-HTTLPR* significantly, albeit modestly, predicts alcohol dependence, with this association greatest among individuals with early-onset and comorbid psychiatric disorders (Feinn et al. 2005).

5-HTTLPR (locus SLC6A4) has a well-studied functional VNTR polymorphism in the promoter region. There are two common functional alleles of *5-HTTLPR*, the short (S) allele and the long (L) allele. The S allele of *5-HTTLPR* contains an attenuated promoter segment and is associated with reduced transcription and functional capacity of the 5-HT transporter relative to the L allele (Lesch et al. 1995).

In studies with nonhuman primates, polymorphic variation in *5-HTTLPR* has been found to moderate the effects of early stress on alcohol consumption later in life. In nonhuman primates, *5-HTTLPR* genotype makes little difference in predicting alcohol preference of primates reared under optimal conditions (e.g., parent reared). However, for primates reared under more stressful conditions (e.g., peer reared), compared with those homozygous for the L allele, heterozygous S/L primates show increased ethanol preference and consumption in young adulthood (Barr et al. 2004). Thus, there appears to be a gene–environment interaction between experiences of stress and the 5-HT transporter gene, with the S allele of *5-HTTLPR* associated with alcohol consumption, but only in primates subjected to early stress. Preliminary gene–environment interactions in predicting alcohol use involving *5-HTTLPR* have also been identified in humans, with good family relations acting as a protective factor and associated with decreased frequency of intoxication in older adolescents with the high-risk S/L genotype (Nilsson et al. 2005) and more stressful life events in the preceding year predictive of greater alcohol use in college students with the S/S and L/S genotypes (Covault et al. 2007).

Because alcohol use before the age of 14 is associated with a 40% risk for the development of alcohol dependence (Grant and Dawson 1997), our group (Kaufman et al. 2007) studied genetic and environmental predictors of drinking behavior in a cohort of maltreated children and community control subjects. The study represented an add-on project to an investigation examining the efficacy of an intervention for maltreated children entering out-of-home care. A total of 219 children were recruited for the original intervention study over 3 consecutive years. Two-year follow-up data, *5-HTTLPR* genotype, and alcohol assessments were available for 127 children: 76 maltreated and 51 demographically matched community control children, 83% of the first two cohorts recruited for the SAFE Homes study. The mean age of the children at follow-up was 12.5 years (SD=2.3; range: 8.1–16.5). Nineteen percent of the sample were 8–10 years, 21% were 10–12 years, 30% were 12–14 years, and 30% were 14–16 years, with no differences between the two groups in the proportion of children in each age group. Predictors of early alcohol use explored included maltreatment, family loading for alcohol/substance use disorders, and 5-HT transporter genotype.

As depicted in Figure 7–2, maltreated children were statistically more likely to have had their first alcoholic beverage and more likely to have had an episode of getting drunk. Of the children who had experimented with alcohol, maltreated children did so on average 2 years earlier than control subjects (mean drinking age: maltreated, 11.2 years; control subjects, 13.5 years), and 9% of the maltreated children who had experimented with alcohol reported weekly intoxication.

In predicting alcohol use, sex and ethnicity were not statistically significant in the model, and age and parental history of alcohol or substance use disorders showed nonsignificant trends in increasing risk of early alcohol experimentation. After these covariates were controlled for, maltreatment, *5-HTTLPR*, and the interaction of maltreatment history by *5-HTTLPR* were potent predictors of early alcohol use, with the presence of the S allele associated with the greatest vulnerability to early alcohol use (see Figure 7–3).

Most adolescent alcohol use prevention programs are school based and universal, targeted toward the general population regardless of risk (Boyd 2005). Although these programs have demonstrated modest efficacy in reducing risk for later alcohol use, intervention effects have predominantly been confined to the baseline nondrinker groups, with no significant effects demonstrated in youth who have already begun drinking (Zucker and Wong 2005).

Although not initially designed to reduce adolescent alcohol use, a child abuse prevention program involving nurse home visitation for the first 2 years of life (Olds et al. 1998) was found not only to reduce child maltreatment and other psychosocial risk factors, but also to be associated with lower rates of antisocial behavior and alcohol use in the adolescent offspring at 15-year follow-up. Preventing the revictimization of children already identified by the child protective services system and utilization of targeted preventive intervention programs appear to be promising strategies to reduce risk of alcohol use in this vulnerable population.

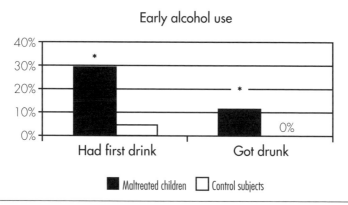

FIGURE 7–2.   Proportion of maltreated and control children who experimented with alcohol.

At the 2-year follow-up, when the mean age of the children was 12.4, maltreated children were statistically more likely than control subjects to have experimented with alcohol. Of the children who had experimented with alcohol, the children in the maltreated group did so, on average, more than 2 years earlier than the children in the control group (11.2 vs. 13.5). In addition, at the 2-year follow-up, maltreated children were statistically more likely to have had an experience of getting drunk.
Source.   Reprinted from Kaufman J, Yang BZ, Douglas-Palumberi H, et al.: "Genetic and Environmental Predictors of Early Alcohol Use." *Biological Psychiatry* 61:1228–1234, 2007. Used with permission.

Depression

Caspi, Moffitt, and colleagues also examined gene–environment interactions in the development of depression (Caspi et al. 2003). They were the first to report that *5-HTTLPR* moderated the influence of early child maltreatment and stressful life events on the development of depression. Individuals with a history of abuse with the S allele of *5-HTTLPR* exhibited more depressive symptoms and diagnosable depression than individuals homozygous for the L allele. This finding has since been replicated in numerous independent investigations with child (Kaufman et al. 2004), adolescent (Eley et al. 2004), and young adult (Kendler et al. 2005) populations.

Figure 7–4 shows the interaction between maltreatment experiences and the *5-HTTLPR* genotype in the one child study (Kaufman et al. 2004). Participants included 101 children: 57 children who had been removed from their parents' care within the past 6 months because of allegations of abuse and/or neglect, and 44 community control subjects with no history of maltreatment or exposure to intrafamilial violence. The children in the control group had relatively low depression scores, regardless of their genotype. Within the maltreated group, the children with L/L or L/S genotype

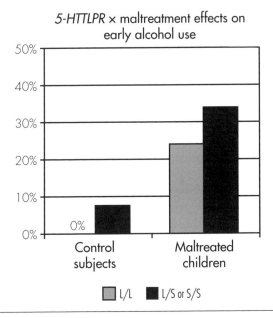

FIGURE 7–3. **Relationship between maltreatment, the serotonin transporter gene (*5-HTTLPR*), and early alcohol use.**

After all the relevant covariates were controlled for, there was a significant interaction between maltreatment and genotype. The presence of the short (S) allele conferred a vulnerability for early alcohol use, with the vulnerability associated with the S allele significantly greater in the maltreated children. Children with the heterozygous S/long (L) genotype showed the greatest vulnerability to early alcohol use. Only 11% of the sample had the less common S/S genotype, and none of these children reported a history of alcohol experimentation.

Source. Reprinted from Kaufman J, Yang BZ, Douglas-Palumberi H, et al.: "Genetic and Environmental Predictors of Early Alcohol Use." *Biological Psychiatry* 61:1228–1234, 2007. Used with permission.

only had slight elevations in their depression scores compared with control subjects, but the children with the S/S genotype, the most vulnerable genotype, had depression scores that were twice as high as the depression scores of the control children with the same genotype.

GENE–GENE INTERACTIONS

Given that gene–gene interactions have been theorized to contribute to the etiology of depression (Holmans et al. 2004; Kendler and Karkowski-Shuman 1997), our group also hypothesized that a polymorphism in the brain-derived neurotrophic factor (BDNF) gene (*BDNF*) might interact with *5-*

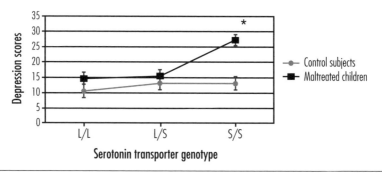

FIGURE 7–4.   Gene–maltreatment interaction in predicting depression in children.

The interaction between serotonin transporter gene (*5-HTTLPR*) genotype and maltreatment history was significant (*P*<0.01). The short (S)/S genotype conferred a significant vulnerability for depression but only in the maltreated children.
Source.   Reprinted from Kaufman J, Yang BZ, Douglas-Palumberi H, et al.: "Social Supports and Serotonin Transporter Gene Moderate Depression in Maltreated Children." *Proceedings of the National Academy of Sciences of the United States of America* 101:17316–17321, 2004. Used with permission.

HTTLPR to further increase risk for depression in maltreated children (Kaufman et al. 2006). *BDNF* genetic variation has recently been associated with child-onset depression in two independent samples (Strauss et al. 2004, 2005). In addition, both BDNF (i.e., the protein product of *BDNF*) and 5-HT have been implicated in the etiology of depression, and they are also known to interact at multiple intra- and intercellular levels (Duman et al. 1997; Malberg et al. 2000).

Our group (Kaufman et al. 2006) studied a sample of 109 maltreated and 87 nonmaltreated demographically matched comparison children and found a significant three-way interaction between *BDNF* genotype, *5-HTTLPR*, and maltreatment history in predicting depression. As depicted in Figure 7–5, children with the met allele of *BDNF* and two S alleles of *5-HTTLPR* had the highest depression scores, but the vulnerability associated with these two genotypes was only evident in the maltreated children (Kaufman et al. 2006).

SOCIAL SUPPORTS

Clinical studies of individuals with a history of abuse suggest that the availability of a caring and stable parent or alternative guardian is one of the most important factors that distinguish abused individuals with good developmental outcomes from those with more deleterious outcomes (Kaufman

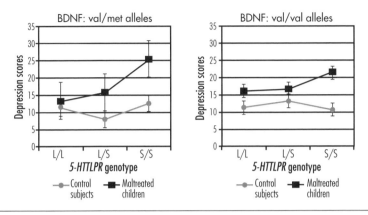

FIGURE 7–5. **Three-way interaction between maltreatment history, brain-derived neurotrophic factor (*BDNF*) genotype, and serotonin transporter genotype (*5-HTTLPR*).**

The graphs above depict the data of the maltreated and normally treated and demograhically matched control children. There was a significant three-way interaction between *BDNF* genotype, *5-HTTLPR* genotype, and maltreatment history in predicting children's depression scores. Children with the Val66Met polymorphism of *BDNF* and the short (S)/S *5-HTTLPR* genotype had the highest depression scores, with the vulnerability associated with these two genotypes only elevated in the maltreated children.

Source. Reprinted from Kaufman J, Yang BZ, Douglas-Palumberi H, et al.: "Brain-Derived Neurotrophic Factor-5-HTTLPR Gene Interactions and Environmental Modifiers of Depression in Children." *Biological Psychiatry* 59:673–680, 2006. Used with permission.

and Henrich 2000). Consequently, in addition to examining gene–gene interactions, our group (Kaufman et al. 2006) also examined the effect of social supports in moderating genetic risk for depression in maltreated children. Children were asked to name people they 1) talk to about personal things, 2) count on to buy the things they need, 3) share good news with, 4) get together with to have fun, and 5) go to if they need advice. The summary social support measure used was the number of positive support categories listed for the child's top support. The children were most likely to name an adult as their primary support. Sixty-one percent of the maltreated children and 83% of the control subjects listed their mothers as their top support, and 30% of the maltreated children and 10% of the control subjects listed alternative parental figures (e.g., father, stepfather, foster mother), grandparents, or other adult relatives as their primary support.

As depicted in Figure 7–6, maltreated children with positive supports had depression scores that were only slightly greater than those of control

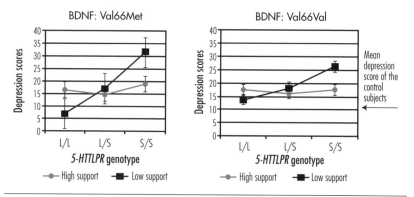

FIGURE 7–6.   **Four-way interaction between maltreatment history, brain-derived neurotrophic factor (*BDNF*) genotype, serotonin transporter gene (*5-HTTLPR*) genotype, and social supports in maltreated children.**

The graphs above depict only the data of the maltreated children. The mean score of the control subjects is indicated on the right as a frame of reference. The depression scores of the maltreated children with high social supports were close to the mean depression score of the control subjects, regardless of genotype. The short (S)/S genotype was associated with an increase in maltreated children's depression scores, which was greatest for the children without positive supports and the additional presence of the met allele of the *BDNF* polymorphism. L/L=long/long genotype; L/S=long/short genotype; S/S=short/short genotype.

Source.   Reprinted from Kaufman J, Yang BZ, Douglas-Palumberi H, et al.: "Brain-Derived Neurotrophic Factor-5-HTTLPR Gene Interactions and Environmental Modifiers of Depression in Children." *Biological Psychiatry* 59:673–680, 2006. Used with permission.

subjects, regardless of genotype. The quality and availability of social supports was an extremely potent factor in determining risk for depression in maltreated children—with the effect greatest for those maltreated children with the most vulnerable genotypes.

There are likely multiple mechanisms by which social supports may ameliorate risk. Data from preclinical (e.g., animal) studies suggest that maternal behavior can produce stable changes in DNA methylation and chromatin structure of the glucocorticoid receptor gene promoter in the hippocampus (Weaver et al. 2004). These epigenetic changes and the subsequent alteration in hypothalamic-pituitary-adrenal (HPA) axis response to stress may be one important mechanism by which variations in maternal behavior/social supports alter risk for stress-related disorders.

A take-home message from the gene–environment studies is that to help promote resiliency in maltreated children we must 1) prevent the re-abuse of children, and 2) facilitate the formation of lasting positive relationships with birthparents or alternative caregivers. An additional take-home message that was highlighted earlier is worth repeating. Neither a history of maltreatment nor the presence of high-risk genes guarantees deleterious outcomes. There are multiple protective factors that can shift the likelihood of these outcomes occurring.

TRANSLATIONAL RESEARCH APPROACHES AND NOVEL THERAPEUTIC TARGETS

Preclinical (e.g., animal) studies of the effects of stress provide a valuable heuristic in understanding the pathophysiology of depression and other stress-related disorders (Gorman et al. 2002; Heim et al. 1997), with many of the biological alterations associated with early stress in preclinical studies reported in adults with these problems. As reviewed elsewhere (Kaufman et al. 2000), there has been extensive preclinical research conducted examining the neurobiological effects of early stress using maternal separation paradigms. These experiences are associated with elevated anxiety, aggressive, and depressive-like behaviors; increased HPA stress axis activity; and decreased binding to glucocorticoid receptor, one of the receptors critical to turning off the stress response. These experiences are also associated with enhanced age-related cell loss in the hippocampus and reduced performance on hippocampal-mediated memory tasks (Meaney et al. 1991, 1993).

There are emerging preclinical data to suggest that the long-term neurobiological and behavioral changes associated with early stress can be modified by the availability of positive supports and optimal subsequent caregiving experiences (Wiedenmayer et al. 2003). Several investigators utilizing mother–infant separation paradigms in rodents, one of the most frequently employed preclinical paradigms to examine the effects of early stress, noted that separation resulted in subtle disruptions in the quality of mother–pup interaction. By providing the mother with a foster litter during the period of pup separation, they were able to prevent the deterioration in maternal care behaviors and subsequently prevent most of the long-term neurobiological changes associated with early separation (Huot et al. 2004). These findings are consistent with the results of studies examining the effects of prenatal stress. In these studies adoption or cross-fostering with optimal parenting has also been found to reverse the HPA axis alterations typically observed in association with these early stress paradigms (Barbazanges et al. 1996).

Environmental enrichment in adolescence has also been found to reverse HPA axis hyperactivity, memory deficits, and other behavioral alterations associated with early nonoptimal rearing, with the reversal of many of these effects apparently mediated by enhancement of glutamate N-methyl-D-aspartate (NMDA) and α-amino-3-hydroxy-5-methyl-4-isoxazolepropionic acid (AMPA) receptor subunit gene expression (Bredy et al. 2003, 2004). Improvement in stress and behavioral measures is associated not with reversal of glucocorticoid receptor changes but with compensatory changes in the glutamate system. It is increasingly becoming evident that there are multiple neurochemical systems that can be altered to modify behavioral and biological sequelae associated with early stress.

For example, Meaney and colleagues (Weaver et al. 2006) recently have also shown that the early life experience–related changes in epigenetic programming of the glucocorticoid receptor gene discussed above can be reversed in adulthood via infusion of L-methionine or trichostatin A, the histone deacetylase inhibitor. With increased knowledge of the mechanism involved in regulating gene expression, novel pharmacological agents will emerge for the treatment of stress-related disorders.

DNA microarray studies also may lead to the identification of novel genes involved in the molecular mechanism of stress susceptibility, psychopathology, and resilience. Microarray analyses are conducted with special chips that permit the simultaneous examination of the expression of thousands of genes (Newton et al. 2005). When applied to rat hippocampal samples to investigate differential gene expression caused by maternal separation during the neonatal period, several genes expressed in the choroid plexus were found to be down regulated (Kohda et al. 2006).

The significance of genes identified through microarray studies can be verified using transgenic knockout mice (i.e., mice lacking the specific gene under investigation). The genes with altered expression following early stress in the choroid plexus have yet to be investigated in behavioral studies using transgenic mice. In one study (Moles et al. 2004) that is potentially relevant for understanding the attachment problems frequently observed in maltreated children, however, opioid receptor knockout mice were found to show no preference toward their mother's cues and to emit fewer vocalizations when separated from her. The failure to exhibit distress upon separation seemed specific to the attachment relationship because the pups did not display fewer vocalizations when exposed to other stressors.

Novel genes identified in preclinical studies can then be tested for significance in clinical samples. Although the study of stress and its consequences is an evolving story, new technologies and emerging findings suggest cause for optimism. Preclinical studies of the effects of stress, when used to guide the design of clinical research investigations, hold significant promise in unraveling the etiology of stress-induced psychopathology—and in identifying mechanisms to help promote resilience.

CONCLUSIONS

The negative effects associated with early stress are not inevitable and need not be permanent. Our understanding of genetic and environmental risk and protective factors is growing. Genetic and environmental factors were previously conceived as distinct influences on child outcome. It is increasingly becoming clear that these two sets of factors are in dynamic interplay. Careful study of both sets of factors will help to elucidate novel targets for intervention efforts that range from the environmental (e.g., social supports, enrichment) to the cellular (e.g., DNA methylation) level.

REFERENCES

Ackard DM, Neumark-Sztainer D: Multiple sexual victimizations among adolescent boys and girls: prevalence and associations with eating behaviors and psychological health. J Child Sex Abuse 12:17–37, 2003

Barbazanges A, Vallee M, Mayo W, et al: Early and later adoptions have different long-term effects on male rat offspring. J Neurosci 16:7783–7790, 1996

Barr CS, Newman TK, Lindell S, et al: Interaction between serotonin transporter gene variation and rearing condition in alcohol preference and consumption in female primates. Arch Gen Psychiatry 61:1146–1152, 2004

Besinger BA, Garland AF, Litrownik AJ, et al: Caregiver substance abuse among maltreated children placed in out-of-home care. Child Welfare 78:221–239, 1999

Boyd G: Prevention, in Alcoholism: Alcohol Problems in Adolescents and Young Adults, Vol 17. Edited by Galanter M. New York, Kluwer Academic/Plenum Publishers, 2005, pp 199–205

Bredy TW, Humpartzoomian RA, Cain DP, et al: Partial reversal of the effect of maternal care on cognitive function through environmental enrichment. Eur J Neurosci 18:571–576, 2003

Bredy TW, Zhang TY, Grant RJ, et al: Peripubertal environmental enrichment reverses the effects of maternal care on hippocampal development and glutamate receptor subunit expression. Eur J Neurosci 20:1355–1362, 2004

Bulik CM, Prescott CA, Kendler KS: Features of childhood sexual abuse and the development of psychiatric and substance use disorders. Br J Psychiatry 179:444–449, 2001

Caldji C, Diorio J, Anisman H, Meaney MJ: Maternal behavior regulates benzodiazepine/GABAA receptor subunit expression in brain regions associated with fear in BALB/c and C57BL/6 mice. Neuropsychopharmacology 29:1344–1352, 2004

Caspi A, McClay J, Moffitt TE, et al: Role of genotype in the cycle of violence in maltreated children. Science 297:851–854, 2002

Caspi A, Sugden K, Moffitt TE, et al: Influence of life stress on depression: moderation by a polymorphism in the 5-HTT gene. Science 301:386–389, 2003

Connelly CD, Hazen AL, Coben JH, et al: Persistence of intimate partner violence among families referred to child welfare. J Interpers Violence 21:774–797, 2006

Cosentino CE, Meyer-Bahlburg HF, Alpert JL, et al: Sexual behavior problems and psychopathology symptoms in sexually abused girls. J Am Acad Child Adolesc Psychiatry 34:1033–1042, 1995

Covault J, Tennen H, Herman AI, et al: Interactive effects of the serotonin transporter 5-HTTLPR polymorphism and stressful life events on college student drinking and drug use. Biol Psychiatry 61:609–616, 2007

Cutrona CE, Cadoret RJ, Suhr JA, et al: Interpersonal variables in the prediction of alcoholism among adoptees: evidence for gene-environment interactions. Compr Psychiatry 35:171–179, 1994

De Bellis MD, Broussard ER, Herring DJ, et al: Psychiatric co-morbidity in caregivers and children involved in maltreatment: a pilot research study with policy implications. Child Abuse Negl 25:923–944, 2001

Drake B, Jonson-Reid M, Way I, et al: Substantiation and recidivism. Child Maltreat 8:248–260, 2003

Dube SR, Anda RF, Felitti VJ, et al: Adverse childhood experiences and personal alcohol abuse as an adult. Addict Behav 27:713–725, 2002

Duman RS, Heninger GR, Nestler EJ: A molecular and cellular theory of depression. Arch Gen Psychiatry 54:597–606, 1997

Eley TC, Sugden K, Corsico A, et al: Gene-environment interaction analysis of serotonin system markers with adolescent depression. Mol Psychiatry 9:908–915, 2004

Famularo R, Kinscherff R, Fenton T: Psychiatric diagnoses of maltreated children: preliminary findings. J Am Acad Child Adolesc Psychiatry 31:863–867, 1992

Famularo R, Fenton T, Kinscherff R, et al: Psychiatric comorbidity in childhood post traumatic stress disorder. Child Abuse Negl 20:953–961, 1996

Feinn R, Nellissery M, Kranzler HR: Meta-analysis of the association of a functional serotonin transporter promoter polymorphism with alcohol dependence. Am J Med Genet B Neuropsychiatr Genet 133B:79–84, 2005

Garland A, Hough R, McCabe K, et al: Prevalence of psychiatric disorders in youths across five sectors of care. J Am Acad Child Adolesc Psychiatry 40:409–418, 2001

Gorman JM, Mathew S, Coplan J: Neurobiology of early life stress: nonhuman primate models. Semin Clin Neuropsychiatry 7:96–103, 2002

Grant BF, Dawson DA: Age at onset of alcohol use and its association with DSM-IV alcohol abuse and dependence: results from the National Longitudinal Alcohol Epidemiologic Survey. J Subst Abuse 9:103–110, 1997

Heim C, Owens MJ, Plotsky PM, et al: The role of early adverse life events in the etiology of depression and posttraumatic stress disorder: focus on corticotropin-releasing factor. Ann N Y Acad Sci 821:194–207, 1997

Holmans P, Zubenko GS, Crowe RR, et al: Genomewide significant linkage to recurrent, early onset major depressive disorder on chromosome 15q. Am J Hum Genet 74:1154–1167, 2004

Huot RL, Gonzalez ME, Ladd CO, et al: Foster litters prevent hypothalamic-pituitary-adrenal axis sensitization mediated by neonatal maternal separation. Psychoneuroendocrinology 29:279–289, 2004

Inoue-Murayama M, Mishima N, Hayasaka I, et al: Divergence of ape and human monoamine oxidase A gene promoters: comparative analysis of polymorphisms, tandem repeat structures and transcriptional activities on reporter gene expression. Neurosci Lett 405:207–211, 2006

Kaplan SJ, Labruna V, Pelcovitz D, et al: Physically abused adolescents: behavior problems, functional impairment, and comparison of informants' reports. Pediatrics 104:43–49, 1999

Kaufman J: Depressive disorders in maltreated children. J Am Acad Child Adolesc Psychiatry 30:257–265, 1991

Kaufman J, Henrich C: Exposure to violence and early childhood trauma, in Handbook of Infant Mental Health. Edited by Zeanah C Jr. New York, Guilford, 2000, pp 195–207

Kaufman J, Zigler E: Child abuse and social policy, in Children, Families and Government: Preparing for the Twenty-First Century. Edited by Zigler E, Kagan S, Hall N. New York, Cambridge University Press, 1996, pp 233–255

Kaufman J, Plotsky P, Nemeroff C, et al: Effects of early adverse experience on brain structure and function: clinical implications. Biol Psychiatry 48:778–790, 2000

Kaufman J, Yang BZ, Douglas-Palumberi H, et al: Social supports and serotonin transporter gene moderate depression in maltreated children. Proc Natl Acad Sci U S A 101:17316–17321, 2004

Kaufman J, Yang BZ, Douglas-Palumberi H, et al: Brain-derived neurotrophic factor-5-HTTLPR gene interactions and environmental modifiers of depression in children. Biol Psychiatry 59:673–680, 2006

Kaufman J, Yang BZ, Douglas-Palumberi H, et al: Genetic and environmental predictors of early alcohol use. Biol Psychiatry 61:1228–1234, 2007

Kendall-Tackett KA, Williams LM, Finkelhor D: Impact of sexual abuse on children: a review and synthesis of recent empirical studies. Psychol Bull 113:164–80, 1993

Kendler KS: "A gene for…": the nature of gene action in psychiatric disorders. Am J Psychiatry 162:1243–1252, 2005

Kendler KS, Karkowski-Shuman L: Stressful life events and genetic liability to major depression: genetic control of exposure to the environment? Psychol Med 27:539–547, 1997

Kendler KS, Bulik CM, Silberg J, et al: Childhood sexual abuse and adult psychiatric and substance use disorders in women: an epidemiological and cotwin control analysis. Arch Gen Psychiatry 57:953–959, 2000

Kendler KS, Kuhn JW, Vittum J, et al: The interaction of stressful life events and a serotonin transporter polymorphism in the prediction of episodes of major depression: a replication. Arch Gen Psychiatry 62:529–535, 2005

Kilpatrick D, Ruggiero K, Acierno R, et al: Violence and risk of PTSD, major depression, substance abuse/dependence, and comorbidity: results from the National Survey of Adolescents. J Consult Clin Psychol 71:692–700, 2003

Kim-Cohen J, Caspi A, Taylor A, et al: MAOA, maltreatment, and gene-environment interaction predicting children's mental health: new evidence and a meta-analysis. Mol Psychiatry 11:903–913, 2006

Kohda K, Jinde S, Iwamoto K, et al: Maternal separation stress drastically decreases expression of transthyretin in the brains of adult rat offspring. Int J Neuropsychopharmacol 9:201–208, 2006

Kolko D: Child physical abuse, in The APSAC Handbook on Child Maltreatment, 2nd Edition. Edited by Myers J, Berliner L, Briere J, et al. Thousand Oaks, CA, Sage, 2002, pp 21–54

Koob GF: Alcoholism: allostasis and beyond. Alcohol Clin Exp Res 27:232–243, 2003

Koob GF, Le Moal M, Barr CS, et al: Drug abuse: hedonic homeostatic dysregulation interaction between serotonin transporter gene variation and rearing condition in alcohol preference and consumption in female primates. Science 278:52–58, 1997

Lanktree C, Briere J, Zaidi L: Incidence and impact of sexual abuse in a child outpatient sample: the role of direct inquiry. Child Abuse Negl 15:447–453, 1991

Lesch KP, Gross J, Franzek E, et al: Primary structure of the serotonin transporter in unipolar depression and bipolar disorder. Biol Psychiatry 37:215–223, 1995

Levy ER, Powell JF, Buckle VJ, et al: Localization of human monoamine oxidase-A gene to Xp11.23–11.4 by in situ hybridization: implications for Norrie disease. Genomics 5:368–370, 1989

Liu IC, Blacker DL, Xu R, et al: Genetic and environmental contributions to age of onset of alcohol dependence symptoms in male twins. Addiction 99:1403–1409, 2004

Malberg JE, Eisch AJ, Nestler EJ, et al: Chronic antidepressant treatment increases neurogenesis in adult rat hippocampus. J Neurosci 20:9104–9110, 2000

McClellan J, Adams J, Douglas D, et al: Clinical characteristics related to severity of sexual abuse: a study of seriously mentally ill youth. Child Abuse Negl 19:1245–1254, 1995

Meaney MJ, Aitken DH, Bhatnagar S, et al: Postnatal handling attenuates certain neuroendocrine, anatomical, and cognitive dysfunctions associated with aging in female rats. Neurobiol Aging 12:31–38, 1991

Meaney MJ, Bhatnagar S, Diorio J, et al: Molecular basis for the development of individual differences in the hypothalamic-pituitary-adrenal stress response. Cell Mol Neurobiol 13:321–347, 1993

Moles A, Kieffer BL, D'Amato FR: Deficit in attachment behavior in mice lacking the mu-opioid receptor gene. Science 304:1983–1986, 2004

Molnar BE, Buka SL, Kessler RC: Child sexual abuse and subsequent psychopathology: results from the National Comorbidity Survey. Am J Public Health 91:753–760, 2001

Moran PB, Vuchinich S, Hall NK: Associations between types of maltreatment and substance use during adolescence. Child Abuse Negl 28:565–574, 2004

Newton SS, Bennett A, Duman RS, et al: Production of custom microarrays for neuroscience research, Gene profile of electroconvulsive seizures: induction of neurotrophic and angiogenic factors. Methods 37:238–246, 2005

Nilsson KW, Sjoberg RL, Damberg M, et al: Role of the serotonin transporter gene and family function in adolescent alcohol consumption. Alcohol Clin Exp Res 29:564–570, 2005

Noll JG, Horowitz LA, Bonanno GA, et al: Revictimization and self-harm in females who experienced childhood sexual abuse: results from a prospective study. J Interpers Violence 18:1452–1471, 2003

Olds D, Henderson CR, Cole R, et al: Long-term effects of nurse home visitation on children's criminal and antisocial behavior. JAMA 280:1238–1244, 1998

Oroszi G, Goldman D: Alcoholism: genes and mechanisms. Pharmacogenomics 5:1037–1048, 2004

Pelcovitz D, Kaplan SJ, DeRosa RR, et al: Psychiatric disorders in adolescents exposed to domestic violence and physical abuse. Am J Orthopsychiatry 70:360–369, 2000

Putnam FW, Helmers K, Horowitz LA, et al: Hypnotizability and dissociativity in sexually abused girls. Child Abuse Negl 19:645–655, 1995

Romans SE, Martin JL, Anderson JC, et al: Sexual abuse in childhood and deliberate self-harm. Am J Psychiatry 152:1336–1342, 1995

Ruggiero K, McLeer S, Dixon J: Sexual abuse characteristics associated with survivor psychopathology. Child Abuse Negl 24:951–964, 2000

Schuck AM, Widom CS: Childhood victimization and alcohol symptoms in women: an examination of protective factors. J Stud Alcohol 64:247–256, 2003

Strauss J, Barr CL, George CJ, et al: Association study of brain-derived neurotrophic factor in adults with a history of childhood onset mood disorder. Am J Med Genet B Neuropsychiatr Genet 131:16–19, 2004

Strauss J, Barr CL, George CJ, et al: Brain-derived neurotrophic factor variants are associated with childhood-onset mood disorder: confirmation in a Hungarian sample. Mol Psychiatry 10:861–867, 2005

U.S. Department of Health and Human Services, Administration for Children and Families: Child Maltreatment 2004. Washington, DC, U.S. Government Printing Office, 2006. Available at: http://www.acf.hhs.gov/programs/cb/pubs/cm04/index.htm. Accessed December 12, 2007.

Weaver IC, Cervoni N, Champagne FA, et al: Epigenetic programming by maternal behavior. Nat Neurosci 7:847–854, 2004

Weaver IC, Meaney MJ, Szyf M: Maternal care effects on the hippocampal transcriptome and anxiety-mediated behaviors in the offspring that are reversible in adulthood. Proc Natl Acad Sci U S A 103:3480–3485, 2006

Widom CS, Ireland T, Glynn PJ: Alcohol abuse in abused and neglected children followed-up: are they at increased risk? J Stud Alcohol 56:207–217, 1995

Widom CS, Brzustowicz LM: MAOA and the "cycle of violence:" childhood abuse and neglect, MAOA genotype, and risk for violent and antisocial behavior. Biol Psychiatry 60:684–689, 2006

Wiedenmayer CP, Magarinos AM, McEwen BS, et al: Mother lowers glucocorticoid levels of preweaning rats after acute threat. Ann N Y Acad Sci 1008:304–307, 2003

Wolfner GD, Gelles RJ: A profile of violence toward children: a national study. Child Abuse Negl 17:197–212, 1993

Yoshimoto K, McBride WJ, Lumeng L, et al: Alcohol stimulates the release of dopamine and serotonin in the nucleus accumbens. Alcohol 9:17–22, 1992

Zeanah CH, Scheeringa M, Boris NW, et al: Reactive attachment disorder in maltreated toddlers. Child Abuse Negl 28:877–888, 2004

Zigler E: Controlling child abuse: do we have the knowledge and/or the will? in Child Abuse: An Agenda for Action. Edited by Gerbner G, Ross CJ, Zigler E. New York, Oxford University Press, 1980, pp 293–304

Zucker RA, Wong MM: Prevention for children of alcoholics and other high risk groups. Recent Dev Alcohol 17:299–320, 2005

Chapter 8

GENETIC AND ENVIRONMENTAL INFLUENCES ON ANXIOUS/DEPRESSION

A Longitudinal Study in 3- to 12-Year-Old Children

Dorret I. Boomsma, Ph.D.

C.E.M. van Beijsterveldt, Ph.D.

Meike Bartels, Ph.D.

James J. Hudziak, M.D.

Pathways of developmental psychopathology have long been of interest to scientists, clinicians, and patients. To date it is unclear why some children are never affected by psychopathological illness, why others become ill and re-

This work was supported by Netherlands Organisation for Scientific Research Grants 575-25-006, 575-25-012, and 904-57-94 (D.I. Boomsma, Principal Investigator); by the Centre for Neurogenomics and Cognition Research of Vrije Universiteit, Amsterdam; and by National Institute of Mental Health Grant MH58799 (J.J. Hudziak, Principal Investigator). We would like to thank Christel Middeldorp for her critical reading of this chapter.

cover, and why still others are impaired across their entire lives. Questions about stability and change over time for common childhood psychopathological conditions must be answered to provide diagnostic, therapeutic, and prognostic guidance to families of children who suffer from these disorders. Anxious/depression (A/D) in childhood, the focus of this chapter, has been poorly studied from a developmental point of view. Studies beginning in early childhood and progressing into adolescence and adulthood are rare.

Unlike some other common child psychiatric disorders (e.g., attention-deficit/hyperactivity disorder [ADHD], autism, conduct disorders), it can be said with certainty that all children experience anxiety. Indeed, it is a normal aspect of development. Severe anxiety, or an anxiety disorder, is thought to occur in over 20% of humans across their lifetime (Greenberg et al. 1999). The relative cost of the morbidity of anxiety is estimated to be approximately 44 billion dollars in the United States annually (Greenberg et al. 1999). Given the prevalence of anxiety disorders, it is surprising that little work has been done on the developmental stability and change across childhood.

Certain disorders, such as ADHD, originally were conceptualized as "going away with puberty." Through careful research it has now become clear that the majority of individuals who have ADHD in childhood still manifest both symptoms and impairment associated with this condition in adulthood (Castellanos et al. 2006; Manuzza et al. 2003). Similarly, pessimism surrounds the perception about the developmental prognosis of oppositional defiant disorder and conduct disorder. It has been repeatedly estimated that 50% of children with oppositional defiant disorder will go on to develop conduct disorder, and 50% of those will go onto develop antisocial personality disorder (Robins 1996). Children with autism and pervasive developmental disorders are predicted to suffer from lifelong impairments associated with these conditions (Rutter 2005).

Anxiety disorders are thought to be stable, but little is known about the stability of early childhood anxiety across development, with avoidance and shyness giving way to generalized anxiety and social anxiety and then later adult anxiety disorders (Kagan et al. 1999).

Major depressive disorder presents a bit more baffling target. Little is known about the developmental outcomes of major depressive disorder. Some have reported that major depressive disorder in childhood places a child at greater risk for later affective disorders, both unipolar and bipolar (Geller et al. 1996). Others argue that major depressive disorder, even in children, is an episodic, and in some cases even seasonal, condition (Klein et al. 2002, 2006). It is difficult to fully understand why so little is known about the developmental stability of major depressive disorder in children. Part of the explanation may well be due to taxonomic problems, including developmental, sex, and informant issues that affect studies of this type.

It is widely accepted that different genetic factors affect core neuro-development processes such as neuronal genesis, synaptogenesis, myelination, and apoptosis. As such, it should be axiomatic that the genetic influences on brain development will have similar and sentinel influences on children's behavioral and emotional problems (such as A/D) and that these influences may vary in their relative importance depending on the age of the child. The influence of environmental factors may also vary with the age and sex of the child. This statement applies not only to the magnitude of these influences (i.e., percentage of variation explained by environmental effects) but also to the type of environmental influence. The influence of the family environment (often referred to as "shared" or "common" environment), which includes the effects of parental education, socioeconomic status of the family, and rearing practices, may depend on the age or sex of the child. For example, it is now well established that as children grow older, the large initial influence of shared family environment disappears, whereas the influence of genetic factors on cognitive abilities increases (Bartels et al. 2002; Posthuma et al. 2002; Rietveld et al. 2003). For childhood psychopathology such changes in genetic and environmental influences across development are much less clear than for cognitive abilities. It has been argued that until confounds (or modifiers), such as phenotypic assessment and rater bias, and interactions between genes and age and between genes and sex can be addressed, the full impact of molecular genetic studies will not be realized (Rutter and Silberg 2002).

Questions regarding age, sex, rater bias, and development can be addressed in twin studies, but only if the samples are large enough, if the phenotypic information is collected from multiple raters, and if the sample is followed across development. Our group has previously reported on the development of both internalizing and externalizing behavioral problems in young children, as well as on aggressive behavior, attention problems, juvenile bipolar disorder, and obsessive-compulsive disorder in a large sample of Dutch twin pairs registered since birth with the Netherlands Twin Register (NTR) (Bartels et al. 2003, 2007; Boomsma et al. 2006; van Beijsterveldt et al. 2003; van Grootheest et al. 2007; van der Valk et al. 2003). Longitudinal parental ratings of these phenotypes were studied using structural equation modeling approaches. The longitudinal modeling allowed the assessment of correlations between phenotypes at one age and subsequent ages (stability), and the participation of twins allowed the decomposition of those correlations into a genetic part and an environmental part. Furthermore, these studies have allowed the evaluation of the impact of age, sex, and information on estimates of environmental and genetic influences (heritability) on these phenotypes. For all phenotypes, the results have implications for clinical medicine. For example, the correlations between aggressive behavior scores at age 3 and at age 7 years are low, but between ages 7 and 10 years, and between ages 10 and 12 years, the correlations are quite high. Such findings demonstrate that early measures of aggressive behavior do not necessarily correlate highly with later measures. However, the correlations from age 7 years forward are highly predictive of later aggression problems. Furthermore, we found, for example, that for internalizing behavior problems there are no sex differences in the magnitude of the variance components and there is a decrease in heritability with an increase in shared environment across age. For externalizing behavior problems, sex differences in the magnitude of genetic and environmental effects are found at ages 10 and 12 years. Furthermore, an increase in the influence of additive genetic influences is observed between ages 3 and 7 years. For attention problems, a constant and rather high influence of genetic factors was found between ages 3 and 12 years. The remaining variance is attributable to nonshared environmental influences.

For A/D, in a previous article, we analyzed maternal and paternal ratings *cross-sectionally* at ages 3, 5, 7, 10, and 12 years. Data were available for more than 9,025 twin pairs at age 3 years and for more than 2,300 pairs at age 12 years (Boomsma et al. 2005). Multivariate genetic models were used to test for rater-independent and rater-specific assessments of A/D. The agreement between parental A/D ratings was between 0.5 and 0.7, with somewhat higher correlations for the youngest group. Disagreement in ratings between the parents was not merely the result of unreliability or rater bias. Both parents provided unique information from their own perspective on the behavior of their children. Heritability estimates for rater-independent A/D were high in 3-year-olds (76%) and decreased in size as children grew up (60% at age 5, 67% at age 7, 53% at age 10 [60% in boys], and 48% at age 12 years). The decrease in genetic influences was accompanied by an increase in the influence of the shared family environment (absent at ages 3 and 7, 16% at age 5, 20% at age 10 [5% in boys], and 18% at age 12 years). Significant influences of genetic and shared environmental factors were found for the unique parental views. At all ages, the contribution of shared environmental factors to variation in rater-specific views was higher for fathers' ratings. Also, at all ages except age 12 years, the heritability estimates for the rater-specific phenotype were higher for mothers' (59% at age 3 and decreasing to 27% at age 12 years) than for fathers' ratings (between 14% and 29%).

The aim of this chapter is to take the analyses of the A/D data one step further and to assess the *stability* of A/D between ages 3 and 12 years in a genetically informative sample. We assess whether stability in A/D depends on the sex of the child and to what extent the stability in A/D is explained by stable genetic and/or environmental factors. A/D in 3- to 12-year-old children was assessed with the Child Behavior Checklist (CBCL) (Achenbach et al. 2003). The A/D syndrome contains items with features of both anxiety and depression. A/D is highly related to both the Somatic Complaints and Withdrawn Behavior syndromes of the CBCL, which are also highly predictive of either childhood anxiety (Somatic Complaints) or childhood depression (Withdrawn Behavior). The choice of the phenotype CBCL-A/D is consistent with the work of others who have demonstrated the high rates of co-occurrence between anxiety and depressive disorders (Gorman 1996–1997). Twin and family studies indicate shared vulnerabilities (Boomsma et al. 2000; Kendler et al. 1992, 2006; Ninan and Berger 2001) for anxiety and depression in adults. Ratings on CBCL-A/D were obtained from both parents of the twins to assess rater bias. The relative contributions of genetic and non-genetic factors were estimated conditional on age and sex of the children. The stability of A/D was modeled as a function of stable genetic and environmental influences. Environmental influences were separated into influences unique to each child and influences shared by children growing up in the same family. A large number of twin pairs (at age 3 years: $N=9,346$ pairs) participated.

METHODS

Sample

The data in this chapter come from a large ongoing longitudinal study that examines the genetic and environmental influences on the development of behavioral and emotional problems in families with 3- to 12-year-old twins. The families are volunteer members of the Netherlands Twin Registry, established by the Department of Biological Psychology at the Free University in Amsterdam (Bartels et al. 2007; Boomsma et al. 2002, 2006). From 1987 onward the NTR has recruited families with twins a few weeks or months after birth. Currently 40%–50% of all multiple births are registered by the NTR. For this study, we included data of 3- and 5-year-old twin pairs from cohorts 1986–1997, of 7-year-old twin pairs from cohorts 1986–1996, of 10-year-old twin pairs from cohorts 1986–1993, and of 12-year-old twin pairs from birth cohort 1986–1990. Both parents of twin pairs were asked to complete questionnaires about problem behaviors for the eldest and youngest twin at ages 3, 5, 7, 10, and 12 years. Because of funding problems, the questionnaire for 3-year-olds was not sent to the fathers of twins born between May 1989 and November 1991. Two months after the questionnaire was mailed out, a reminder was sent to the nonresponders. After 4 months those who still had not responded were telephoned, if resources for telephone follow-up were available at the time. This procedure resulted in a response rate (at least one parental questionnaire returned) of 77% at age 3 years. From ages 3 to 7, ages 7 to 10, and ages 10 to 12 years, the continued participation was 80%. Nonresponders also include twin families who changed addresses. Some families who did not participate at one age entered the study again at subsequent ages. Families in which one of the twins had a disease or handicap that interfered severely with normal daily functioning (about 2%) were excluded.

Table 8–1 describes the number of twin pairs by sex and zygosity at each age. The smaller sample size for the higher ages reflects the fact that this is an ongoing longitudinal study in which we add newborn twins annually. Thus, only families with twins born in 1986–1991 could have completed all surveys. A total of 1,513 families have completed all questionnaires. For 3,065, 5,353, and 7,516 twin families, there were data for respectively four, three, and two time points. The sample size was always smaller for father data, with an average response of 76%.

In order to test whether attrition has an effect on A/D, scores were compared between continuing and noncontinuing participants. At age 7 years A/D scores were somewhat larger in the noncontinuing group compared with the continuing group ($F_{1,4061}=6.426$; $P=0.011$). For all other ages, the means of the anxiety scores did not differ between the continuing and noncontinuing group.

Zygosity determination was based on blood/DNA polymorphisms and on questionnaires. For 854 same-sex twin pairs, zygosity was based on blood group ($n=436$ pairs) or DNA polymorphisms ($n=418$ pairs). For the remaining twins, zygosity was determined by questionnaire items about physical similarity and frequency of confusion of the twins by family and strangers (Goldsmith 1991; Rietveld et al. 2000) obtained at ages 3, 5, 7, 10, and 12 years. The classification of zygosity was based on a discriminant analysis, relating the questionnaire items to zygosity based on blood/DNA typing in a group of same-sex twin pairs. According to this analysis, the zygosity was correctly classified by questionnaire in nearly 95% of the cases. If a discrepancy in zygosity status appeared across ages, then the most frequent zygosity status was used.

Instruments

At age 3 years, problem behavior was measured with the CBCL/2–3, a questionnaire comprising 100 items that describe specific behavioral, emotional, and social problems. Parents were asked to rate the behavior that the child displayed currently or in the past 2 months on a 3-point scale: 0 if the problem item was not true, 1 if the item was somewhat or sometimes true, and 2 if it was very true or often true. The A/D scale is based on factor analyses of data from several Dutch population samples (see Koot et al. 1997)

TABLE 8–1. Number of families with at least one parental report on Anxious/Depression at ages 3, 5, 7, 10, and 12 years

	3 years, *n*	5 years, *n*	7 years, *n*	10 years, *n*	12 years, *n*
Monozygotic, male	1,478	1,495	1,239	771	437
Dizygotic, male	1,576	1,561	1,248	693	384
Monozygotic, female	1,711	1,757	1,423	926	503
Dizygotic, female	1,463	1,453	1,166	672	356
Dizygotic, opposite sex, male and female	1,602	1,539	1,211	746	379
Dizygotic, opposite sex, female and male	1,516	1,450	1,133	691	344
Total	9,346	9,225	7,420	4,499	2,403

Note. Only twin pairs with known zygosity are included.

and is compatible with the syndrome scale as developed by Achenbach (1991). The A/D scale derived from the CBCL/2–3 contains 9 items. Anxiety at age 5 years was measured with a shortened version of the Devereux Child Behavior (DCB) Rating Scale (Spivack and Spotts 1966) that consisted of 42 items (van Beijsterveldt et al. 2004). Parents were asked to rate the behavior of their child in the last 2 months. Items were scored on a 5-point scale, with 1 = never and 5 = very frequently. The anxiety scale included 6 items. At ages 7, 10, and 12 years, A/D behavior was measured with the CBCL/4–18 (Achenbach 1991; Verhulst et al. 1996), a questionnaire of 113 items developed to measure problem behavior in 4- to 18-year-old children. Again parents were asked to rate the behavior of the child in the preceding 2 months on a 3-point scale. The A/D scale derived from the CBCL/4–18 contained 14 items. Table 8–2 summarizes the means and standard deviations for A/D at each age (average scores of mother and father).

STATISTICAL ANALYSES

Phenotypic Stability

Correlations across time within individuals (phenotypic stability coefficients) and twin cross-correlations were calculated by using the statistical software program Mx (Neale et al. 1997). To test for sex differences in correlation structure, the stability coefficients were constrained to be equal across boys and girls, and the fit of this model was compared with the fit of the previous model.

Next, twin cross-correlations (i.e., the correlation of first-born twin at time 1, with the second-born twin at time 2 and vice versa) were calculated. For each age and zygosity group, cross-correlations between oldest youngest and youngest oldest twins were constrained to be the same. The cross-correlations provide a first indication of the importance of genetic and environmental influences on the stability of a trait. If cross-correlations are higher for monozygotic (MZ) than for dizygotic (DZ) twin pairs, then genetic factors influence the stability of the trait.

Genetic Analyses

The essence of genetic model fitting is the decomposition of the observed variance in a univariate or multivariate phenotype (here A/D measured at multiple time points) due to additive genetic effects (A), shared or common environment effects (C), and nonshared environment (E) factors. A represents the additive effects of alleles at multiple loci; C represents common environment effects shared by children growing up in the same family such

TABLE 8–2. Means and standard deviation (SD) for untransformed Child Behavior Checklist (CBCL) Anxious/Depression (at ages 3, 7, 10, and 12 years) and Devereux Child Behavior (DCB) Anxiety (age 5 years): average scores from mother and father

	3 years		5 years		7 years		10 years		12 years	
	Mean	SD	Mean	SD	Mean	SD	Mean	SD	Mean	SD
Monozygotic, male	3.43	2.8	10.69	2.9	1.88	2.3	2.39	2.7	2.00	2.6
Dizygotic, male	3.45	2.9	10.99	3.0	2.22	2.5	2.55	3.0	2.16	2.8
Monozygotic, female	3.71	2.9	11.29	3.0	2.05	2.4	2.43	2.9	2.30	2.6
Dizygotic, female	3.71	2.9	11.38	3.1	2.31	2.5	2.54	3.0	2.20	2.7
Dizygotic, opposite sex, males	3.53	2.9	10.75	3.0	1.85	2.4	2.23	2.9	1.89	2.6
Dizygotic, opposite sex, females	2.98	2.8	10.96	3.0	2.00	2.4	2.30	2.8	2.05	2.6
Males	3.49	2.9	10.81	3.0	1.99	2.4	2.39	2.8	2.02	2.7
Females	3.48	2.9	11.21	3.0	2.12	2.4	2.42	2.9	2.20	2.6

as parental rearing practices, parental income, or socioeconomic status; and E represents all nonshared environmental influences, including measurement error. In model fitting of twin data the influences of A, C, and E are inferred through their effects on the covariances of relatives. The twin design compares the resemblance of MZ twins with DZ twins. MZ twins are nearly always genetically identical, and DZ twins share, on average, 50% of their segregating genes. If genetic variation affects trait variation, the phenotypic resemblance should be larger for MZ twins. If the degree of resemblance of traits is the same in MZ and DZ twins, shared environment mainly determines trait variation. Nonshared environmental effects are a source of phenotypic differences. The same reasoning applies to the analysis of multivariate and longitudinal data: if cross-correlations in MZ twins are higher than those in DZ twins, the covariance between traits is caused by genetic covariance. Application of longitudinal developmental models to the MZ and DZ data allows inferences about the underlying genetic and environmental effects of stability and change to be drawn (Boomsma and Molenaar 1987; Boomsma et al. 1989).

In the first series of longitudinal genetic analyses, we examined which developmental model give the best description of the developmental pattern. For these first series of analyses, the mean of the mother and father A/D ratings were used. If a value was missing for one of the parents, then the value was replaced by the rating of the other parent. By using the mean of the parental ratings, it is assumed that mothers and fathers rate the same underlying phenotype with a shared common understanding of the behavioral descriptions. Next, we combined the rater bias model with the longitudinal model and analyzed all available longitudinal maternal and paternal ratings.

Model Selection

To explore the influence of genetic and environmental factors over time, we started the longitudinal analyses with a triangular, or Cholesky, decomposition. A *Cholesky decomposition* is a fully saturated model in which the number of estimated parameters is equal to the number of independent variances and covariances. For each latent structure (A, C, and E) the number of factors is equal to the number of time points. The first factor influences all phenotypes at all five ages. The second factor influences the phenotype at the subsequent age plus all later ages. The following three factors operate in the same manner, with every factor starting one time point later. The model does not make any strong developmental assumptions, but it provides a general description of the contribution of genetic and environmental factors to developmental processes of stability and change. From the Cholesky decomposition the genetic and environmental correlations between the A/D ratings across time can be obtained (as well as the heritabilities and other parameters at each time point). Next, we fitted two developmental models to the data that explicitly take into account the nature of developmental processes. The first approach is called a *common factor model*. This model contains one latent genetic (environmental) factor that accounts for the co-variance among the five time points. The impact of a genetic (environmental) factor on A/D is the same at each age. To account for new influences, an age-specific factor is included for each age. The second model is called a *simplex model*, and in this model the latent factors that influence A/D scores at successive ages are causally linked. For example, genetic factors affecting A/D at age 3 years influence genetic factors affecting A/D at age 5 years (see Figure 8–1). The model also allows for genetic and environmental innovations (Neale and Cardon 1992) that introduce new variation at a time point. Because at the first time point the first latent factor cannot be explained by previous factors, these factors are handled as an innovation. Both developmental mechanisms predict different patterns of age-to-age correlations. A factor model predicts a correlational pattern across measures at different ages in which the size of the correlations does not depend on the time interval between measures. The simplex model predicts correlations that decrease with increasing time (Boomsma and Molenaar 1987). To test the fit of the two developmental models, we used the unconstrained Cholesky decomposition as a reference model.

The Rater Model

After the best longitudinal model is found, we combine this model with a multiple rater model. The psychometric model (Hewitt et al. 1992) estimates the influence of a genetic (A), a shared environmental (C), and a non-shared environmental (E) factor common to the phenotypes of the twins as rated by both parents. In addition, three rater specific factors—genetic ($A_{m/f}$), shared environmental ($C_{m/f}$), and nonshared environmental ($E_{m/f}$)—are estimated for the ratings of mother/father. Disagreement between parents in this model can be caused by rater specific behavioral views, leading to different but valid information from each rater. These rater-specific behavioral views can have their own unique influences, estimated in the rater-specific A, C, and E factors. Disagreements can also be caused by rater bias, which will confound the rater-specific shared environmental effects, or by unreliability, which will confound the rater-specific nonshared environmental effects. The three common factors loading on the twins' phenotypes contain only reliable variance, causing the common nonshared environmental factor to contain only pure independent environmental effects

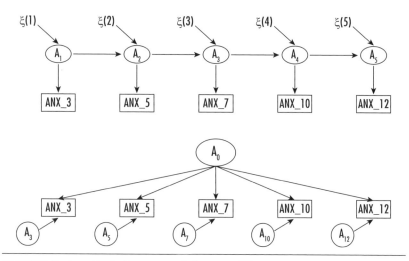

FIGURE 8–1. Path diagrams of the two different models used to investigate the underlying developmental mechanism in the latent factors across five time points (Anx_3, Anx_5, Anx_7, Anx_10, and Anx_12).

The upper figure represents a simplex model, and the lower figure represents a common factor model with age-specific effects. The two models are given for additive genetic (A) factors. The same models were applied to common environmental (C) and nonshared environmental (E) factors.

(McArdle and Goldsmith 1990) and the common shared environmental factor to contain only pure shared environmental effects.

Model-Fitting Procedures

Using raw data, Mx provides the possibility of handling missing data and allowed us to retain twin pairs who have missing data at one or more assessments. In this procedure the likelihood is calculated separately for each pedigree and the product of these likelihoods (i.e., the sum of the log likelihood) is maximized. This procedure assumes that the data are at least missing at random (Wothke 2000), meaning that the probability of missing depends on the observed data but not on the unobserved data, given the observed data (Little and Rubin 1987). From previous studies that used the same data set as the present one, it is tenable that the pattern of missing data in our study is at least missing at random (Rietveld et al. 2004; van Beijsterveldt et al. 2003).

The use of maximum likelihood estimation requires that the data be approximately normally distributed. The A/D scales of the CBCL and DCB showed a positively skewed distribution. Therefore, prior to the genetic analyses the normalizing procedure of PRELIS (Jöreskog and Sörbom 1993) was applied to the data to approximate a normal distribution.

Goodness of fit was assessed by likelihood-ratio χ^2 tests. These tests compare the differences between −2-log likelihood of a full model with that of a restricted nested model. This difference is distributed as a χ^2, and the degrees of freedom (*df*) for this test are equal to the difference between the number of estimated parameters in the full model and that in a restricted model. A large χ^2 value in comparison to the number of degrees of freedom suggest that the simpler model does not fit to the data as well as the more complex models. To select the best model, we used Akaike's information criterion (AIC). The AIC is the χ^2 minus twice the degrees of freedom (Akaike 1987). The model with the lowest AIC value is considered as the most parsimonious model.

RESULTS

Phenotypic Stability

Table 8–3 displays the phenotypic stability coefficients for the different time intervals. The stability coefficients did not differ between girls and boys ($\Delta\chi^2 = 16.33$, $df = 10$, $P = 0.091$). It can be seen that the degree of stability depends on age of the child and length of time interval. The stability is lower at younger ages and lower for longer time intervals. Moderate stability coefficients were found for age 7 years and older. From ages 3 and 5 years the continuity of A/D is low, but after age 7 years A/D becomes more stable. At first sight, the pattern of coefficients does not provide a clear insight in the nature of the underlying developmental processes. The correlation pattern did not point to a common factor model, which predicts a stable pattern of correlations, or to a simplex model, which predicts a decreasing correlation with increasing time intervals. This unclear picture could be a result of a mixture of developmental processes for the genetic and environmental factors.

Genetic Analyses

The lower part of Table 8–3 presents the twin correlations (at the diagonal) and twin cross-correlations for A/D. At each age, the MZ correlations were larger than the DZ correlations, suggesting additive genetic influences. The cross-correlations provide insight into the involvement of genes and environment in the observed stability of A/D across age. At first sight, it seems that at younger ages MZ cross-correlations were only slightly higher than the DZ cross-correlations and suggested that both genetic and environmental influences contributed to the stability. From age 7 years, the differences

TABLE 8–3. Phenotypic (within-person) correlations across age for Anxious/Depression (average rater score), cross-sectional twin correlations (on diagonal), and across-age twin correlations in males (below diagonal) and females (above diagonal) for monozygotic and dizygotic male and female same-sex twin pairs and dizygotic opposite-sex twin pairs

	Age 3 years	Age 5 years	Age 7 years	Age 10 years	Age 12 years
All twins					
Age 3 years	—	—	—	—	—
Age 5 years	0.30	—	—	—	—
Age 7 years	0.30	0.39	—	—	—
Age 10 years	0.30	0.36	0.59	—	—
Age 12 years	0.27	0.33	0.53	0.67	—
Monozygotic males and females					
Age 3 years	0.69/0.73	0.29	0.27	0.23	0.21
Age 5 years	0.26	0.74/0.74	0.31	0.3	0.24
Age 7 years	0.22	0.34	0.64/0.65	0.44	0.42
Age 10 years	0.24	0.31	0.47	0.61/0.69	0.49
Age 12 years	0.22	0.29	0.4	0.45	0.61/0.63
Dizygotic males and females					
Age 3 years	0.34/0.36	0.24	0.25	0.24	0.2
Age 5 years	0.22	0.44/0.46	0.21	0.26	0.23
Age 7 years	0.22	0.27	0.39/0.40	0.33	0.27
Age 10 years	0.18	0.31	0.28	0.40/0.47	0.35
Age 12 years	0.2	0.27	0.28	0.35	0.39/0.41

TABLE 8–3. Phenotypic (within-person) correlations across age for Anxious/Depression (average rater score), cross-sectional twin correlations (on diagonal), and across-age twin correlations in males (below diagonal) and females (above diagonal) for monozygotic and dizygotic male and female same-sex twin pairs and dizygotic opposite-sex twin pairs *(continued)*

	Age 3 years	Age 5 years	Age 7 years	Age 10 years	Age 12 years
Dizygotic opposite-sex twin pairs					
Age 3 years	0.38/0.31	0.19	0.17	0.22	0.25
Age 5 years	0.21	0.52/0.49	0.21	0.24	0.24
Age 7 years	0.22	0.26	0.41/0.41	0.31	0.27
Age 10 years	0.25	0.25	0.28	0.37/0.48	0.4
Age 12 years	0.26	0.28	0.28	0.3	0.43/0.51

between MZ and DZ cross-correlations seemed to be larger, suggesting that genetic factors became more important. However, the DZ correlations were still larger than expected on the basis of genetic influences alone, and it is expected that environmental factors play a role in the stability of anxiety in the older ages.

Next, a series of model-fitting analyses were conducted to test which developmental model best described the data. Each variance component (A, C, and E) was tested to see which developmental model best explains the data. The analyses started with a general developmental model, a Cholesky decomposition, which served also as the reference for evaluating of the fit of the other models. In all models the estimates of the parameters were allowed to differ across sex. Table 8–4 presents the fitting results of the various models. For the genetic component, neither the common factor model nor the simplex model provided a better fit than the Cholesky decomposition. Thus, it seems that a common factor or a simplex model alone is not a sufficient model to explain the developmental processes. For the shared environmental influences, a common factor model provided a better fit. This model contains one common factor loading on all five age groups and age-specific influences at each age. For the nonshared environmental influences neither the simplex nor the common factor model provided an adequate fit. Thus, a model with a common factor for shared environmental influences and a Cholesky decomposition for genetic and nonshared environmental influences provided the best description of the data. As a last step, we tested whether the parameter estimates in the best model differed between males and females. In contrast to the model with sex differences, the fit did not deteriorate after constraining the parameters to be equal across sex.

On the diagonal of Table 8–5, the proportion of explained variance by genetic and environmental factors is given for A/D at each age. Genetic factors explained 63% of the variance of anxiety at age 3 years and declined slowly to 41% at age 12 years. The contribution of shared environment at a specific age consisted of age-specific shared environment and environmental influences shared with all ages. The role of age-specific shared environment was low at all ages (ranging from 0 to 5). The total variance explained by shared environment factors was 8% at age 3 years and increased to 23% at age 12 years. The contribution of nonshared environmental factors remained quite stable and ranged from 26% to 36%.

Because our focus was on developmental processes, of special interest are the contributions of genetic and environmental factors on the stability of anxiety as reported on the off-diagonal in Table 8–5 and the genetic and environmental correlations in the lower part. At younger ages (3 and 5 years), the genetic and environmental factors contributed to stability to the same degree. Genetic factors accounted for, on average, 48%, and shared

TABLE 8–4. Model fitting results for longitudinal developmental models of anxious/depression (average rater scores)

	–2 LL	df	Compared with model	χ^2	df	P	AIC	Critical value χ^2
1. Triangular decomposition for A, C, E	301164.9	65655						
2. A simplex	301250.4	65667	1	85.501	12	0.000	61.501	21.026
3. A common factor	301201.2	65665	1	36.276	10	0.000	16.276	18.307
4. C simplex	301174.7	65667	1	9.777	12	0.636	–14.223	21.026
5. C common factor	301166.4	65665	1	1.478	10	0.999	–18.522	18.307
6. E simplex	301221.8	65667	1	56.928	12	0.000	32.928	21.026
7. E common factor	301198.8	65665	1	33.905	10	0.000	13.905	18.307
8. Model 5 without sex differences	301216.4	65705	5	50.051	40	0.133	–29.949	55.758

Note. AIC=Akaike's information criterion (c^2; df=2); LL=log likelihood; $\chi^2 = -2$ (difference in log likelihood) between models; df=degrees of freedom; P=probability value associated with χ^2.

TABLE 8–5. Upper part: relative contribution of genetic and environmental factors to the total variance (i.e., heritability on diagonal of first matrix) and covariances of Anxious/Depression (based on the across-rater score). Lower part: correlations between genetic and environmental factors for Anxious/Depression (based on the across-rater score)

Additive genetic

Age	3 years	5 years	7 years	10 years	12 years
3 years	0.63				
5 years	0.50	0.52			
7 years	0.67	0.51	0.51		
10 years	0.56	0.34	0.58	0.49	
12 years	0.47	0.27	0.55	0.47	0.41

Age	3 years	5 years	7 years	10 years	12 years
3 years	1.00				
5 years	0.26	1.00			
7 years	0.35	0.39	1.00		
10 years	0.27	0.24	0.69	1.00	
12 years	0.24	0.20	0.63	0.70	1.00

Common environment

Age	3 years	5 years	7 years	10 years	12 years
3 years	0.00/0.08[a]				
5 years	0.43	0.00/0.22[a]			
7 years	0.27	0.35	0.05/0.09[a]		
10 years	0.43	0.54	0.21	0.01/0.17[a]	
12 years	0.46	0.60	0.24	0.27	0.04/0.19[a]

Age	3 years	5 years	7 years	10 years	12 years
3 years	1.00				
5 years	1.00	1.00			
7 years	0.79	0.79	1.00		
10 years	0.99	0.99	0.78	1.00	
12 years	0.91	0.91	0.72	0.90	1.00

Unshared environment

Age	3 years	5 years	7 years	10 years	12 years
3 years	0.29				
5 years	0.08	0.26			
7 years	0.06	0.13	0.35		
10 years	0.01	0.11	0.21	0.33	
12 years	0.07	0.13	0.21	0.26	0.36

Age	3 years	5 years	7 years	10 years	12 years
3 years	1.00				
5 years	0.08	1.00			
7 years	0.06	0.17	1.00		
10 years	0.01	0.14	0.37	1.00	
12 years	0.05	0.14	0.32	0.50	1.00

[a]Effect of shared or common environment effects (C) is partitioned into age-specific C (first number) and to C common to all ages (second number).

environmental factors accounted for 44%, of the phenotypic stability across ages. From age 7 years the contribution of genetic influences to the stability was comparable (53%), but the contribution of shared environmental influences was reduced (24%). The contribution of nonshared environmental factors to stability was small in the younger ages (8%) and became more important after age 7 years (on average 23%).

The lower part of Table 8–5 presents the correlations among the genetic and environmental factors, which represent the extent to which the same genes or same environmental factors contribute to the phenotypic stability. A high correlation suggests that the same factors play a role, whereas a low correlation points to processes of change. The genetic correlations between the younger ages and older ages were low, suggesting that different genes operate at these ages. The genetic correlations were substantially higher at ages 7–12 years but still were suggestive for change processes. The correlations among the shared environmental correlations were high and indicated that the same shared environmental factors were important during childhood. The correlations among the unique nonshared environmental correlations were very low at the younger ages but were higher between the factors at the higher ages. Thus it seems that nonshared environmental influences were mainly age specific at younger ages, but after age 7 years some influence of the nonshared factors persisted over time.

Longitudinal Rater Models

Finally, we combined the best-fitting longitudinal model with a psychometric rater model. In the previous models, the assumption was that both parents rate the same underlying phenotype. From previous results it is known that the parents indeed assess the same behavior in their twins but that there is also a component specific to each rater (Boomsma et al. 2005). This rater-specific part contains rater-specific views but also rater bias and may lead to biased estimates of the genetic and environmental components. To get insight into the contribution of rater-specific factors to the total variance of anxiety, a model was applied that takes into account the effects of the specific rater part. The model decomposes the variance into a part that is similarly assessed by both raters and into a part that is specific for each rater. Table 8–6 and Figure 8–2 show the age-specific parameter estimates of A, C, and E accounted by the common parental part and by the specific rater part. Genetic factors accounted for 61% (43% [common]+18% [specific]) at age 3 years to 35% (22%+13%) at age 12 years of the total variance of anxiety as rated by the mother. For anxiety rated by the father, genetic factors explained 56% (47%+9%) of the variance at age 3 years and 42% (31%+11%) at age 12 years. The largest part of the genetic variance was accounted

TABLE 8–6. Proportion of variance and covariance explained by genetic factors common to raters (father and mother), by environmental factors common to raters, and by rater-specific genetic and environmental factors

	Mother rating					Father rating				
Age	3 years	5 years	7 years	10 years	12 years	3 years	5 years	7 years	10 years	12 years
A common										
3 years	0.43					0.47				
5 years	0.42	0.32				0.51	0.34			
7 years	0.50	0.42	0.28			0.65	0.58	0.41		
10 years	0.45	0.32	0.37	0.25		0.60	0.45	0.57	0.37	
12 years	0.36	0.24	0.38	0.31	0.22	0.54	0.33	0.55	0.48	0.31
C common										
3 years	0.04					0.05				
5 years	0.24	0.11				0.29	0.11			
7 years	0.15	0.18	0.04			0.19	0.25	0.06		
10 years	0.25	0.29	0.10	0.09		0.33	0.40	0.16	0.13	
12 years	0.28	0.34	0.14	0.16	0.11	0.42	0.48	0.19	0.24	0.16
E common										
3 years	0.16					0.18				
5 years	0.07	0.14				0.08	0.14			
7 years	0.03	0.10	0.16			0.04	0.13	0.24		
10 years	0.00	0.08	0.16	0.16		0.00	0.11	0.24	0.23	
12 years	0.04	0.10	0.14	0.16	0.17	0.05	0.14	0.20	0.26	0.24

TABLE 8–6. Proportion of variance and covariance explained by genetic factors common to raters (father and mother), by environmental factors common to raters, and by rater-specific genetic and environmental factors *(continued)*

		Mother rating					Father rating				
	Age	3 years	5 years	7 years	10 years	12 years	3 years	5 years	7 years	10 years	12 years
A rater-specific	3 years	0.18					0.09				
	5 years	0.13	0.19				-0.02	0.11			
	7 years	0.10	0.08	0.19			-0.05	-0.08	0.07		
	10 years	0.06	0.05	0.15	0.17		-0.02	-0.06	0.00	0.09	
	12 years	0.15	0.14	0.13	0.14	0.13	-0.28	-0.15	-0.07	0.00	0.11
C rater-specific	3 years	0.04					0.09				
	5 years	0.16	0.11				0.15	0.16			
	7 years	0.20	0.19	0.12			0.15	0.12	0.10		
	10 years	0.24	0.22	0.17	0.13		0.13	0.10	0.06	0.08	
	12 years	0.16	0.17	0.13	0.11	0.15	0.25	0.18	0.11	0.07	0.07
E rater-specific	3 years	0.15					0.13				
	5 years	-0.01	0.14				-0.01	0.13			
	7 years	0.02	0.03	0.21			0.03	0.01	0.13		
	10 years	0.01	0.05	0.06	0.21		-0.03	0.01	-0.03	0.11	
	12 years	0.01	-0.01	0.07	0.12	0.21	0.01	0.02	0.01	-0.04	0.12

Note. A=additive genetic effects; C= shared or common environment effects; E = nonshared environment effects.

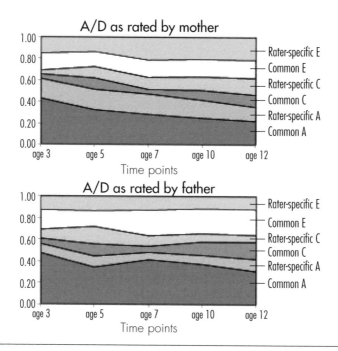

FIGURE 8–2.   **Relative influence of additive genetic effects (A) and environmental effects, common (C) and nonshared (E), across ages 3–12 years, separately for father and mother ratings of Anxious/Depression (A/D).**

by the common parental view. Averaged over 5 ages, 66% (80% for fathers) of the genetic variance could be explained by a common parental view. The rater-specific genetic part of the mother accounted for 13%–19% of the total variance and was somewhat lower for the father (7%–11%). The total variance explained by shared environmental factors ranged between 8% (4%+4%) at age 3 years and 26% (11%+15%) at age 12 years, and the largest part of the shared environmental variance was accounted by rater-specific factors. The variance accounted by nonshared environmental factors was around 30%, and about the half of this variance was accounted for by rater-specific factors. The same picture emerged for the estimates of stability. The largest part of the covariance between ages was explained by the factors representing the common view of both parents. The rater-specific factors contributed only to a small part of the total variance.

DISCUSSION

We analyzed longitudinal data on A/D in a large sample of young twins ages 3–12 years who had been rated by both their parents. The purpose of the study was to determine the relative stability and change of genetic and environmental influences on common child A/D. Such research can be seen as providing a view on possible windows of development when environmental factors may be of greater importance than at other ages. Similar ideas about genetic influences can also be considered. By employing a longitudinal design it was possible to investigate how genes and environmental factors contribute to the processes of stability and change across development. Because our study included five time points we could also test the structure of the developmental process. By applying the longitudinal model to both mother and father ratings, we were able to disentangle the rater-specific views from that part of the phenotype upon which both parents agree.

As suggested by the results of the cross-sectional study of A/D in the same sample of twins, the influence of genetic factors declined with increasing age (Boomsma et al. 2005). The heritability was around 60% at age 3 years and declined to about 40% at age 12 years. The decrease in heritability when children grew older was accompanied by an increase in the influence of the shared environment (8% at age 3 years and 23% at age 12 years). Although not directly addressed in the analyses, findings such as these argue for shared environmental factors as playing a major role in protecting children from or putting them at risk for the expression of A/D. The contribution of nonshared environmental factors ranged from 26% to 36%. These data indicate that nonshared environment—or environmental influences that contribute to differences between siblings—plays a substantial role across development when considering the expression of A/D.

The results showed that the stability of A/D was relatively low between age 3 years and later ages (correlations around 0.30) but became higher after age 7 years (up to 0.67 between ages 10 and 12 years). Both genetic and shared environmental factors accounted for the phenotypic stability of A/D. Across all ages, genetic factors accounted for about 50% of the phenotypic stability. The genetic correlations between A/D assessed at 3 years and other ages were modest, suggesting a small overlap of genes that influence A/D in preschool children and in middle childhood (genetic correlations between 0.24 and 0.35 for A/D at age 3 years with other ages). These results raise the possibility of different genetic influences of genes across development, either by variable expression patterns, variable response to environmental mediators and modifiers, or simply evidence of developmental genetic processes. After age 7 years, the genetic correlations were larger (0.63–0.70), indicating that the extent to which the same genes operate across ages 7–12 years was increased.

The influence of common environmental factors shared by twins from the same family on the stability of A/D was highest in early childhood (around 50% for the preschool children) and was reduced after age 7 years. Across ages, the same common environmental factors were suggested, because a single C factor could explain the covariance pattern across age. Family variables such as parental conflict, negative familial environments, and separation are likely candidates for these shared environmental influences. Future genetic research should include such environmental variables (e.g., parental divorce) to specify the role of these environmental factors.

Nonshared environmental factors operate mainly in a time-specific manner. At younger ages, the role of nonshared environmental factors in stability of A/D is nearly nil but is somewhat increased (up to 26%) between ages 10 and 12 years. When children grow up they have a greater chance to experience life events outside the family. These individual outside experiences could promote A/D in one twin and not in the other.

It should be mentioned that a part of the shared environmental factors reflects parental bias. Because the same rater was used at two or more points, the prediction of A/D could reflect some shared rater bias. If this is the case, the observed stability is not only a reflection of stability of children's problem behavior but also a reflection of the stability of the mother's or father's perception. However, when the longitudinal model is applied to both father and mother ratings, it is possible to disentangle the effects caused by "real" environment and the effect caused by rater bias. As indicated by the results, there is still evidence for shared environmental influences on the stability of A/D when data from father and mother are analyzed simultaneously. However, results indicate also that the rater-specific shared environment contributes to stability of A/D. This could point to possible rater bias that is persistent and affects the stability of A/D.

In general the stability of A/D was lower than reported for the externalizing behaviors in the same sample of twins across all ages (Bartels et al. 2004; Rietveld et al. 2004; van Beijsterveldt et al. 2003). For example, the stability coefficient of aggression was 0.48 between ages 3 and 7 years and 0.42 between ages 3 and 12 years. The stability coefficients of aggression ranged from 0.67 to 0.77 for the shorter time intervals (between ages 7 and 10 years). The stability coefficients of attention problems were in between the coefficients of aggression and A/D. One possible explanation for the lower stability of A/D, compared with externalizing behaviors, is that preschool children have a limited ability to express feelings of anxiety and that parents have more difficulties recognizing A/D problems. In accordance with the externalizing problem behaviors, the stability of A/D became a more stable characteristic as children age. However, we cannot exclude that the lower stability of preschool A/D is due to the use of different assessment instruments. Anxiety is measured with the CBCL/2–3 at age 3 years, with the DCB at age 5 years, and with the CBCL/4–18 at age 7 years. Although the items of the CBCL/2–3 and the CBCL/4–18 have some overlap, they may not measure the same underlying construct.

The developmental pattern of changing genetic and environmental influences of A/D during childhood also differed from externalizing problem behaviors as measured in the same sample of twins (Bartels et al. 2004; Rietveld et al. 2004; van Beijsterveldt et al. 2003). For aggression we found that the heritability increased from ages 3 to 12 years and that the relative influence of shared environmental influences decreased. For attention problems the heritability remained constant over the years, and shared environmental influences were of no importance at all.

This departure from the findings for aggressive behavior and ADHD is of tremendous importance from both a clinical and a research point of view. From our cross-sectional and longitudinal work on A/D, it appears that early in life the expression of an anxious phenotype is influenced significantly by genetic factors. These data are consistent with a wide literature on infant anxiety, behavioral inhibition, and temperament. From research in humans (Kagan and Snidman 1999) and animals (Suomi 2005), it is clear that life experience can affect both positively and negatively the childhood, adolescent, and adult outcomes of anxious children. Perhaps most importantly, with the evidence that the influence of shared environment increases with age comes the possibility that children at risk for anxiety can be influenced away from the expression of severe expression of A/D or, sadly, influenced toward the expression of the same phenotype. Recent, remarkable findings from association studies of the serotonin transporter gene and tryptophan hydroxylase gene provide evidence that children with different genotypes have variable responses to different environmental stimuli and are at highly variant risk for negative outcomes. For a review of this work, see Chapter 7, "Genetic and Environmental Modifiers of Risk and Resiliency in Maltreated Children," in this book.

Further support that childhood A/D has a different developmental profile than disruptive or externalizing disorders is provided by the study of childhood obsessive-compulsive behavior. The developmental pattern was comparable with that of anxiety: from ages 10 to 12 years a threefold increase in the shared environmental influences was reported (van Grootheest et al. 2007). These various developmental patterns of genetic and environmental influences have implications for parenting, clinical medicine, and ultimately research. For parents, it is important to know that having a child with early anxiety does not necessarily indicate a lifelong problem with this phenotype or outcome. Clinically, a commitment to behavioral (e.g., shared environmental mediation) therapies such as those embodied by cognitive-behavioral therapy may yield robust, stable wellness outcomes. Indeed, research by Kendall and Panichelli-Mindel (1995; Kendall et al. 2004) reported that 90% of children who received cognitive-behavioral therapy at an index visit for child anxiety disorders no longer suffered from that disorder at 3.5 and 7 years posttreatment (and without any ongoing treatment other than the original course of cognitive-behavioral therapy). Other forms of therapy, such as exposure response prevention, for childhood anxiety disorders have consistently resulted in robust improvement in children who suffer from these disorders. A commitment to these treatments is at the very least supported by our findings.

Taking these results to the research community via translational research is already under way. Alleles of common candidate genes have been shown to place individuals at differential risk for the development of anxiety and depressive disorders on the basis of the genetic makeup of the individual and whether he or she has been exposed to stressful life events. As research identifies more candidate genes for anxiety and depressive disorders, it may well be that we will reconceptualize these genes as reactivity genes rather than as genes of illness. Such a perception could directly lead to a frameshift in how wellness medicine could be practiced. Children with certain genotypes may well benefit from different types of (therapeutically designed) environments.

CONCLUSIONS

With the evidence from family studies that affective and anxiety disorders are familial, combined with the evidence that parental psychopathology increases the risk of offspring psychopathology (perhaps by creating a more toxic shared environment), we may need to consider more robustly assessing for and treating parental psychopathology as a direct clinical intervention for children with A/D. This perception is supported at least in part by the recent study of Weissman et al. (2005, 2006), which demonstrates that with the successful treatment of maternal depression, children in that family will have a reduction in their internalizing psychopathology syndrome scores of a full standard deviation. To put it succinctly, by treating mothers, children's A/D scores improved without directly treating the children.

As we move into the generation of genomic and wellness medicine, combining consideration of the etiopathologic contributions to A/D throughout development invites us to consider how we can use traditional therapies (e.g., Kendall and Panichelli-Mindel 1995; Kendall et al. 2004) with greater confidence in at-risk populations. In addition, generalizing these lessons to educational programs for the better public health of all children could well lead to a reduction in the morbidity and mortality associated with anxiety and affective disorders.

REFERENCES

Achenbach TM: Manual for the Child Behavior Checklist/4–18 and 1991 profile. Burlington, VT, University of Vermont, Department of Psychiatry, 1991

Achenbach TM, Dumenci L, Rescorla LA: DSM-oriented and empirically based approaches to constructing scales from the same item pools. J Clin Child Adolesc Psychol 32:328–340, 2003

Akaike H: Factor analysis and AIC. Psychometrika 52:317–322, 1987

Bartels M, Rietveld MJH, Van Baal GCM, et al: Genetic and environmental influences on the development of intelligence. Behav Genet 32:237–249, 2002

Bartels M, Hudziak JJ, Boomsma DI, et al: A study of parent ratings of internalizing and externalizing problem behavior in 12-year-old twins. J Am Acad Child Adolesc Psychiatry 42:1351–1359, 2003

Bartels M, van den Oord EJCG, Hudziak JJ, et al: Genetic and environmental mechanisms underlying stability and change in problem behaviors at ages 3, 7, 10, and 12. Dev Psychol 40:852–867, 2004

Bartels M, van Beijsterveldt CE, Derks EM, et al: Young Netherlands Twin Register (Y-NTR): a longitudinal multiple informant study of problem behavior. Twin Res Hum Genet 10:3–11, 2007

Boomsma DI, Molenaar PCM: The genetic analysis of repeated measures, I: simplex models. Behav Genet 17:111–123, 1987

Boomsma DI, Martin NG, Molenaar PCM: Factor and simplex models for repeated measures: application to two psychomotor measures of alcohol sensitivity in twins. Behav Genet 19:79–96, 1989

Boomsma DI, Beem AL, van den Berg M, et al: Netherlands twin family study of anxious depression (NETSAD). Twin Res 3:323–334, 2000

Boomsma DI, Vink JM, van Beijsterveldt CE, et al: Netherlands Twin Register: a focus on longitudinal research. Twin Res 5:1–6, 2002

Boomsma DI, van Beijsterveldt CE, Hudziak JJ: Genetic and environmental influences on Anxious/Depression during childhood: a study from the Netherlands Twin Register. Genes Brain Behav 4:466–481, 2005

Boomsma DI, de Geus EJ, Vink JM, et al: Netherlands Twin Register: from twins to twin families. Twin Res Hum Genet 9:849–857, 2006

Castellanos FX, Glaser PE, Gerhardt GA: Towards a neuroscience of attention-deficit/hyperactivity disorder: fractionating the phenotype. J Neurosci Methods 151:1–4, 2006

Geller B, Todd RD, Luby J, et al: Treatment-resistant depression in children and adolescents. J Psychiatr Clin North Am 19:253–267, 1996

Goldsmith HH: A zygosity questionnaire for young twins: a research note. Behav Genet 21:257–270, 1991

Gorman JM: Comorbid depression and anxiety spectrum disorders. Depress Anxiety 4(4):160–168, 1996–1997

Greenberg PE, Sisitsky T, Kessler RC, et al: The economic burden of anxiety disorders in the 1990s. J Clin Psychiatry 60(7):427–435, 1999

Hewitt JK, Silberg JL, Neale MC, et al: The analysis of parental ratings of children's behavior using LISREL. Behav Genet 22:293–317, 1992

Jöreskog KD, Sörbom D: New features in PRELIS 2. Chicago, IL, Scientific Software International, 1993

Kagan J, Snidman N: Early childhood predictors of adult anxiety disorders. Biol Psychiatry 46:1536–1541, 1999

Kagan J, Snidman N, Zentner M, et al: Infant temperament and anxious symptoms in school age children. Dev Psychopathol 11:209–224, 1999

Kendall PC, Panichelli-Mindel SM: Cognitive-behavioral treatments. J Abnorm Child Psychol 23:107–123, 1995

Kendall PC, Safford S, Flannery-Schroeder E, et al: Child anxiety treatment: outcomes in adolescence and impact on substance use and depression at 7.4-year follow-up. J Consult Clin Psychol 72:276–287, 2004

Kendler KS, Neale MC, Kessler RC, et al: Major depression and generalized anxiety disorder: some genes, (partly) different environments? Arch Gen Psychiatry 49:716–722, 1992

Kendler KS, Gardner CO, Gatz M, et al: The sources of comorbidity between major depression and generalized anxiety disorder in a Swedish national twin sample. Psychol Med 23:1–10, 2006

Klein DN, Lewinsohn PM, Rohde P, et al: Clinical features of major depressive disorder in adolescents and their relatives: impact on familial aggregation, implications for phenotype definition, and specificity of transmission. J Abnorm Psychol 111:98–106, 2002

Koot HM, Van Den Oord EJ, Verhulst FC, et al: Behavioral and emotional problems in young preschoolers: cross-cultural testing of the validity of the Child Behavior Checklist/2–3. J Abnorm Child Psychol 25:183–196, 1997

Little RJA, Rubin DB: Statistical Analysis With Missing Data. New York, Wiley, 1987

Mannuzza S, Klein RG, Moulton JL 3rd: Persistence of attention-deficit/hyperactivity disorder into adulthood: what have we learned from the prospective follow-up studies? J Atten Disord 7:93–100, 2003

McArdle JJ, Goldsmith HH: Alternative common factor models for multivariate biometric analyses. Behav Genet 20:569–608, 1990

Neale MC, Cardon LR (eds): Methodology for Genetic Studies of Twins and Families (NATO ASI Series, Vol 25). Dordrecht, the Netherlands, Kluwer Academic Publishers, 1992, p. 496

Neale MC, Boker SM, Xie G, et al: Mx; Statistical Modeling, 5th Edition. Richmond, VA, Department of Psychiatry, Virginia Commonwealth University, 1997

Ninan PT, Berger J: Symptomatic and syndromal anxiety and depression. Depress Anxiety 14:79–85, 2001

Posthuma D, de Geus EJ, Boomsma DI: Genetic contributions to anatomical, behavioral, and neurophysiological indices of cognition, in Behavioral Genetics in the Postgenomic Era. Edited by Plomin R, Defries JC, Craig IW, et al. Washington, DC, American Psychological Association, 2002, pp 141–161

Rietveld MJH, van der Valk JC, Bongers IL, et al: Zygosity diagnosis in young twins by parental report. Twin Res 3:134–141, 2000

Rietveld MJH, Dolan CV, van Baal GCM, et al: A twin study of differentiation of cognitive abilities in childhood. Behav Genet 33:367–381, 2003

Rietveld MJH, Hudziak JJ, Bartels M, et al: Heritability of attention problems in children: longitudinal results from a study of twins, age 3 to 12. J Child Psychol Psychiatry 45:577–588, 2004

Robins LN: Deviant children grown up. Eur Child Adolesc Psychiatry 1:44–46, 1996

Rutter M: Genetic influences and autism, in Handbook of Autism and Pervasive Developmental Disorders, 3rd Edition. Edited by Volkmar FR, Paul R, Klin A, et al. New York, Wiley, 2005, pp 425–452

Rutter M, Silberg J: Gene-environment interplay in relation to emotional and behavioral disturbance. Annu Rev Psychol 53:463–490, 2002

Spivack G, Spotts J: The Devereux Child Behavior (DCB) Rating Scale. Devon, PA, The Devereux Foundation, 1966

Suomi SJ: Aggression and social behaviour in rhesus monkeys. Novartis Found Symp 268:216–253, 2005

van Beijsterveldt CE, Bartels M, Hudziak JJ, et al: Causes of stability of aggression from early childhood to adolescence: a longitudinal genetic analysis in Dutch twins. Behav Genet 33:591–605, 2003

van Beijsterveldt CE, Verhulst FC, Molenaar PCM, et al: The genetic basis of problem behavior in 5-year-old Dutch twin pairs. Behav Genet 34:229–242, 2004

van der Valk JC, van den Oord EJ, Verhulst FC, et al: Genetic and environmental contributions to stability and change in children's internalizing and externalizing problems. J Am Acad Child Adolesc Psychiatry 42:1212–1220, 2003

van Grootheest DS, Bartels M, Cath DC, et al: Genetic and environmental contributions underlying stability in childhood obsessive-compulsive behavior. Biol Psychiatry 61:308–315, 2007

Verhulst FC, van der Ende J, Koot HM: [Manual for the CBCL/4–18]. Rotterdam, the Netherlands, Sophia Children's Hospital/Erasmus University, Department of Psychiatry, 1996

Weissman MM, Wickramaratne P, Nomura Y, et al: Families at high and low risk for depression: a three-generation study. Arch Gen Psychiatry 62:29–36, 2005

Weissman MM, Pilowsky DJ, Wickramaratne PJ, et al: Remissions in maternal depression and child psychopathology: a STAR-D Child Report. STAR-D Child Team. JAMA 295:1389–1398, 2006. Erratum in JAMA 296:1234, 2006

Wothke W: Longitudinal and multigroup modeling with missing data, in Modeling Longitudinal and Multilevel Data: Practical Issues, Applied Approaches and Specific Examples. Edited by Little TD, Schnabel KU, Baumert J. Mahwah, NJ, Erlbaum, 2000, pp 219–240

Chapter 9

INTERSECTION OF AUTISM AND ADHD

Evidence for a Distinct Syndrome Influenced by Genes and by Gene–Environment Interactions

Angela M. Reiersen, M.D., M.P.E.

Rosalind J. Neuman, Ph.D.

Wendy Reich, Ph.D.

John N. Constantino, M.D.

Heather E. Volk, Ph.D., M.P.H.

Richard D. Todd, Ph.D., M.D.

Two of the most commonly studied forms of early onset psychopathology are the attention-deficit/hyperactivity disorder (ADHD) and autistic spectrum disorder (ASD) syndromes. Although there is substantial controversy over whether there are one or multiple forms of each of these disorders (see, e.g., Thapar et al. 2006 for discussion of ADHD), population-based studies have demonstrated the presence of distinct, genetically independent forms of ADHD (Rasmussen et al. 2004; Todd et al. 2001c). They have also found that the core symptoms of autism and related disorders can be described as a quantitative trait in the general population (Constantino and Todd 2000, 2005; Constantino et al. 2000, 2003a, 2004, 2006). The goal of this chapter is to describe our recent studies demonstrating that a particular form of

ADHD characterized by severe inattention and hyperactivity symptoms is associated disproportionately with clinically significant autism symptoms and diagnoses in the general population. The prevalence of this combined ADHD/autism syndrome is affected by prenatal exposure to smoking and particular alleles of candidate genes in the dopaminergic pathway.

EVIDENCE FOR DISTINCT ADHD SUBTYPES

ADHD, however defined, is a common and highly heritable syndrome (Faraone and Doyle 2001). The vast majority of genetic studies of ADHD use the DSM-IV classification system (American Psychiatric Association 1994). Although the DSM criteria are very relevant to the clinical treatment of ADHD and to the identification of children who are impaired, the current diagnostic nomenclature has limitations for etiologic studies. For example, a functionally impaired child with 10 ADHD symptoms may be classified as predominantly inattentive if there are 6 inattentive and 4 hyperactive/impulsive symptoms, predominantly hyperactive/impulsive subtype if there are 6 hyperactive/impulsive and 4 inattentive symptoms, or unaffected if there are 5 inattentive plus 5 hyperactive/impulsive symptoms. Such criteria for ADHD subtype definition, developed predominantly using clinically referred samples, can lead to confusion in twin and family studies testing for independent transmission of subtypes. Additionally, in the DSM framework a diagnosis of ADHD cannot be made in the presence of an ASD. To the degree that ADHD and ASD syndromes co-occur, etiologic studies that follow the DSM exclusion approach may generate misleading conclusions.

Over the last 10 years we have adopted population-based approaches to defining ADHD subtypes by collecting complete symptom information on community-based samples of twins and using clustering procedures such as principal component analysis and latent class analysis to identify naturally occurring subtypes. Using parental report of child ADHD symptoms, we have demonstrated the presence of multiple types of ADHD that have family and genetic specificity (Neuman et al. 1999; Todd et al. 2001c). These subtypes, originally defined in girls, have been replicated across sexes and in several populations, including studies from Australia (Rasmussen et al. 2004) and the state of Missouri (Volk et al. 2005). The more severe and clinically relevant ADHD subtypes defined by these criteria include a severe attention problems class and a severe combined problems class (Figure 9–1) that are elicited from maternal, paternal, and teacher reports (Althoff et al. 2006).

These population-based ADHD subtypes have consistent patterns of comorbidity (Neuman et al. 2001; Volk et al. 2005), are differentially asso-

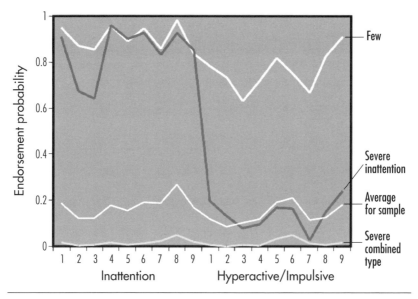

FIGURE 9–1. **Attention-deficit/hyperactivity disorder (ADHD) symptom prevalences for population-based types.**

Three ADHD type endorsement patterns are shown for the 18 DSM-IV ADHD symptoms (the few, severe inattention, and severe combined-type latent classes). The average endorsement probability for the sample as a whole is also shown. *Source.* Neuman et al. 2007.

ciated with candidate gene polymorphisms (Todd et al. 2003b, 2005), and have different patterns of problems with academic progress and cognitive performance (Todd et al. 2002). In contrast to the recent conclusions of other investigators (e.g., see Thapar et al. 2006), we believe these studies considered in total strongly argue that such population-derived ADHD subtypes have particular relevance for etiologic studies of ADHD.

EPIDEMIOLOGY OF AUTISTIC SYMPTOMS

As our efforts to define population-based autistic syndromes are described in detail in Chapter 10 ("Genetic Epidemiology of Pervasive Developmental Disorders") of this book, we review only briefly here evidence that the core symptoms of autism represent a quantitative trait forming a continuum of severity in the general population (rather than autism representing a distinct syndrome or group of syndromes). Using a well-validated 65-item parent- or teacher-rated questionnaire that was designed to assess naturalistically the severity of autistic traits in a quantitative manner (the Social Responsiveness Scale [SRS]), Constantino and colleagues have conducted a series of studies demonstrating that subsyndromal autistic traits are continuously distributed in the general population and are highly heritable (Constantino and Todd 2000, 2003, 2005). SRS scores are also highly correlated with scores on the gold standard autism assessment instruments, the Autism Diagnostic Interview—Revised (ADI-R) (Constantino et al. 2003a) and the Autism Diagnostic Observational Scale (ADOS; see Chapter 10). Factor and latent class analyses of population-derived SRS scores find little or no evidence for discrete subtypes and are consistent with a single quantitative factor explaining approximately 70% of the variance in SRS scores (Constantino et al. 2000). SRS cutoff scores can be used to identify youth with DSM-IV diagnoses of ASD (Constantino et al. 2003a). Hence, our population-based studies have come to opposite conclusions for the ADHD and ASD syndromes, with there being evidence for discrete ADHD subtypes and evidence for an autistic continuum in the general population.

CO-OCCURRENCE OF AUTISM AND ADHD

As noted previously, the DSM framework prohibits dual diagnoses of ADHD and ASD. However, a variety of clinic-based studies have demonstrated the presence of clinically significant ADHD symptoms in the majority of children with pervasive developmental disorder (see, e.g., Goldstein and Schwebach 2004; Sturm et al. 2004; Yoshida and Uchiyama 2004) and the presence of clinically significant symptoms of autism in children with ADHD (Clark et al. 1999; Santosh and Mijovic 2004). There is also evidence from genetic linkage studies for overlapping linkage peaks for the two disorders, suggesting some genes may influence risk for both ADHD and autism (Smalley et al. 2005). In our twin studies of the SRS, a significant association of SRS scores was also found with the Child Behavior Checklist (CBCL) Attention Problems scale (Constantino et al. 2003b); elevated scores on this scale were highly correlated with a clinical diagnosis of ADHD. These clinical, genetic linkage, and population-based studies demonstrate the presence of youth with significant impairment from both ADHD and autism-related problems. Whether this association represents selection artifacts, simple comorbidity of two independent disorders, or a true syndrome representing dysfunction in multiple domains is unknown. The goal of this chapter is to present an argument that a specific subtype of ADHD (severe combined problems) is significantly associated with ASD and that the two disorders represent a true syndrome with specific prenatal and genetic predispositions.

INFLUENCE OF PRENATAL EXPOSURES ON THE DEVELOPMENT OF ADHD

A variety of studies suggest that maternal tobacco smoking and alcohol use during pregnancy increase the risk for ADHD (Brookes et al. 2006; Hill et al. 2000; Kahn et al. 2003; Knopik et al. 2005; Mick et al. 2002; Milberger et al. 1996, 1998; Thapar et al. 2003; reviewed in Linnet et al. 2003). When studies control for the presence of drinking when testing for the effects of smoking and vice versa, various outcomes have been reported for increased risk for ADHD. Part of the problem stems from the high occurrence of both smoking and drinking when one or the other substance is used during pregnancy. In addition, no studies have adequately controlled for other sources of exposure to tobacco smoke such as paternal smoking or other household exposures in a satisfactory way. Hence, though the focus in this chapter is on prenatal smoking, we recognize that there may be interactions with other substances ingested during pregnancy or with other potential sources of prenatal exposure to smoke through passive environmental mechanisms. It may be that self-report of smoking during pregnancy indexes a toxic prenatal/early life environment rather than a discrete toxic exposure.

Although prenatal smoking has been associated with a variety of undesirable outcomes, the mechanism of action for this association is unclear. Interestingly, during development dopamine affects neuronal maturation and branching (Todd 1992). Dopamine levels are increased following activation of high-affinity neural nicotinic acetylcholine receptors (nACHRs) by as little as a few cigarette puffs (see, e.g., Brody et al. 2006a, 2006b; Cao et al. 2005). These observations suggest that there may be significant interactions between early exposure to nicotine and particular candidate genes of the dopaminergic system that affect neuronal maturation and circuitry in the developing brain.

Two studies have investigated the interaction of child genetic polymorphisms with prenatal exposure to smoking or alcohol. Kahn et al. (2003) demonstrated that children who were homozygous for the 480–base pair (bp) allele of the dopamine transporter gene (*DAT*) and had been exposed to prenatal smoking had significantly elevated levels of hyperactive-impulsive symptoms and oppositional defiant symptoms. The largest association was with oppositional defiant behavior. Recently, Brookes et al. (2006) demonstrated an increased risk of ADHD in children who had been exposed to prenatal alcohol but not tobacco if they possessed the 480-bp allele of *DAT*. The prevalence of maternal drinking in this study was unusually high (57.8%).

CO-OCCURRENCE OF AUTISM AND COMBINED-TYPE ADHD

In order to test whether the association between SRS scores and the CBCL Attention Problems scale scores represented a true association of ASD with ADHD, we obtained parent-report SRS scales on a birth records–based cohort of twins (Missouri Twin Study [MOTWINS]) who had been studied with a semistructured, standardized DSM-IV diagnostic interview in which there were no symptom skipouts (the MAGIC interview; Todd et al. 2003a). (The prevalence of ADHD and the representativeness of the sample are described in detail in Neuman et al. 2005.) In total, complete SRS data, in addition to diagnostic interviews, were available for 946 twins. Subjects were assigned to DSM-IV ADHD subtypes and our population-derived latent-class ADHD subtypes based on parent report of the 18 DSM-IV ADHD symptoms. Figure 9–2 shows the distribution of SRS scores for various ADHD subtypes. Linear regression and logistic regression approaches were used to evaluate whether there was a difference in the prevalence of autistic symptoms and diagnoses between the ADHD subtypes. Combined-type ADHD, whether defined by DSM-IV or by latent-class population-based criteria, had the highest mean SRS score of all the ADHD subtypes (Reiersen et al. 2005, 2007). There was no significant elevation of SRS scores in children who had predominantly hyperactive-impulsive ADHD defined by either criteria, and there were only intermediate elevations of scores in children with primarily inattentive ADHD or severe inattention problems. SRS subscale scores based on the three DSM-IV autism domains (social impairment, communication impairment, and stereotyped behaviors) were also highest for DSM-IV combined-type ADHD and the severe combined latent-class subtype.

When SRS scores associated with formal ASD diagnoses (≥91 for male twins and ≥74 for female twins) were used to determine the prevalence of clinically significant ASD across these subtypes, nearly 30% of boys and more than 70% of girls in the population-defined severe combined-type ADHD class had clinically significant scores. These levels of comorbidity are much higher than would be expected by chance (1%–5%). None of the children with predominantly hyperactive-impulsive forms of ADHD met the threshold for clinically significant ASD. Depending on the diagnostic nomenclature used, only 12%–14% of boys and 24%–33% of girls with predominantly inattentive ADHD or severe inattention problems had clinically significant autistic symptom scores on their SRS (Reiersen et al. 2007). On the basis of a multinomial logistic regression analysis that controlled for covariates (sex, age, zygosity, and Wechsler Intelligence Scale for

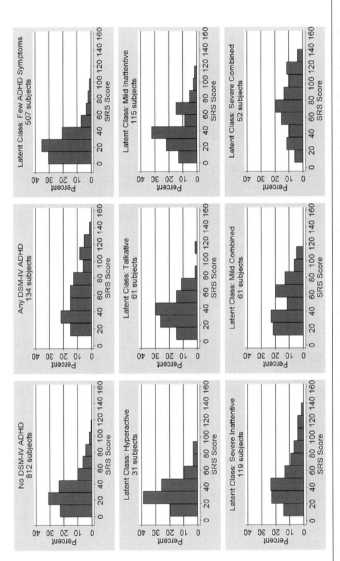

FIGURE 9–2. **Distribution of Social Responsiveness Scale (SRS) scores in DSM-IV- and population-defined attention-deficit/hyperactivity disorder (ADHD) diagnostic groups (*N*=946).**

Note. No DSM-IV ADHD=subjects who did not meet DSM-IV criteria for ADHD. Any DSM-IV ADHD=subjects with any DSM-IV ADHD diagnosis.

Children–III Vocabulary score), a clinically significant SRS score increased the likelihood of having severe combined ADHD by nearly 25-fold (odds ratio [OR]=24.46; 95% confidence interval [CI]=8.72–68.58).

This birth records–based cohort study provides population-based evidence for clinically significant elevations of autistic traits and ASDs in children with combined-type ADHD and, given the prevalence of ASDs in this group, suggests this may represent a distinct disorder rather than a comorbid condition. These findings also call into question the exclusionary clause in DSM-IV prohibiting the diagnosis of both disorders.

INFLUENCE OF PRENATAL EXPOSURES ON COMBINED-TYPE ADHD

In a previous study of a birth records–based cohort of female twins born in the state of Missouri, we identified increased risk of ADHD in offspring exposed prenatally to either tobacco smoking or alcohol consumption (Knopik et al. 2005). When considered together in this cohort, alcohol consumption and parental diagnoses of alcohol-related disorders appeared to have the most significant association with risk for offspring ADHD. In the mixed-sex MOTWINS birth records–based twin study of ADHD described previously for copresence of ASDs and ADHD (Reiersen et al. 2005), we found maternal smoking during pregnancy had a more substantial impact on risk for ADHD than did maternal drinking during pregnancy (Neuman et al. 2007). In part, this finding may reflect that 18% of mothers endorsed smoking sometime during pregnancy, whereas only 5% of mothers endorsed drinking.

When the data were examined by ADHD subtype, the only significant association of prenatal smoking with risk for ADHD was for the latent-class–defined severe combined type (OR=1.92; 95% CI=1.04–3.47, adjusted for sex of child, presence of conduct disorder or oppositional defiant disorder, and negative home environment) (Neuman et al. 2007). In this study, we also collected genomic DNA and tested for the potential impact of several candidate genes for ADHD, including the dopamine D_4 receptor gene (*DRD4*) and *DAT*. For the two most frequently reported risk polymorphisms (the *DRD4* exon 3 seven-repeat expansion allele and the *DAT* 3′440-bp and 3′480-bp variable number of tandem repeats [VNTR] alleles), there was no main effect on risk for ADHD in any ADHD subtype in this sample (Todd et al. 2001a, 2001b).

Attempting to replicate and expand on the previous findings of Kahn et al. (2003), we tested for a possible gene–environment interaction increasing risk for ADHD on the basis of *DRD4* and *DAT* genotype and maternal ex-

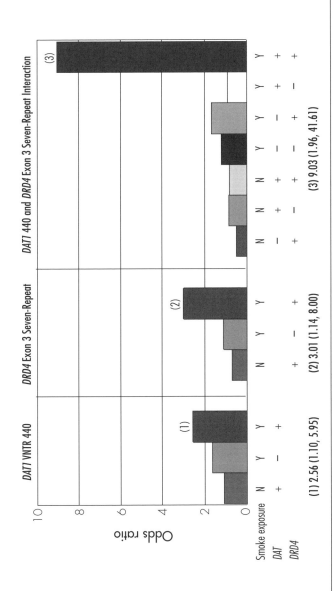

FIGURE 9–3. **Adjusted odds ratios for the association between population-defined attention-deficit/hyperactivity disorder (ADHD) combined subtype and in utero maternal smoking exposure and dopamine pathway genotypes.**

Note. Reference group: No smoking exposure and genotype without risk allele. VNTR=variable number of tandem repeats.

Source. Data redrawn from Neuman et al. 2007.

posure to smoking. In the presence of maternal smoking, we found a significant gene–environment effect for combined-type ADHD defined by either DSM-IV or latent class criteria and the *DAT* 3′440-bp allele (OR= 2.5–3.0) (Neuman et al. 2007). There was no effect for the *DAT* 3′480-bp allele. For the *DRD4* exon 3 seven-repeat expansion allele there was a significant increase in the risk of ADHD among offspring exposed to maternal smoking in combined-type ADHD defined by either criteria (OR=2.8–3.0) (Neuman et al. 2007). These results are shown for the population-defined combined-type ADHD in Figure 9–3. Because we had a main effect of smoking and two possible gene–environment effects for the *DAT* and *DRD4* receptor polymorphisms, we also completed analysis of the possible interaction of both candidate genes with prenatal smoking on increasing risk for ADHD. The only significant subtype effects were for population-defined combined-type ADHD. As shown in Figure 9–3, if a child had a *DAT* 3′440-bp allele and a *DRD4* exon 3 seven-repeat expansion allele, there was an approximate ninefold increased risk of combined-type ADHD in the presence of prenatal maternal smoking (95% CI=1.96–41.61) (Neuman et al. 2007).

This remarkable increase in risk for ADHD mediated by both maternal behavior and child genotype effects is specific to the same type of ADHD that showed the highest elevations in autistic symptoms and the highest frequency of clinically significant ASD (population-defined combined-type ADHD).

INFLUENCE OF CANDIDATE GENES ON SRS SCORES IN COMBINED-TYPE ADHD

To explore whether the observed gene–environment interactions for combined-type ADHD also lead to elevated SRS scores, we tested whether there were any main or interaction effects of maternal smoking during pregnancy and *DAT* and *DRD4* genotype for risk for ASD in this same sample. There were no main effects of maternal smoking and *DAT* genotype on risk for having clinically significant SRS scores in the total sample or in the individual ADHD subtypes. For the *DRD4* exon 3 seven-repeat allele there was a marginally significant OR of 1.6 for the total sample for association with high SRS scores (*P*=0.09), and there was a significant association with *DRD4* seven-repeat allele status and high SRS score in the population-defined severe combined ADHD subtype (OR=3.27; 95% CI=1.25–8.56; *P*=0.016). There was no evidence for gene–environment interactions between maternal smoking and either candidate gene polymorphism in producing ASD within the severe combined latent class.

HYPOTHESES ON MECHANISMS CONTRIBUTING TO CO-OCCURRENCE OF ADHD AND AUTISM

Considering the findings presented in this chapter, clinically significant ADHD and autistic symptoms co-occur more frequently than expected by chance and may represent a distinct syndrome. The mechanisms of this association and the implications of these findings for clinical practice and future research studies are less clear but point to the importance of assessing symptoms of both ADHD and autism in children with either disorder. Here we propose several hypotheses regarding the association between ADHD and autism that could be tested in future studies.

One potential mechanism of association between ADHD and autistic traits is nongenetic phenotypic interaction within individuals. In fact, a prior study by Constantino et al. (2003b) suggested this mechanism. For example, it is possible that a child with ADHD symptoms might have an exacerbation of ADHD symptoms due to the influence of autistic symptoms that result from a completely separate set of genes. There are a number of possible mechanisms for interaction between autism symptoms and ADHD symptoms within an individual. Children with ADHD may have some social deficits simply due to impulsivity, which might produce inappropriate social behaviors. Also, children with ADHD may have associated cognitive problems that make it more difficult to assess social situations or pay attention to social cues, even if they have a normal desire for social interaction. A child who has a true ASD in addition to inattentiveness may pay even less attention to social cues as a result of less motivation to act in a socially appropriate manner. Also, if a child has repetitive stereotypic behaviors due to ASD, these behaviors might be increased because of impulsiveness and lack of inhibition if the child has co-occurring hyperactive-impulsive symptoms.

Previous work by Smalley et al. (2005) and preliminary genetic findings described in this chapter suggest that there may be common genetic influences that affect both ADHD and ASDs. However, except for *DRD4*, the specific genes and gene–environment interactions associated with severe combined ADHD do not appear to be associated with ASD in this sample. Given this information, one might hypothesize that there is a set of genes that can increase the risk for both autism and ADHD and that different gene–gene and gene–environment interactions will lead to either no diagnosis, ADHD, ASD, or ADHD plus ASD in these individuals. The form of ADHD that has the strongest association with ASDs is a disorder characterized by a high degree of both inattentive and hyperactive symptoms. Perhaps most individuals with this relatively severe form of ADHD have a very high genetic loading for ADHD and abnormal social development.

With such a high genetic loading of "ADHD genes," the addition of one additional risk allele that sometimes leads to autistic symptoms (i.e., *DRD4* seven-repeat allele) might be enough to result in an ASD. This could explain why we do not see a significant association between this allele and ASD in the entire sample, but we do see an association when we look at the group of subjects with the severe combined subtype of ADHD. If this mechanism is correct, it illustrates how a single gene may sometimes cause a drastic shift in the degree of autistic symptoms even though multiple genes of small effect account for most of the genetic variance of SRS score in the general population.

In order to facilitate eventual elucidation of disease pathways that could be targeted in treatment interventions, it is also important to consider how genetic and environmental influences might affect brain function at a molecular level. Appreciating the functional interactions between molecules that are expressed by dopaminergic neurons can generate hypotheses regarding the mechanism of gene–gene and gene–environment interactions that may be relevant to the development of treatment and prevention strategies as well as suggesting avenues for further genetic research.

There have been more than 100 candidate gene studies of ADHD (reviewed in Faraone et al. 2005). Because the stimulant medications effective in treating ADHD increase synaptic dopamine concentration, most of these studies have been directed at gene polymorphisms relevant to the dopaminergic system. The finding most strongly supported by existing genetic studies is the association between ADHD and the seven-repeat polymorphism in exon 3 of the *DRD4* receptor gene, which codes for a D_2 family dopamine receptor. Somewhat fewer studies support an association of ADHD with the 480-bp or 440-bp polymorphisms of a 40-bp repeat VNTR in the 3′ untranslated region of the dopamine transporter gene *DAT1*. All of these polymorphisms are thought to be functional (Vanness et al. 2005). Interestingly, stimulation of high-affinity neuronal nACHRs increases dopamine release at synapses within the striatum and cortical regions (see, for example, Cao et al. 2005), and stimulation of *DRD4* receptors alters the branching and outgrowth of neurites (Swarzenski et al. 1994; Todd 1992). Considering the above, the effects of prenatal nicotine on ventral dopaminergic system development may be dependent on the child's genotype at *DRD4, DAT,* and *CHRNA4/CHRNB2* loci. The locations of these proteins are schematically shown in Figure 9–4. Of note, *DAT1* and *DRD4* genetic variations have been shown to modify human frontostriatal gray matter volumes (Durston et al. 2005). Our own findings demonstrating the interaction of *DRD4* and *DAT* polymorphisms with prenatal smoke exposure may be mediated by changes in *DRD4* and *DAT* function that interact with changes in dopamine release induced by nACHR stimulation. The resulting disrup-

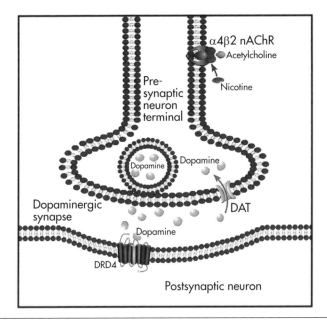

FIGURE 9–4. **Diagram of a dopaminergic synapse, illustrating the functional interaction of DRD4 (a D$_2$ class dopamine receptor), DAT (dopamine transporter), and α4β2 nAChR (high-affinity neural nicotinic acetylcholine receptor complex) in dopaminergic neurotransmission.**

Note. Polymorphisms of *DAT* and *DRD4* may interact to influence the degree and quality of dopaminergic neurotransmission at the synapse. Nicotine can also influence dopaminergic neurotransmission by increasing the amount of dopamine released into the synapse. The effect of nicotine is mediated through α4β2 nAChR, located at the dopaminergic neuron cell body and neuron terminal.

tion of dopaminergic system development may contribute to the development of ADHD and autistic symptoms.

CONCLUSIONS

Overall, these findings demonstrate in a general community sample that there is a frequent and meaningful co-occurrence of clinically significant ASD in combined-type ADHD. Moreover, risk for combined-type ADHD is markedly influenced by both maternal behavior and child genotype. At least one of these genotypic associations with combined-type ADHD risk also predicts ASD risk within this type of ADHD. Obviously, these complex findings require replication and refinement in larger samples before definitive conclusions can be made, and the exact mechanisms that produce co-occurrence of severe combined-type ADHD and autism spectrum disorders remain to be elucidated. However, the concurrence of results from clinical and population-based studies on the true association of ADHD and autism argues strongly that the current exclusion of codiagnoses in DSM is inappropriate and may lead to misleading conclusions in etiologic and biological studies of both disorders.

REFERENCES

Althoff RR, Rettew DC, Faraone SV, et al: Latent class analysis shows strong heritability of the Child Behavior Checklist-juvenile bipolar phenotype. Biol Psychiatry 60:903–911, 2006

American Psychiatric Association: Diagnostic and Statistical Manual of Mental Disorders, 4th Edition. Washington, DC, American Psychiatric Association, 1994

Brody AL, Mandelkern MA, London ED, et al: Cigarette smoking saturates brain alpha 4 beta 2 nicotinic acetylcholine receptors. Arch Gen Psychiatry 63:907–915, 2006a

Brody AL, Mandelkern MA, Olmstead RE, et al: Gene variants of brain dopamine pathways and smoking-induced dopamine release in the ventral caudate/nucleus accumbens. Arch Gen Psychiatry 63:808–816, 2006b

Brookes KJ, Mill J, Guindalini C, et al: A common haplotype of the dopamine transporter gene associated with attention-deficit/hyperactivity disorder and interacting with maternal use of alcohol during pregnancy. Arch Gen Psychiatry 63:74–81, 2006

Cao YJ, Surowy CS, Puttfarcken PS: Different nicotinic acetylcholine receptor subtypes mediating striatal and prefrontal cortical [3H]dopamine release. Neuropharmacology 48:72–79, 2005

Clark T, Feehan C, Tinline C, et al: Autistic symptoms in children with attention deficit-hyperactivity disorder. Eur Child Adolesc Psychiatry 8:50–55, 1999

Constantino JN, Todd RD: Genetic structure of reciprocal social behavior. Am J Psychiatry 157:2043–2045, 2000

Constantino JN, Todd RD: Autistic traits in the general population: a twin study. Arch Gen Psychiatry 60:524–530, 2003

Constantino JN, Todd RD: Intergenerational transmission of subthreshold autistic traits in the general population. Biol Psychiatry 57:655–660, 2005

Constantino JN, Przybeck T, Friesen D, et al: Reciprocal social behavior in children with and without pervasive developmental disorders. J Dev Behav Pediatr 21:2–11, 2000

Constantino JN, Davis SA, Todd RD, et al: Validation of a brief quantitative measure of autistic traits: comparison of the Social Responsiveness Scale with the Autism Diagnostic Interview—Revised. J Autism Dev Disord 33:427–433, 2003a

Constantino JN, Hudziak JJ, Todd RD: Deficits in reciprocal social behavior in male twins: evidence for a genetically independent domain of psychopathology. J Am Acad Child Adolesc Psychiatry 42:458–467, 2003b

Constantino JN, Gruber CP, Davis S, et al: The factor structure of autistic traits. J Child Psychol Psychiatry 45:719–726, 2004

Constantino JN, Lajonchere C, Lutz M, et al: Autistic social impairment in the siblings of children with pervasive developmental disorders. Am J Psychiatry 163:294–296, 2006

Durston S, Fossella JA, Casey BJ, et al: Differential effects of DRD4 and DAT1 genotype on fronto-striatal gray matter volumes in a sample of subjects with attention deficit hyperactivity disorder, their unaffected siblings, and controls. Mol Psychiatry 10:678–685, 2005

Faraone S, Doyle AE: The nature and heritability of attention-deficit/hyperactivity disorder. Child Adolesc Psychiatr Clin N Am 10:299–316, 2001

Faraone SV, Perlis RH, Doyle AE, et al: Molecular genetics of attention-deficit/hyperactivity disorder. Biol Psychiatry 57:1313–1323, 2005

Goldstein S, Schwebach AJ: The comorbidity of pervasive developmental disorder and attention deficit/hyperactivity disorder: results of a retrospective chart review. J Autism Dev Disord 34:329–339, 2004

Hill SY, Lowers L, Locke-Wellman J, et al: Maternal smoking and drinking during pregnancy and the risk for child and adolescent psychiatric disorders. J Stud Alcohol 61:661–668, 2000

Kahn RS, Khoury J, Nichols WC, et al: Role of dopamine transporter genotype and maternal prenatal smoking in childhood hyperactive-impulsive, inattentive, and oppositional behaviors. J Pediatr 143:104–110, 2003

Knopik VS, Sparrow EP, Madden PA, et al: Contributions of parental alcoholism, prenatal substance exposure, and genetic transmission to child ADHD risk: a female twin study. Psychol Med 35:625–635, 2005

Linnet KM, Dalsgaard S, Obel C, et al: Maternal lifestyle factors in pregnancy risk of attention deficit hyperactivity disorder and associated behaviors: review of the current evidence. Am J Psychiatry 160:1028–1040, 2003

Mick E, Biederman J, Faraone SV, et al: Case-control study of attention-deficit hyperactivity disorder and maternal smoking, alcohol use, and drug use during pregnancy. J Am Acad Child Adolesc Psychiatry 41:378–385, 2002

Milberger S, Biederman J, Faraone SV, et al: Is maternal smoking during pregnancy a risk factor for attention deficit hyperactivity disorder in children? Am J Psychiatry 153:1138–1142, 1996

Milberger S, Biederman J, Faraone SV, et al: Further evidence of an association between maternal smoking during pregnancy and attention deficit hyperactivity disorder: findings from a high-risk sample of siblings. J Clin Child Psychol 27:352–358, 1998

Neuman RJ, Todd RD, Heath AC, et al: Evaluation of ADHD typology in three contrasting samples: a latent class approach. J Am Acad Child Adolesc Psychiatry 38:25–33, 1999

Neuman RJ, Heath AC, Reich W, et al: Latent class analysis of ADHD and comorbid symptoms in a population sample of adolescent female twins. J Child Psychol Psychiatry 42:933–942, 2001

Neuman RJ, Sitdhiraksa N, Reich W, et al: Estimation of prevalence of DSM-IV and latent class-defined ADHD subtypes in a population-based sample of child and adolescent twins. Twin Res Hum Genet 8:392–401, 2005

Neuman RJ, Lobos E, Reich W, et al: Prenatal smoking exposure and dopaminergic genotypes interact to cause a severe ADHD subtype. Biol Psychiatry 61:1320–1328, 2007

Rasmussen ER, Neuman RJ, Heath AC, et al: Familial clustering of latent class and DSM-IV defined attention-deficit/hyperactivity disorder (ADHD) subtypes. J Child Psychol Psychiatry 45:589–598, 2004

Reiersen AM, Constantino JN, Todd RD: Autistic traits in heritable ADHD subtypes. Am J Med Genet B Neuropsychiatr Genet 138B:60, 2005

Reiersen AM, Constantino JN, Volk HE, et al: Autistic traits in a population-based ADHD twin sample. J Child Psychol Psychiatry 45:464–472, 2007

Santosh PJ, Mijovic A: Social impairment in hyperkinetic disorder—relationship to psychopathology and environmental stressors. Eur Child Adolesc Psychiatry 13:141–150, 2004

Smalley SL, Loo SK, Yang MH, et al: Toward localizing genes underlying cerebral asymmetry and mental health. Am J Med Genet B Neuropsychiatr Genet 135:79–84, 2005

Sturm H, Fernell E, Gillberg C: Autism spectrum disorders in children with normal intellectual levels: associated impairments and subgroups. Dev Med Child Neurol 46:444–447, 2004

Swarzenski BC, Tang L, Oh YJ, et al: Morphogenic potentials of D2, D3, and D4 dopamine receptors revealed in transfected neuronal cell lines. Proc Natl Acad Sci U S A 91:649–653, 1994

Thapar A, Fowler T, Rice F, et al: Maternal smoking during pregnancy and attention deficit hyperactivity disorder symptoms in offspring. Am J Psychiatry 160:1985–1989, 2003

Thapar A, Langley K, O'Donovan M, et al: Refining the attention deficit hyperactivity disorder phenotype for molecular genetic studies. Mol Psychiatry 11:714–720, 2006

Todd RD: Neural development is regulated by classical neurotransmitters: dopamine D2 receptor stimulation enhances neurite outgrowth. Biol Psychiatry 31:794–807, 1992

Todd RD, Jong YJ, Lobos EA, et al: No association of the dopamine transporter gene 3' VNTR polymorphism with ADHD subtypes in a population sample of twins. Am J Med Genet 105:745–748, 2001a

Todd RD, Neuman RJ, Lobos EA, et al: Lack of association of dopamine D4 receptor gene polymorphisms with ADHD subtypes in a population sample of twins. Am J Med Genet 105:432–438, 2001b

Todd RD, Rasmussen ER, Neuman RJ, et al: Familiality and heritability of subtypes of attention deficit hyperactivity disorder in a population sample of adolescent female twins. Am J Psychiatry 158:1891–1898, 2001c

Todd RD, Sitdhiraksa N, Reich W, et al: Discrimination of DSM-IV and latent class attention-deficit/hyperactivity disorder subtypes by educational and cognitive performance in a population-based sample of child and adolescent twins. J Am Acad Child Adolesc Psychiatry 41:820–828, 2002

Todd RD, Joyner CA, Heath AC, et al: Reliability and stability of a semistructured DSM-IV interview designed for family studies. J Am Acad Child Adolesc Psychiatry 42:1460–1468, 2003a

Todd RD, Lobos EA, Sun LW, et al: Mutational analysis of the nicotinic acetylcholine receptor alpha 4 subunit gene in attention deficit/hyperactivity disorder: evidence for association of an intronic polymorphism with attention problems. Molecular Psychiatry 8:103–108, 2003b

Todd RD, Huang H, Smalley SL, et al: Collaborative analysis of DRD4 and DAT genotypes in population-defined ADHD subtypes. J Child Psychol Psychiatry 46:1067–1073, 2005

Vanness SH, Owens MJ, Kilts CD: The variable number of tandem repeats element in DAT1 regulates in vitro dopamine transporter density. BMC Genet 6:55, 2005

Volk HE, Neuman RJ, Todd RD: A systematic evaluation of ADHD and comorbid psychopathology in a population-based twin sample. J Am Acad Child Adolesc Psychiatry 44:768–775, 2005

Yoshida Y, Uchiyama T: The clinical necessity for assessing attention deficit/hyperactivity disorder (AD/HD) symptoms in children with high-functioning pervasive developmental disorder (PDD). Eur Child Adolesc Psychiatry 13:307–314, 2004

Chapter 10

GENETIC EPIDEMIOLOGY OF PERVASIVE DEVELOPMENTAL DISORDERS

John N. Constantino, M.D.
Richard D. Todd, Ph.D., M.D.

Pervasive developmental disorders (PDDs)—the most common of which are autistic disorder, Asperger's disorder, and PDD not otherwise specified (PDD-NOS)—have been characterized as discrete disorders in the DSM-IV-TR diagnostic classification system (American Psychiatric Association 2000). Recent genetic epidemiologic studies have revealed that the symptoms of these conditions are common, substantially overlap across disorders, and are continuously distributed in both clinical and nonclinical populations such that it may be arbitrary where distinctions are drawn between the statuses of being "affected" versus "unaffected." Moreover, factor analysis, latent-class analysis, and cluster analysis of these data have suggested that the DSM-IV-TR symptom domains for autism—which constitute the current criteria for differentiating the PDDs—are *not* empirically separable. These findings underscore the central role of quantitative deficiencies in reciprocal social behavior in PDD and have led us to reconceptualize PDDs as extreme manifestations of a quantitative trait or traits that are continuously distributed in the general population. This quantitative characterization has important implications for research exploring the genetic and neurobiological causes of this family of disorders, for diagnosis, for measuring response to treatment, for our understanding of normal social development, and for understanding the multiplier effects of subthreshold autistic traits on other psychopathological conditions in comorbidly affected individuals.

PDDs are conditions that are characterized primarily by deficits in reciprocal social behavior, for which the prototype is autism. According to DSM-IV-TR, a diagnosis of autistic disorder is made on the basis of deficits in three domains: 1) reciprocal social behavior (RSB), 2) language development, and 3) repetitive/stereotypic behaviors (or a restricted range of interests). A diagnosis of Asperger's disorder requires impairment in RSB and restricted range of interests but is excluded if there are significant delays in the development of language. PDD-NOS is a condition defined by impairment in the development of RSB, coupled with language impairment and/or repetitive/stereotypic behavior whose severity is subthreshold or atypical and does not fulfill the criteria for a full diagnosis of autistic disorder. There are two other PDDs that are much less common than the others: Rett's disorder and childhood disintegrative disorder.

All PDDs, with the possible exception of some cases of childhood disintegrative disorder, appear to be highly genetically determined (Cook 2001; Le Couteur et al. 1996; Pickles et al. 2000). A specific genetic locus has been confirmed only for Rett's disorder, a rare condition in the autism spectrum caused by a point mutation in the *MECP2* gene on the X chromosome, which is usually fatal in the homozygous condition in boys (Amir et al. 1999). Best estimates from family studies and international genome-wide scans suggest that autism is an oligogenic disorder, with 3 to as many as 20 or more genes contributing to genetic susceptibility to the disorder (Pickles et al. 1995; Risch et al. 1999). For autistic disorder, monozygotic twin concordance is at least 75%, but dizygotic twin concordance is only 10%–15% (Le Couteur et al. 1996). Several replicated linkage regions have been reported for autistic disorder, but only a limited share of the variance in autistic symptoms in the population would be explainable on the basis of single genes lying in these regions (Cantor et al. 2005; International Molecular Genetic Study of Autism Consortium 2001; Shao et al. 2003).

Whether the various entities within the autism spectrum (autistic disorder, Asperger's disorder, and PDD-NOS) might share specific genetic susceptibility loci is unknown. However, these conditions are now believed to cluster together in families (Lauritsen et al. 2005; Le Couteur et al. 1996; Pickles et al. 2000). Lauritsen et al. (2005) examined data from a recent Danish national register–based study ($N=943,664$ children), which showed elevated rates of autistic disorder among both the siblings of autistic probands and the siblings of children with other PDDs, including Asperger's disorder.

In general, PDDs are more common than previously believed. This conclusion has been reached by several large independent epidemiologic studies. Conservative estimates from these studies (Chakrabarti and Fombonne 2001; Fombonne 2003; Fombonne et al. 2001; Yeargin-Allsopp et al. 2003) place the prevalence of autistic disorder at approximately 1–3 per 1,000, with a male to female ratio of 4:1 (the prevalence of PDD-NOS is approximately 5 per 1,000 in boys and 1 per 1,000 in girls in the general population). Up to one-half of children meeting diagnostic criteria for PDDs have some level of cognitive impairment; among those for whom cognitive impairment is severe, the male to female ratio drops to as low as 4:3.

In the current DSM-IV-TR taxonomy, distinctions between the common PDDs (autistic disorder, Asperger's disorder, PDD-NOS) rest on judgments about the relative severity of symptoms and the presence or absence of symptomatology reaching threshold criteria within the various criterion domains for autism (social deficits, language deficits, stereotypic behaviors/restricted interests). Thus, disagreement about the diagnosis of PDD occurs both within and across clinical disciplines (pediatrics, psychiatry, psychology, education) (see Klin et al. 2005), stemming from at least three important problems: 1) the diagnostic criteria for the disorder set out in DSM-IV-TR are vague and difficult to interpret, 2) mild autistic symptoms can be difficult to distinguish from the symptoms of other psychiatric conditions, and 3) it is unclear where to draw the line between clinical and nonclinical levels of impairment. Furthermore, factor analyses of autistic symptoms in clinical and nonclinical populations have not consistently supported the existence of separable subdomains of symptoms along the three DSM-IV-TR criterion domains (which are used in differentiating the disorders). Spiker et al. (2002) studied a large number of affected sibling pairs with autism and found that empirically derived clusters of sibling pairs differed not by specific symptom sets but by the degree of impairment that existed (mild, moderate, or severe) across all three DSM-IV-TR criterion domains for autism. Their findings were most consistent with the possibility that autism results from a single, heritable, continuously distributed deficit that might influence dysfunction in all three symptom domains (i.e., RSB, language development, and repetitive/stereotypic behaviors). Dawson et al. (2005) examined features of the broader autism phenotype in the relatives of autistic probands and found evidence for highly heritable social deficits aggregating in the families. In other family studies (Constantino et al. 2006; Pickles et al. 2000; Piven et al. 1997; Wolff et al. 1988), subthreshold impairments in all three DSM-IV-TR criterion domains for autism have been found to aggregate among the family members of autistic probands, suggesting common genetic underpinnings for clinical level and subthreshold symptomatology.

DEVELOPMENT OF A QUANTITATIVE MEASURE OF AUTISTIC TRAITS FOR USE IN CLINICAL SETTINGS

If the true defining features of PDDs are social deficiencies that vary in severity, breed true in families (even in their subtlest form), and are shared across PDDs, it is potentially important to have a method for characterizing them as quantitative traits (as is the case for blood pressure, weight, or IQ). Previously established rating scales for autism primarily were designed to assign "case-ness" in a categorical sense. For this reason, in the later 1990s, our research group began the task of developing a quantitative measure of autistic symptoms in children in an attempt to capture the continuous nature of this spectrum of impairments for clinical assessment and to test specific hypotheses about autistic symptoms as quantitative traits.

The quantitative measure that we developed is known as the Social Responsiveness Scale (SRS; Constantino 2002). The SRS is a 15-minute parent- and/or teacher-report questionnaire that inquires about a child's capacity for RSB based on day-to-day observations in naturalistic social settings. Interrater agreement between mothers, fathers, and teachers is on the order of 0.7 (Constantino et al. 2003a; Pine et al. 2006). The SRS includes items that ascertain autistic impairment in social awareness, social information processing, the capacity for reciprocal social responses (including language and purposeful social communication), motivational aspects of social behavior (including social anxiety/avoidance), and characteristic autistic preoccupations/traits. There are versions of the SRS for 3-year-olds, 4- to 18-year-olds, and adults; other brief instruments, such as the Checklist for Autism in Toddlers (Robins et al. 2001), are available for the purpose of screening younger children. The SRS generates a singular scale score that serves as an index of severity of social deficits in the autism spectrum; higher scores on the SRS indicate greater severity of social impairment. Details regarding its psychometric properties are described elsewhere (Constantino et al. 2000, 2003a, 2004).

The use of a single-scale score is supported by the observation that factor analysis, cluster analysis, and latent-class analysis of SRS data in large clinical and nonclinical samples have failed to support the existence of separable domains of dysfunction within the autism spectrum (Constantino et al. 2003a, 2003b, 2004). Recent analyses of data from the Autism Diagnostic Observation Schedule have confirmed strong interrelations between language deficits and social deficits in affected children and have prompted a revision of the instrument's scoring to reflect a combined social-communication domain. New research in very young children is exploring, from a developmental perspective, how core social deficits in a given individual might interact with variations in his or her sensorimotor systems, temperament, language development, and cognitive development to result in the wide variety of clinical manifestations seen in children with autism spectrum conditions. The interrelatedness of social development and language development are further demonstrated by long-term follow-up studies of children diagnosed with specific language impairment (revealing substantial social impairment in a majority of these individuals in adulthood) (Howlin et al. 2000) and by studies of early language development highlighting the crucial role of social interaction (Dawson et al. 2005; Kuhl 2000).

In initial studies involving more than 500 school-age children with and without PDDs (Constantino et al. 2000, 2003a), scores for autistic traits measured by the SRS were generally unrelated to IQ, and distinguished (by 3 standard deviations) patients with autism spectrum disorders (including PDD-NOS) from children with other psychiatric disorders and from control subjects. Scores are highly stable over time; test-retest reliability up to 5 years between assessments is on the order of 0.80 (Constantino et al. 2003a, in press). Moreover, scores on the instrument exhibited continuous (rather than bimodal) distributions, indicating that it may be arbitrary where cutoffs are made between the status of being affected versus unaffected with an autism spectrum condition.

EPIDEMIOLOGY AND GENETIC STRUCTURE OF QUANTITATIVE AUTISTIC TRAITS

In order to determine the developmental stability of heritable social deficits measured by the SRS, we subsequently examined the longitudinal course of SRS scores in boys with and without PDD. To date we have analyzed follow-up assessments of several hundred children and adolescents assessed on the SRS at two time points, spaced 1–5 years apart. Interindividual variation in SRS scores is highly preserved over time, with test-retest correlation of 0.80 for our entire sample (Constantino et al., in press). Despite an absence of age effects in SRS scores when cross-sectionally obtained, we have observed modest general improvement over time (on the order of 0.1 standard deviation per year) in the subjects in our longitudinal study. Such improvements have suggested the presence of period effects possibly relating to improvements in educational interventions for socially impaired children.

We next recruited an epidemiologic sample of twins in order to examine the genetic structure of autistic traits across the entire range of the distribution of autistic symptoms that occurs in nature. In this sample of 1,576 twins, the distribution was again found to be continuous, essentially a slightly skewed normal distribution (Constantino and Todd 2003). The prevalence of individuals with SRS scores at or above the mean for children with PDD-NOS closely matched prevalence figures for individuals with PDD-NOS derived from the large epidemiologic studies described earlier (see Chakrabarti and Fombonne 2001; Fombonne et al. 2001; Yeargin-Allsopp et al. 2003).

SRS scores were highly correlated within twin pairs, consistent with there being important familial determinants for RSB. To examine the extent to which this familial clustering was caused by genetic versus environmental factors, structural equation modeling (SEM) was implemented. SEM involves the use of path models that represent mathematically the totality of causal influences on a trait of interest; variation in twin–twin concordance is examined as a function of zygosity (i.e., whether the twins share all or only half of their genetic variance), and the data are tested for its goodness of fit to competing models of causation. For male twins, scale scores for RSB were strongly influenced by additive genetic factors (accounting for approximately 76% of the total trait variance), exhibited minimal measurement error, and were not significantly influenced by age, rater bias, or rater contrast effects (Constantino and Todd 2000). For females, the best-fitting model incorporated both common environment influences and additive genetic influences, and the magnitude of additive genetic influences was somewhat lower than that observed in boys (Constantino and Todd 2003).

To ascertain whether gender-specific genetic effects accounted for the discrepancy in genetic influences between boys and girls, SRS reports on 300 pairs of opposite-sex dizygotic twins were utilized. Opposite-sex twin pairs are uniquely suited for testing hypotheses about gender-specific genetic influences because they represent a gender-comparison condition in which common environmental influences are controlled. The results of SEM applied to this data indicated that the genes influencing autistic traits appear to be the same for males and females. Lower prevalence (and severity) of autistic traits in females was found not to be a function of sex-linked genetic influences but rather to possibly result from increased sensitivity to early environmental influences (in females), which operate to reduce the phenotypic expression of genetic susceptibility factors and promote social competency (Constantino and Todd 2003).

If the same genetic structure holds true for autistic traits in the clinical range of severity, it would indicate that given similar levels of genetic susceptibility, girls are relatively protected (compared with boys) from phenotypically expressing this liability. This would constitute an intriguing, but as yet only preliminary, explanation for the gender disparity (male more prevalent than female) observed across all autism spectrum conditions as well as for gender differences in social development in unaffected children.

The question next arose whether the strong genetic influences on subthreshold autistic traits in boys in the general population were the same as or different from genetic influences involved in other domains of psychopathology. Twin designs are capable of answering such questions about genetic overlap as long as the various traits of interest are all measured in the subjects in a given genetically informative sample. Parent-report data from the Child Behavior Checklist (CBCL; Achenbach 1991) was collected on the epidemiologic sample of male twins. The CBCL is a 113-item checklist that covers a broad range of child psychopathological domains that correlate strongly with DSM-IV-TR diagnoses. Regression analysis indicated that scores for Internalizing behavior and Externalizing behavior explained only a minority of the variance in SRS scores. SEM supported the results of the regression analysis and revealed that the majority of causal influences on SRS scores (55%; 90% confidence interval=0.45–0.70) were genetic influences specific to the SRS and unrelated to the causes of psychopathology measurable on the CBCL (Constantino et al. 2003b). Other than the expected association of SRS score with the CBCL Social Problems subscale, the only significant association was with the Attention Problems subscale. This association had also been observed in the original clinic-based twin sample studied with the SRS (Constantino et al. 2000). In the general population-based twin sample, bivariate modeling of SRS and Attention Problems subscale scores was most consistent with SRS scores increasing Attention Problems scores. In the clinical sample, many CBCL subscale scores were significantly correlated with SRS scores, suggesting that subsyndromal autistic symptoms may exacerbate a variety of problems. In Chapter 9 ("Intersection of Autism and ADHD") of this book we present evidence for a discrete interaction of clinically significant SRS scores with severe combined-type attention-deficit/hyperactivity disorder (ADHD). In this case there is evidence for genetic overlap of both types of behaviors and for the presence of a distinct ADHD/autistic syndrome.

Taken together, these results indicate that even *subthreshold* autistic traits represent a unique, genetically determined component of development that is substantially independent of other domains of child psychopathological traits. When autistic traits are present—even at a level that is subthreshold for a diagnosis of autism, Asperger's disorder, or PDD-NOS (which occurs commonly in the general population)—they may operate to make other types of comorbid psychopathology worse. Whether this worsening is at the level of shared genes or within individual independent genetic efforts will likely vary with the specific comorbidity (see Chapter 9, "Intersection of Autism and ADHD," of this book for discussion of models). It should be noted, however, that such SRS score–related increases in severity of other psychopathological domains may result in false causative inferences when selecting extreme phenotypes for study (such as families with more than one classically defined case of autism) (Todd 2005).

We next examined the *intergenerational* transmission of subthreshold autistic traits in the general population. For this effort, the SRS was completed on 285 pairs of twins (by maternal report) and on their parents (by spouse report). Correlation for social impairment or competence was on the order of 0.4 for associations 1) between parents and their children and 2) between spouses. In families in which both parents scored in the upper quartile for social impairment on the SRS, mean SRS score of offspring was significantly elevated (effect size=1.0). Estimated assortative mating explained approximately 30% of the variation in parent SRS scores. This raised the possibility that societal trends in the extent to which assortative mating is facilitated could be responsible for shifts in genotype frequency that result in changes in prevalence of the disorder. As was the case for children, subthreshold autistic impairments measured in the adults (parents of epidemiologically ascertained twins) appeared continuously distributed.

To determine whether the genetic influences on subthreshold autistic traits affecting social development in nonclinically affected children might overlap with those responsible for most cases of clinically defined PDDs, we next investigated subsyndromal autistic impairments among the siblings of autistic probands.

We studied three groups of proband–sibling pairs: 1) fully autistic children from multiple-incidence families and their closest-in-age nonautistic brothers (N=49 pairs); 2) children with any PDD, including autism, and their closest-in-age brothers (N=100 pairs); and 3) children with psychopathology unrelated to autism and their closest-in-age brothers (N=45 pairs). *Sibling* SRS scores were continuously distributed and substantially elevated for both the autistic and PDD groups. Highest scores (i.e., greatest impairment) were seen among siblings of autistic probands from multiple-incidence families, followed by siblings of probands with any PDD, then siblings of probands with psychopathology unrelated to autism. Furthermore, the proband–sibling correlation for this clinical sample was identical to that observed among nonidentical twins in the general population (r=0.35). Scatterplots of proband versus sibling SRS score for each diagnostic group were positioned along the same regression line, which overlaps with that derived for unaffected nonidentical twin pairs, as shown in Figure 10–1.

Thus, siblings of children with PDDs, who have a 10-fold increase in risk for affected PDD status, are also more likely than their counterparts in unaffected families to exhibit subthreshold levels of autistic social impairment. This increased liability was observed among siblings of autistic probands from multiple-incidence autism families and to a lesser (but still highly significant) extent among siblings of probands with any PDD. These

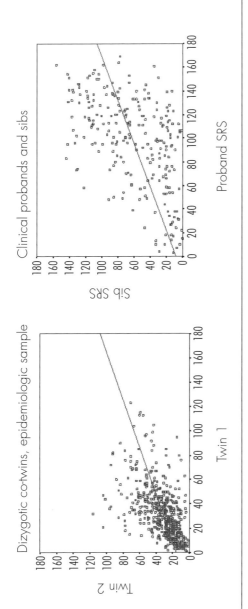

FIGURE 10–1.   Sibling correlations for general population and clinical samples.

Note.   Scatterplots lie along a uniform regression line. SRS=Social Responsiveness Scale.

findings support the notion that the specific genetic susceptibility factors responsible for PDDs may also be responsible for more common social impairments observed in "unaffected" family members and in children in the general population.

Only when the specific genetic and environmental factors causing autism are elucidated will it be possible to confirm whether specific genetic underpinnings of normal social development are shared with those of the PDDs or whether the specific developmental disorders share genetic causes with one another. In pursuing the molecular genetic determinants of autism and in collaboration with the laboratory of Dr. Daniel Geschwind at UCLA and the Autism Genetic Resource Exchange (AGRE), we recently conducted the first genome-wide scan for the continuously distributed social endophenotype measured by the SRS. In this study, which involved a sample of 105 sibling pairs affected by autism, their parents, and their unaffected siblings, we obtained SRS data from all siblings in each family (affected and unaffected) and conducted linkage analysis using this phenotypic information from *all* siblings rather than restricting the analysis to the traditional affected sibling pair method.

The SRS genome scan identified two loci, on chromosomes 11 and 17, that had linkage signals reaching a nominal statistical threshold of $P<0.01$, with the highest score on chromosome 11 ($Z=3.2$; $P=0.00068$). In contrast to these SRS linkage results, no linkage signals reached a significance of $P<0.01$ when the traditional affected sibling pair method for linkage analysis was implemented in this same sample. The linkage signals on chromosomes 11 and 17 closely matched those derived from qualitative linkage analysis involving a much larger sample ($N=345$) of affected AGRE sibling pairs and their parents (Duvall et al. 2007).

Thus, this study demonstrated the power of the SRS quantitative endophenotype to enhance detection of autism-related genetic loci by using quantitative behavioral information from both affected and unaffected members of families.

A RECONCEPTUALIZATION OF PERVASIVE DEVELOPMENTAL DISORDER NOT OTHERWISE SPECIFIED

An intriguing feature of autistic disorder is its association with impairment in general cognition and with language delay. There is clearly a higher prevalence of cognitive impairment (including mental retardation) among children with autism spectrum conditions, but many children with autistic social impairments—even when those impairments are very severe—do not have superimposed intellectual deficits, and some of these children (e.g., those with Asperger's disorder) are spared the binds of general language impairments that characterize autism. Among fully autistic subjects, language impairment and IQ are arguably the most important factors in determining long-term functional outcome in autism (Stevens et al. 2000) and are strongly intercorrelated. Furthermore, in both clinical (Constantino et al. 2003a; Fombonne 2003) and nonclinical populations (Constantino et al. 2000, 2003b) it has been shown that the *degree* of autistic social impairment (in the continuum from subthreshold to severe) generally predicts degree of impairment in the other two criterion domains of autism (language impairment and stereotypic behaviors/restricted interests), even though there are individual exceptions to these trends. It is possible that exceptions in both directions represent manifestations of the effects of superimposed factors on the expression of autistic social impairments or in some cases represent entirely separate genetic pathways to social dysfunction.

Given a general lack of evidence for differentiating PDD subtypes on the basis of the factor structure of autistic symptoms, the lack of evidence for "true-breeding" patterns of familial aggregation for any PDD subtype, and the fact that autistic social impairments are continuously distributed in the general population, we propose a modified conceptualization of autism spectrum conditions in children until such time as specific syndromes can be more precisely differentiated on the basis of genetic, neurobiological, or neuropsychological markers. A parsimonious approach might entail a three-axis configuration incorporating 1) degree of core impairment in reciprocal social interaction as an independent variable, 2) nonverbal IQ as a separate independent variable, and 3) the capacity for verbal language as a variable that is substantially dependent on the first two axes. Figure 10–2 provides a schematic depiction of this reconceptualization that shows how current diagnostic entities within the autism spectrum might fall into this modified conceptual framework. Essentially, rather than subdividing autism spectrum conditions based on categorical notions of presence versus absence of language development (as in the case of differentiating Asperger's disorder from autism) or presence versus absence of criteria whose underlying distribution is actually continuous in the population, this conceptual framework characterizes the pathology on the basis of the confluence of two continuously distributed variables—reciprocal social behavior (RSB) and nonverbal IQ—and a third variable, verbal language, which may exhibit a more dichotomous distribution and has complex associations with the other two variables.

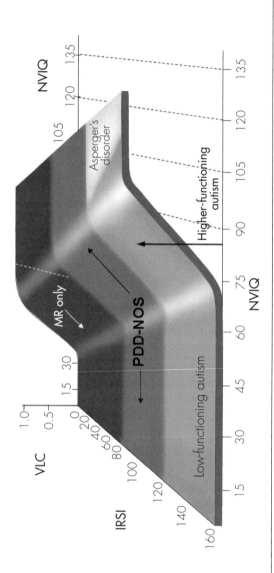

FIGURE 10–2.   Surface plot of current DSM-IV-TR diagnoses of the pervasive developmental disorders.

Note.   This surface plot depicts the manner in which current DSM-IV-TR diagnoses would map onto a new schema based on two continuously distributed variables: impairment in reciprocal social interaction (IRSI) and nonverbal IQ (NVIQ). The *z*-axis represents a third variable, verbal language capacity (VLC), substantially (though not completely) dependent on the first two. Its incorporation into the surface plot indicates that as IRSI intensifies, higher levels of IQ are required for an individual to develop purposeful verbal communication. Generally, autistic subjects with IQ less than 65 are likely to be nonverbal and have a significantly poor functional prognosis (Stevens et al. 2000). MR=mental retardation; PDD–NOS=pervasive developmental disorder not otherwise specified.

IMPLICATIONS OF THE MODEL FOR QUANTITATIVE GENETICS

We suggest that autistic traits may have similar genetic structures across the entire range of severity with which they are manifested in nature (from subthreshold to severe) and that the genetic underpinnings of the PDDs may be related to genetic mechanisms that underlie normal social development. An intriguing corollary to our findings of the familial aggregation of such threshold autistic traits is the recent finding that abnormal event-related potentials commonly observed in autistic subjects are also observed in their unaffected relatives (Dawson et al. 2005). What emerges from these findings (and from our knowledge of the oligogenic patterns of inheritance observed for PDDs) is the notion that autistic social impairment may result from the co-occurrence of multiple quantitative heritable abnormalities any of which is insufficient by itself seriously to disrupt social development. It is thus possible that the severity of any PDD is a stochastic function of the degree of affectedness across such contributing domains. In its subclinical form, an autistic trait may actually be adaptive (and thereby evolutionarily preserved), but in a more severe form or when combined with extremes in other psychopathological domains it may became highly maladaptive. We have shown that subthreshold autistic traits are transmitted intergenerationally and that for the parental generation of our current subjects there are substantial influences of preferential mating based on the expression of these traits in adults (Constantino and Todd 2005).

IMPLICATIONS FOR CLINICAL CARE

There is no known cure for any autism spectrum condition, and the effectiveness of treatment can only be measured in terms of symptom improvement. Use of repeated quantitative measurements of core deficits in RSB should aid in the assessment of candidate therapies and in the clinician's management of individual patients. In addition to rapid quantitative measures such as the SRS, methods for deriving quantitative scores from the more labor-intensive diagnostic instruments for autism (the Autism Diagnostic Interview and the Autism Diagnostic Observation Schedule) are being developed (Gotham et al. 2007; Lord et al. 2001).

Treatments of demonstrated benefit in controlled trials involving autistic youth include therapeutic nursery interventions (Jocelyn et al. 1998), other specific early childhood interventions (Kasari et al. 2006; Lovaas and Smith 1989), and pharmacological interventions, most recently including risperidone (McCracken et al. 2002). What is not yet known is whether application of these interventions to less severely affected children, such as those with PDD-NOS or subsyndromal manifestations of autistic traits, might result in even greater impact on outcome than occurs when the treatments are reserved for more severely affected children (i.e., those with full-blown autism). Answering this question should be a research priority and may ultimately inform difficult decisions regarding how to allocate limited educational, therapeutic, and financial resources for children with pervasive developmental disorders.

REFERENCES

Achenbach TM: Manual for the Child Behavior Checklist/4–18 and 1991 profile. Burlington, VT, University of Vermont, Department of Psychiatry, 1991

American Psychiatric Association: Diagnostic and Statistical Manual of Mental Disorders, 4th Edition, Text Revision. Washington, DC, American Psychiatric Association, 2000

Amir RE, Van den Veyver IB, Wan M, et al: Rett syndrome is caused by mutations in X-linked MECP2, encoding methyl-CpG-binding protein 2. Nat Genet 23:185–188, 1999

Cantor RM, Kono N, Duvall JA, et al: Replication of autism linkage: fine-mapping peak at 17q21. Am J Hum Genet 76:1050–1056, 2005

Chakrabarti S, Fombonne E: Pervasive developmental disorders in preschool children. Jama 285:3093–3099, 2001

Constantino JN: Social Responsiveness Scale. Los Angeles CA, Western Psychological Services, 2002

Constantino JN, Todd RD: Genetic structure of reciprocal social behavior. Am J Psychiatry 157:2043–2045, 2000

Constantino JN, Todd RD: Autistic traits in the general population: a twin study. Arch Gen Psychiatry 60:524–530, 2003

Constantino JN, Todd RD: Intergenerational transmission of subthreshold autistic traits in the general population. Biol Psychiatry 57:655–660, 2005

Constantino JN, Przybeck T, Friesen D, et al: Reciprocal social behavior in children with and without pervasive developmental disorders. J Dev Behav Pediatr 21:2–11, 2000

Constantino JN, Davis SA, Todd RD, et al: Validation of a brief quantitative measure of autistic traits: comparison of the Social Responsiveness Scale with the Autism Diagnostic Interview–Revised. J Autism Dev Disord 33:427–433, 2003a

Constantino JN, Hudziak JJ, Todd RD: Deficits in reciprocal social behavior in male twins: evidence for a genetically independent domain of psychopathology. J Am Acad Child Adolesc Psychiatry 42:458–467, 2003b

Constantino JN, Gruber CP, Davis S, et al: The factor structure of autistic traits. J Child Psychol Psychiatry 45:719–726, 2004

Constantino JN, Lajonchere C, Lutz M, et al: Autistic social impairment in the siblings of children with pervasive developmental disorders. Am J Psychiatry 163:294–296, 2006

Constantino JN, Abbacchi A, LaVesser P, et al: Developmental course of autistic social impairment in males. Dev Psychopathol (in press)

Cook EH Jr: Genetics of autism. Child Adolesc Psychiatr Clin N Am 10:333–350, 2001

Dawson G, Webb SJ, Wijsman E, et al: Neurocognitive and electrophysiological evidence of altered face processing in parents of children with autism: implications for a model of abnormal development of social brain circuitry in autism. Dev Psychopathol 17:679–697, 2005

Duvall JA, Lu A, Cantor RM, et al: A quantitative trait locus analysis of social responsiveness in multiplex autism families. Am J Psychiatry 164:656–662, 2007

Fombonne E: The prevalence of autism. JAMA 289:87–89, 2003

Fombonne E, Simmons H, Ford T, et al: Prevalence of pervasive developmental disorders in the British nationwide survey of child mental health. J Am Acad Child Adolesc Psychiatry 40:820–827, 2001

Gotham K, Risi S, Pickles A, et al: The Autism Diagnostic Observation Schedule: revised algorithms for improved diagnostic validity. J Autism Dev Disord 37:613–627, 2007

Howlin P, Mawhood L, Rutter M: Autism and developmental receptive language disorder—a follow-up comparison in early adult life. II: social, behavioural, and psychiatric outcomes. J Child Psychol Psychiatry 41:561–578, 2000

International Molecular Genetic Study of Autism Consortium (IMGSAC): A genomewide screen for autism: strong evidence for linkage to chromosomes 2q, 7q, and 16p. Am J Hum Genet 69:570–581, 2001

Jocelyn LJ, Casiro OG, Beattie D, et al: Treatment of children with autism: a randomized controlled trial to evaluate a caregiver-based intervention program in community day-care centers. J Dev Behav Pediatr 19:326–334, 1998

Kasari C, Freeman S, Paparella T: Joint attention and symbolic play in young children with autism: a randomized controlled intervention study. J Child Psychol Psychiatry 47:611–620, 2006

Klin A, Pauls D, Schultz R, et al: Three diagnostic approaches to Asperger syndrome: implications for research. J Autism Dev Disord 35:221–234, 2005

Kuhl PK: A new view of language acquisition. Proc Natl Acad Sci U S A 97:11850–11857, 2000

Lauritsen MB, Pedersen CB, Mortensen PB: Effects of familial risk factors and place of birth on the risk of autism: a nationwide register-based study. J Child Psychol Psychiatry 46:963–971, 2005

Le Couteur A, Bailey A, Goode S, et al: A broader phenotype of autism: the clinical spectrum in twins. J Child Psychol Psychiatry 37:785–801, 1996

Lord C, Leventhal BL, Cook EH Jr: Quantifying the phenotype in autism spectrum disorders. Am J Med Genet 105:36–38, 2001

Lovaas OI, Smith T: A comprehensive behavioral theory of autistic children: paradigm for research and treatment. J Behav Ther Exp Psychiatry 20:17–29, 1989

McCracken JT, McGough J, Shah B, et al: Risperidone in children with autism and serious behavioral problems. N Engl J Med 347:314–321, 2002

Pickles A, Bolton P, Macdonald H, et al: Latent-class analysis of recurrence risks for complex phenotypes with selection and measurement error: a twin and family history study of autism. Am J Hum Genet 57:717–726, 1995

Pickles A, Starr E, Kazak S, et al: Variable expression of the autism broader phenotype: findings from extended pedigrees. J Child Psychol Psychiatry 41:491–502, 2000

Pine E, Luby J, Abbacchi A, et al: Quantitative assessment of autistic symptomatology in preschoolers. Autism 10:344–352, 2006

Piven J, Palmer P, Jacobi D, et al: Broader autism phenotype: evidence from a family history study of multiple-incidence autism families. Am J Psychiatry 154:185–190, 1997

Risch N, Spiker D, Lotspeich L, et al: A genomic screen of autism: evidence for a multilocus etiology. Am J Hum Genet 65:493–507, 1999

Robins DL, Fein D, Barton ML, et al: The Modified Checklist for Autism in Toddlers: an initial study investigating the early detection of autism and pervasive developmental disorders. J Autism Dev Disord 31:131–144, 2001

Shao Y, Cuccaro ML, Hauser ER, et al: Fine mapping of autistic disorder to chromosome 15q11-q13 by use of phenotypic subtypes. Am J Hum Genet 72:539–548, 2003

Spiker D, Lotspeich LJ, Dimiceli S, et al: Behavioral phenotypic variation in autism multiplex families: evidence for a continuous severity gradient. Am J Med Genet 114:129–136, 2002

Stevens MC, Fein DA, Dunn M, et al: Subgroups of children with autism by cluster analysis: a longitudinal examination. J Am Acad Child Adolesc Psychiatry 39:346–352, 2000

Todd RD: Genetic advances in autism hinge on the method of measuring symptoms. Current Psychiatry Reports 7:133–137, 2005

Wolff S, Narayan S, Moyes B: Personality characteristics of parents of autistic children: a controlled study. J Child Psychol Psychiatry 29:143–153, 1988

Yeargin-Allsopp M, Rice C, Karapurkar T, et al: Prevalence of autism in a US metropolitan area. JAMA 289:49–55, 2003

Chapter 11

THE FOURTEEN-YEAR PREDICTION OF ANTISOCIAL BEHAVIOR

Frank C. Verhulst, M.D.

It is important to study violence and other antisocial behaviors within a developmental context, because these behaviors do not arise anew but are assumed to be the result of the development of such behaviors in some ordered fashion. It is believed that the development of antisocial behaviors is influenced by genetic factors, training, or the culmination of neurological, psychological, or social damage to the child. Understanding the course of such development can provide better insight into factors that are responsible for the emergence of violent and other antisocial behaviors, and this may aid in developing effective prevention or intervention strategies. Especially large-scale, prospective, longitudinal studies of general population samples are useful types of study for untangling the roots and consequences of antisocial behaviors across the lifespan (Rutter et al. 1998).

There are different definitions for describing antisocial behaviors. In criminology, the terms *delinquency* and *criminality* are used to describe behaviors that potentially can lead to conviction. In psychiatry and psychology, the term *antisocial behavior* is used to describe behaviors that violate the rights of others or that violate societal norms appropriate for a certain age. These behaviors need not be necessarily within the realm of the law. Clinicians tend to consider diagnostic categories such as oppositional defiant disorder, conduct disorder, and antisocial personality disorder. Although these disorders involve engaging in delinquent activities, the criteria for these diagnoses include behaviors that do not involve breaking the law (Rutter et al. 1998). Another approach in psychology and psychiatry is the use of continuous scales to quantify the level of antisocial behavior. A distinction can be made between overt or defiant acts and covert or sneaky acts. The former type of behavior tends to be directly aggressive or rule-breaking defiance of authority, whereas the latter type involves acts such as stealing and lying (Loeber et al. 1993). This distinction is reflected in the two Externalizing scales of the Child Behavior Checklist (CBCL; Achenbach 1991a), designated as Delinquent Behavior and Aggressive Behavior. Another distinction can be made on the basis of how overt/covert an act is on one dimension and how destructive or serious an act is on the other dimension (Frick et al. 1992).

DEVELOPMENT OF CHILDREN WITH CONDUCT DISORDER

A consistent finding in the literature is that conduct disorder in children is persistent (Offord et al. 1992) and increases the risk of antisocial personality disorder in adulthood (Farrington 1999; Rutter 1995; Zoccolillo et al. 1992) in both clinical and nonclinical samples (Cohen et al. 1993; Robins 1991).

One of the few long-term, prospective cohort studies into the development of psychopathology in the general population from birth into adulthood is the Dunedin Longitudinal Birth Cohort Study (Caspi et al. 1996; Feehan et al. 1993; Moffit 1990). In this study, conduct disorder was associated with the highest risk for later psychopathology measured across the interval from ages 15–18 years. Attention-deficit/hyperactivity disorder (ADHD) was associated with the lowest risk for later disorder. In another study of the same sample, but with measurements across a much larger time interval, it was found that children at age 3 years with undercontrolled behavior, such as impulsive, restless, and distracted behavior, had a greater probability of having antisocial personality disorder at age 21 years and of committing criminal acts than children who showed normal behavior at age 3 years (Caspi et al. 1996).

Studies that describe the development of children with behaviors that resemble, but are not equivalent to, conduct disorder criteria, clearly showed that these children are at increased risk for later antisocial behaviors, even as adults (Farrington 1991a, 1991b, 1999).

STABILITY OF AGGRESSION

Olweus (1979), in an early overview of studies investigating the stability of aggression in boys, found that the stability of aggression measured with continuous scales is considerable and comparable to the stability of intelligence measures. This finding indicates that those individuals who could be regarded as the most aggressive within the study population could still be regarded as the most aggressive at later measurements of the same population. Other studies looking at the stability of overt aggressive behaviors not only confirmed the considerable stability of these behaviors in boys but also showed that the stability of overt aggression in girls was high (Achenbach et al. 1995).

DEVELOPMENTAL THEORIES OF ANTISOCIAL BEHAVIOR

So far, studies have been discussed that reported the overall association between measures of antisocial behavior assessed at two time points without taking into account factors such as age at onset, type of behavior, and the developmental trajectory individuals followed during the interval between the first and the last measurement. If we know more about which developmental trajectories will lead to later antisocial behavior, which factors increase the likelihood of following such trajectories, and which individuals run the greatest risk, then we may more effectively develop strategies for preventing and treating these deviant developmental pathways. The two most widely cited theoretical frameworks for describing developmental trajectories of antisocial behavior are the ones described by Moffitt (1993) and Loeber and Hay (1994).

Moffit (1993) hypothesized two developmental trajectories: the life-course persistent pattern consisting of antisocial behavior spanning childhood and adolescence into adulthood, and the adolescence-limited pattern with antisocial behavior, which usually starts in early adolescence and desists in late adolescence. The life-course persistent group is characterized, at young age, by adverse temperamental features such as restlessness, inattention, and negativism; by cognitive, motor, and language deficits; and, at later age, by reading difficulties, aggressiveness, impulsivity, adverse family contexts, and a lack of social closeness. There seems to be an interaction between neuropsychological dysfunction and adverse environmental influences. This group of children is characterized both by an unusually early age at onset of antisocial behavior and a tendency to persist into adult life. The adolescence-limited pattern is characterized by an onset of antisocial behavior in adolescence and a lack of persistence into adult life. This pattern arises from a teenager's attempt to escape the "maturity gap" by adopting the behavioral styles of antisocial peers, who seem older. Their behavior is more or less normative, and they do not show high levels of psychopathology.

Loeber and Hay (1994) describe a three-pathway model to antisocial behavior in boys by splitting overt acts into those that represent aggression and those that represent authority defiance. The overt pathway begins with childhood aggression, such as annoying and bullying others as the first step, followed by physical fighting, and then violent crime. The covert pathway begins with minor covert behaviors such as shoplifting and lying and then progresses to property damage such as vandalism and fire setting, and then to moderate to serious delinquency such as fraud, burglary, and serious theft. The authority conflict pathway progresses from stubborn behavior in childhood to acts of defiance and open disobedience, to more serious acts such as truancy, running away, and staying out late, and applies to juveniles below age 12 years. This model combines age at onset of antisocial behavior, type of behavior, and the involvement in a sequence of behavior. The Loeber and Hay model, like the model by Moffitt, indicate that the earlier the onset of problems, the worst the prognosis will be. In addition, Loeber and Hay state that the more types of problems seen, the greater the likelihood of serious and long-standing delinquency.

THE ZUID-HOLLAND PROSPECTIVE LONGITUDINAL STUDY

To determine the development of psychopathology from childhood/adolescence into adulthood, we conducted a 14-year prospective longitudinal study starting in 1983 with a random sample of 2,076 4- to 16-year-old subjects from the general population (Verhulst et al. 1985a, 1985b). The sample was assessed with 2-year intervals across an 8-year period from 1983 to 1991 and again 6 years later in 1997, 14 years after the first assessment. At the last assessment, 1,578 subjects participated, which is nearly 80% of the original sample after correction for deceased, handicapped, or emigrated subjects (Hofstra et al. 2000a, 2000b, 2001, 2002).

Problem behavior of children younger than 18 years was assessed with the CBCL (Achenbach 1991a; Verhulst et al. 1996), a parent questionnaire for quantifying a broad range of psychopathology. For children between the ages of 11 and 18 years, a self-report version of the CBCL, the Youth Self-Report (YSR; Achenbach 1991b; Verhulst et al. 1997), was used. At the last assessment, psychopathology was assessed with a version of the CBCL to be completed by parents of their adult son or daughter, the Young Adult Behavior Checklist (YABCL; Achenbach 1997), and the extension of the YSR to be completed for ages over 18 years, the Young Adult Self-Report (YASR; Achenbach 1997). In addition, during the last assessment, subjects were interviewed using a standardized psychiatric interview, the Composite

International Diagnostic Interview (CIDI) (World Health Organization 1992).

The CBCL and related instruments can be scored on the following scales: Anxious/Depressed, Withdrawn, and Somatic Complaints (together constituting the Internalizing scale); Aggressive Behavior and Delinquent Behavior (together constituting the Externalizing scale); and Social Problems, Thought Problems, and Attention Problems. The sum of all problem scores is the Total Problems scale.

CONTINUITY OF ANTISOCIAL BEHAVIOR

To determine the continuity of antisocial behaviors across the 14-year time interval, we determined the proportion of subjects who scored in the deviant range at time 1 on the Externalizing, the Aggressive Behavior, and the Delinquent Behavior scales, and who could still be regarded as deviant 14 years later on the corresponding scale. Table 11–1 shows the percentages of subjects who scored in the deviant range on the CBCL at time 1 and who continued scoring in the deviant range on the YABCL (parent information at both times of assessment) or the YASR (parent information at time 1 and self-report information at time 2).

As can be seen, the percentage of subjects who were scored in the deviant range of the problem scales representing antisocial behaviors and who could still be regarded as deviant 14 years later was considerable for most scales and for both sexes and age groups. For example, the percentage of subjects who were in the deviant range of the Externalizing scale at time 1 and who were still deviant at the last assessment 14 years later ranged from 37% to 52%. There is a scarcity of information regarding the stability of antisocial behaviors in girls as compared with boys. Therefore, a remarkable finding was that the stability of antisocial behaviors was greater for females than for males for the majority of scales. Another finding was that the stability for more overt behaviors exemplified by the Aggressive Behavior scale was not much different than that for more covert behaviors represented by the Delinquent Behavior scale.

PREDICTION OF DSM-IV DIAGNOSES

The CIDI was used to assess DSM-IV diagnoses (American Psychiatric Association 1994) in the total sample of 1,578 18- to 30-year-old subjects. We used the modules for the diagnoses antisocial personality disorder, oppositional disorder, and ADHD of the Diagnostic Interview Schedule (DIS; Robins et al. 1997) because these diagnoses were not included in the CIDI.

TABLE 11–1. Percentage of subjects who were deviant at both assessments across the 14-year interval for the scales Externalizing, Delinquent Behavior, and Aggressive Behavior

	Externalizing				Delinquent Behavior				Aggressive Behavior			
	Male		Female		Male		Female		Male		Female	
Age at onset, years	4–11	12–16	4–11	12–16	4–11	12–16	4–11	12–16	4–11	12–16	4–11	12–16
CBCL×YABCL	44	37	42	52	17	22	27	33	18	5	23	33
CBCL×YASR	30	26	34	33	16	17	0	27	17	14	14	19

Note. CBCL=Child Behavior Checklist; YABCL=Young Adult Behavior Checklist; YASR=Young Adult Self-Report.

Because of the small numbers in each separate diagnostic category, we placed the DSM-IV diagnoses into four main categories: anxiety disorders (11.7%), mood disorders (5.4%), substance use disorders (4.1%), and disruptive disorders (3.7%). The disruptive disorders group consisted of antisocial personality disorder (3.0%), oppositional disorder (0.4%), and ADHD (0.4%). The diagnosis of antisocial personality disorder occurred more frequently in males (5.5%) than females (0.8%).

We determined associations between CBCL scale scores at time 1, with DSM-IV diagnoses 14 years later in males and females separately. We used odds ratios to determine the strength of the association. CBCL scales were dichotomized into scores in the deviant range and scores in the normal range (see Hofstra et al. 2000a).

We first looked at the predictive associations of the CBCL scales that are related to antisocial behavior: Delinquent Behavior and Aggressive Behavior (for associations of the other CBCL scales, see Hofstra et al. 2000a). That is, we looked at parent-reported problem behavior in childhood or adolescence and determined its power to predict DSM-IV diagnoses in adulthood 14 years later.

Next we looked at adult DSM-IV diagnoses of disruptive disorders and determined which CBCL scale scores were associated with the presence of these disruptive disorders. That is, we started in adulthood and looked at which problems in childhood/adolescence assessed 14 years earlier predicted adult antisocial behaviors. Logistic regression analyses were performed to determine the strength of the associations. First, univariate logistic regressions were performed between each CBCL scale and each DSM-IV group of disorders separately. Next, we controlled for the intercorrelations between CBCL scales by performing multivariate logistic regression analyses. In the multivariate analyses, possible interactions with age at initial assessment were determined (age groups 4–11 and 12–16 years). The figures in this chapter give the significant associations in univariate analyses. Associations that were not significant (and for Figure 11–4 those associations that remained significant) in multivariate analyses are indicated with an asterisk.

ASSOCIATIONS FROM CHILDHOOD/ ADOLESCENCE INTO ADULTHOOD

Figure 11–1 gives the associations between the parent-reported CBCL Delinquent Behavior problem scale for the sample ages 4–16 years at initial assessment, with DSM-IV diagnoses determined 14 years later for the same sample. For males, the Delinquent Behavior scale predicted both mood dis-

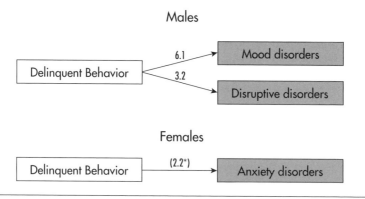

FIGURE 11–1. Associations between the Child Behavior Checklist Delinquent Behavior scale and later DSM-IV diagnoses.

*Not significant in multivariate analysis.

orders and disruptive disorders. Both associations remained significant in the multivariate analysis. Apparently, the covert antisocial behaviors reflected by the Delinquent Behavior scale, such as stealing, lying, truancy, and vandalism, persist into adulthood. From this study it is not possible to determine what the reasons for this persistence are. It is possible that the persistence of antisocial behavior is an autonomic process in which the same kind of antisocial behavior persists or in which one type of antisocial behavior is succeeded by another more or less independent of environmental influences. Also, it is possible that the persistence of antisocial behavior is the result of persisting negative environmental influences. Finally, it is possible that both influences interact. For example, it is possible that antisocial behavior in childhood has a negative effect on school functioning or on the relationships with significant adults, which in turn strengthens the antisocial behavior.

Males who were scored in the deviant range on Delinquent Behavior not only had a higher probability of having a DSM-IV diagnosis of disruptive behavior, they were also more likely to have a mood disorder 14 years later. Females who were scored in the deviant range on Delinquent Behavior were more likely to have an anxiety disorder 14 years later. However, this association did not remain significant when the other CBCL scales in the multivariate analysis were controlled for. It was thus striking that covert antisocial behavior in females ages 4–16 years was not predictive of disruptive disorders in adulthood.

In another study with the same sample, we determined the ability of the Delinquent Behavior scale to predict a number of poor outcomes 14 years later, including arrest by police, expulsion from school or job, alcohol abuse,

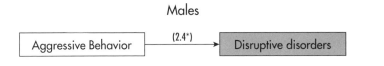

FIGURE 11–2. Association between Child Behavior Checklist Aggressive Behavior scale and later DSM-IV diagnoses.

*Not significant in multivariate analysis.

and no formal education beyond elementary school. Delinquent behavior did not predict any of these poor outcomes in females, whereas in males delinquent behavior predicted arrest, alcohol abuse, and absence of formal education beyond elementary school 14 years later. In conclusion, covert antisocial behaviors reflected by the Delinquent Behavior scale were a clear predictor of antisocial behavior in males but not in females across a 14-year time span.

Figure 11–2 gives the only association between the Aggressive Behavior scale and later DSM-IV diagnoses. Only for males was it found that aggressive behavior predicted disruptive disorders. However, this association did not remain significant in the multivariate analysis. Aggressive behavior did not predict DSM-IV diagnoses in females. It did predict later alcohol abuse in females, but not in males, and in males it predicted the absence of formal education beyond elementary school. In conclusion, overt behaviors as reflected by the Aggressive Behavior scale were not a strong independent predictor of adult antisocial behaviors.

It is striking that covert behaviors represented by the Delinquent Behavior scale in childhood and adolescence seem more predictive of later antisocial behaviors than overt behaviors represented by the Aggressive Behavior scale. This difference in prediction of DSM-IV diagnoses and other poor outcome variables was present despite the fact that the persistence for aggressive behavior is not much less than that for delinquent behavior (Table 11–1). Genetic studies showed that the genetic component is stronger for the Aggressive Behavior scale than for the Delinquent Behavior scale (Edelbrock et al. 1995; van den Oord et al. 1994). For the Delinquent Behavior scale, the influence of environmental factors was larger. It may be that overt aggressive behaviors in childhood and adolescence as measured by the CBCL Aggressive Behavior scale represent genetically determined temperamental features that may cause problems with the environment when they are present but do not as such greatly increase the risk for antisocial behaviors.

Figure 11–3 gives the only association for the Attention Problems scale with later DSM-IV disorders. Only in males did this scale predict disruptive

Males

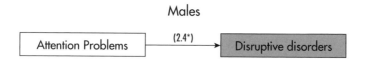

FIGURE 11–3. Association between Child Behavior Checklist Attention Problems scale and later DSM-IV diagnoses.

*Not significant in multivariate analysis.

disorders. It should be noted that this association did not remain significant when the effects of the other "comorbid" scales were controlled for in the multivariate analysis. This negative finding supports the finding by Fergusson et al. (1997), who found that attention problems at age 8 years were not predictive of criminal behavior or substance abuse at age 18 years in a birth cohort when the effects of comorbid antisocial behavior were controlled for. Attention problems in the Fergusson et al. (1997) study were associated with later school failure. Studies reporting on the adult outcome of childhood ADHD diagnoses often pertain to clinical samples (Rutter et al. 2006). These studies show that childhood ADHD is the precursor of later antisocial disorder, even in the absence of co-occurring disruptive behaviors in childhood. However, factors other than comorbidity that are associated with referral may influence the course of childhood ADHD.

There were no significant interactions between the CBCL scales and age group in the prediction of disruptive disorders. The hypothesis by Loeber and Hay (1994) and Moffitt (1993) that the earlier the onset of antisocial behaviors, the greater its impact on later functioning, could not be confirmed by these analyses of the 14-year prediction of DSM-IV diagnoses. It may be, however, that our sample, despite the fact that it contained 1,578 individuals from the general population, was too small to capture enough young individuals with highly problematic behaviors.

PRECURSORS OF DSM-IV DIAGNOSES IN ADULTHOOD

Figure 11–4 shows which CBCL scales predicted later DSM-IV disruptive disorders. In the univariate analyses, five CBCL scales were associated with later disruptive disorders in males. After correction for intercorrelations of the CBCL scales, only the Anxious/Depressed and Delinquent Behavior scales remained independent predictors of later disruptive disorders. For boys who were scored in the deviant range at initial assessment on both scales, the odds ratio indicating the risk for later disruptive disorder was $3.2 \times 2.5 =$

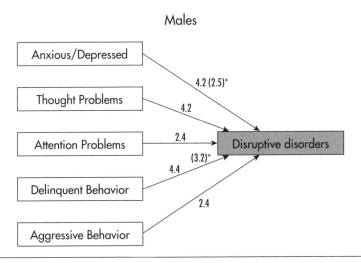

FIGURE 11–4. **Child Behavior Checklist scales predicting later DSM-IV disruptive disorders.**

Note. Multivariate odds ratios are in parentheses.
*Scales that stayed significant in multivariate analysis.

8.0. This corroborates findings that depressed children who also showed antisocial behaviors had a greater risk for criminality in adulthood than depressed children who did not show antisocial behavior (Harrington et al. 1991). No CBCL scales were found to predict disruptive behaviors in adult females.

DEVELOPMENTAL TRAJECTORIES OF ANTISOCIAL BEHAVIORS

To test major developmental pathways models as described by Moffitt (1993) and Loeber and Hay (1993) in a more direct way, Bongers et al. (2004) computed group-based developmental trajectories of CBCL problem scores, using the semi-parametric mixture model-fitting procedure as proposed by Nagin and Tremblay (1999). Analyses were performed on the four measurements with 2-year intervals across an 8-year period in the Zuid-Holland longitudinal sample. Trajectories covered developmental changes from ages 4 to 18 years. Associations between developmental trajectories and psychiatric or criminal outcomes assessed at 14 years from initial assessment were computed. To organize the CBCL Externalizing items, Bongers et al. used the following four clusters of behaviors proposed by Frick et al. (1992): aggression, opposition, property violations, and status violations.

The trajectories for the scales designated as Aggression, Opposition, and Property Violations showed an overall decrease in severity from childhood to adolescence, whereas Status Violations showed a developmental increase from childhood to adolescence.

Within each of the four behavioral problem clusters, three to six different group-based developmental pathways could be determined, and most of these different trajectories followed the shape of the average trajectories at various levels of severity. Within each cluster the largest group of individuals followed a developmental trajectory at a low level, indicating that most individuals showed very little externalizing problems during their development from ages 4 to 18 years as reported by their parents.

Because much less is known about the development of antisocial behaviors in girls versus boys, it was important to find that despite the fact that more boys than girls could be assigned to the higher (more problematic) trajectories, the shape of the trajectories did not differ for boys versus girls.

The high-level trajectories indicated that the most troublesome children tended to be the most troublesome adolescents. Individuals who persistently showed high levels of antisocial behaviors from childhood into young adulthood followed a developmental pattern that was designated as "life-course persistent" by Moffitt (1993). However, we could not identify the developmental pattern of antisocial behaviors referred to as "adolescence limited" by Moffitt (1993). We did identify within the clusters Opposition and Status Violations a group with increasingly high levels in adolescence, but the severity of these problems did not level off until the upper limit of age 18 years in this study.

Another finding was that, contrary to the results of studies indicating that oppositional behaviors become less common after the transition from childhood to adolescence, behaviors represented by the Opposition cluster in this study remained more common than those represented by the other clusters. Of course, it should be stressed that this study used parent information, and it may well be that parents were largely unaware of externalizing behaviors exhibited by their adolescent son or daughter.

It will not come as a surprise that individuals in the most problematic trajectories run the highest risk for a variety of psychiatric disorders, including antisocial personality disorder and mood disorders. However, it was a surprise to find that, despite the recent emphasis on physically aggressive behavior as a precursor of later violent delinquency, we found deviant trajectories of physically aggressive behaviors to be the least problematic. Only in combination with deviant trajectories of opposition or status violations did they show adverse outcomes.

CONCLUSIONS

The stability of antisocial behaviors across the 14-year time span of the Zuid-Holland prospective longitudinal study from ages 4–16 to 18–30 years was considerable. A remarkable finding was that the stability of antisocial behaviors for females was not smaller than that found for males. A different picture emerged when we looked at the prediction of adult disruptive disorders from CBCL scores obtained in childhood/adolescence. The CBCL scales predicted later disruptive disorders in males but not in females. This may be caused by the fact that the prevalence of DSM-IV disruptive disorders in females was very low. However, the diagnostic criteria for antisocial personality disorder—the most prevalent diagnosis in the disruptive behavior category—reflect antisocial behavior that is more typical for males than for females. If the criteria for antisocial personality disorder had been more representative of female antisocial behavior, then the prevalence and possibly the prediction of antisocial behavior in adult women from childhood/adolescent problem behavior would have been different. The inclusion of relational aggression in the diagnostic criteria for antisocial personality disorder especially might have resulted in different findings.

The findings of the Zuid-Holland study correspond with those reviewed by Loeber and Farrington (1998). Antisocial behavior in childhood or adolescence is a predictor of antisocial behavior in adulthood, even across the long follow-up interval of 14 years, as in our study. The combination of covert antisocial behavior and affective problems in childhood/adolescence is an especially potent predictor of adult antisocial behavior.

There were also findings that did not correspond with what one would expect. Despite its persistence, physically aggressive behavior at a young age was only weakly associated with later disruptive disorders after correction for the influence of other problems. The same was true for attention problems, which did not independently predict later disruptive disorders. Most research showing poor long-term prognosis of childhood ADHD, even after taking comorbid antisocial behaviors into account, pertains to clinical samples. However, referred children differ in many ways from children with the same type and level of problems from the general population, including the presence of negative environmental factors that may negatively influence development.

Using statistical techniques (semi-parametric mixture model–fitting procedures) that take full advantage of the multiple assessments in the Zuid-Holland study, we determined developmental trajectories that reflected developmental changes from ages 4 to 18 years. On the basis of these analyses we confirmed a number of findings that can be found in the literature, including the poor long-term prognosis of persistently high levels of antisocial behaviors in childhood and adolescence. However, some of our findings could not confirm what other people found or theorized. For example, our findings showed that the prognosis of adolescent antisocial behaviors is about as problematic as the prognosis for childhood antisocial behaviors that persisted across adolescence; we could not find a developmental trajectory of antisocial behaviors that started in early adolescence and ended by the beginning of young adulthood. Another finding that surprised us was that physically aggressive behaviors in childhood or adolescence had a much better prognosis than other types of disruptive behaviors such as oppositional behaviors or status violations.

More research is needed to gain more insight into the different developmental trajectories toward antisocial behavior into which children can go. Such knowledge may help us identify children at risk at an early age. It may also help us understanding which factors put children at risk and which factors protect them from going into deviant pathways. This kind of knowledge may aid us developing more effective prevention and treatment programs. This kind of research should aim at multiple risk and protective factors, multiple assessments, using multiple informants, including the child him- or herself, parents, and teachers. Teachers especially are an important source, and not only for information that may help identifying children at risk at a young age. Teachers are also important for implementing preventive and treatment programs to prevent children at risk from going into developmental trajectories that are detrimental to themselves, their families, and to society at large. Another area in which progress can be made is in the methodology of identifying individuals who show developmental trajectories that deviate from pathways followed by normally developing children. Longitudinal screening—that is, the identification of individuals who are at risk for showing long-lasting problem behaviors based on multiple measurements—may be a more accurate approach than the identification of at-risk children through cross-sectional screening. It is important that more experience be gained in the identification of children who are most at risk for serious deviant development.

REFERENCES

Achenbach TM: Manual for the Child Behavior Checklist/4–18 and 1991 Profile. Burlington, University of Vermont, Department of Psychiatry, 1991a

Achenbach TM: Manual for the Youth Self-Report and 1991 Profile. Burlington, University of Vermont, Department of Psychiatry, 1991b

Achenbach TM: Manual for the Young Adult Self Report and Young Adult Behavior Checklist. Burlington, University of Vermont, Department of Psychiatry, 1997

Achenbach TM, Howell C, McConaughy S, et al: Six-year predictors of problems in a national sample, III: transitions to young adult syndrome. J Am Acad Child Adolesc Psychiatry 34:658–669, 1995

American Psychiatric Association: Diagnostic and Statistical Manual of Mental Disorders, 4th Edition. Washington, DC, American Psychiatric Association, 1994

Bongers IL, Koot HM, van der Ende J, et al: Developmental trajectories of externalizing behaviors in childhood and adolescence. Child Dev 75:1523–1537, 2004

Caspi A, Moffitt TE, Newman DL, et al: Behavioral observations at age 3 years predict adult psychiatric disorders. Arch Gen Psychiatry 53:1033–1039, 1996

Cohen P, Cohen J, Brook J: An epidemiological study of disorders in late childhood and adolescence: 2. Persistence of disorders. J Child Psychol Psychiatry 34:869–877, 1993

Edelbrock C, Rende R, Plomin R, et al: A twin study of competence and problem behavior in childhood and early adolescence. J Child Psychol Psychiatry 36:775-785, 1995

Farrington DP: Antisocial personality from childhood to adulthood. Psychologist 4:389–394, 1991a

Farrington DP: Childhood aggression and adult violence: early precursors and later-life outcomes, in The Development and Treatment of Childhood Aggression. Edited by Pepler DJ, Rubin KH. Hillsdale, NJ, Erlbaum, 1991b, pp 5–29

Farrington DP: Conduct disorder and delinquency, in Risks and Outcomes in Developmental Psychopathology. Edited by Steinhausen HC, Verhulst FC. Oxford, UK, Oxford University Press, 1999, pp 165–192

Feehan M, McGee R, Williams S: Mental health disorders from age 15 to age 18 years. J Am Acad Child Adolesc Psychiatry 32:1118–1126, 1993

Fergusson DM, Lynskey MT, Horwood LJ: Attentional difficulties in middle childhood and psychosocial outcomes in young adulthood. J Child Psychol Psychiatry 38:633–644, 1997

Frick PJ, Lahey BB, Loeber R, et al: Familial risk factors to oppositional defiant disorder and conduct disorder: parental psychopathology and maternal parenting. J Consult Clin Psychol 60:49–55, 1992

Harrington R, Fudge H, Rutter M, et al: Adult outcomes of childhood and adolescent depression: 2. Links with antisocial disorders. J Am Acad Child Adolesc Psychiatry 30:434–439, 1991

Hofstra MB, Van der Ende J, Verhulst FC: Child and adolescent problems predict DSM-IV disorders in adulthood: a 14-year follow-up of a Dutch epidemiological sample. J Am Acad Child Adolesc Psychiatry 41:182–189, 2000a

Hofstra MB, Van der Ende J, Verhulst FC: Continuity and change of psychopathology from childhood into adulthood: a 14-year follow-up study. J Am Acad Child Adolesc Psychiatry 39:850–858, 2000b

Hofstra MB, Van der Ende J and Verhulst FC: Adolescents' self-reported problems as predictors of psychopathology in adulthood: 10-year follow-up study. Br J Psychiatry 179:203–209, 2001

Hofstra MB, Van der Ende J and Verhulst FC: Pathways of self-reported problem behaviors from adolescence into adulthood. Am J Psychiatry 159:401–407, 2002

Loeber R, Farrington DP (eds): Serious and Violent Juvenile Offenders: Risk Factors and Successful Interventions. Thousand Oaks, CA, Sage, 1998

Loeber R, Hay DF: Developmental approaches to aggression and conduct problems, in Development Through Life: A Handbook for Clinicians. Edited by Rutter M, Hay DF. Oxford, UK, Blackwell Scientific, 1994, pp 488–515

Loeber R, Wung P, Kennan K, et al: Developmental pathways in disruptive child behavior. Dev Psychopathol 5:101–132, 1993

Moffitt TE: Juvenile delinquency and attention deficit disorder: boys' developmental trajectories from age 3 to age 15. Child Dev 61:893–910, 1990

Moffitt TE: Adolescence-limited and life-course-persistent antisocial behavior: a developmental taxonomy. Psychol Rev 100:674–701, 1993

Nagin D, Tremblay RE: Trajectories of boys' physical aggression, opposition, and hyperactivity on the path to physically violent and nonviolent juvenile delinquency. Child Dev 70:1181–1196, 1999

Offord DR, Boyle MH, Racine YA, et al: Outcome prognosis and risk in a longitudinal follow-up study. J Am Acad Child Adolesc Psychiatry 31:919–923, 1992

Olweus D: Stability of aggressive reaction patterns in males: a review. Psychol Bull 86:852–875, 1979

Robins LN: Conduct disorder. J Child Psychol Psychiatry 32:193–212, 1991

Robins LN, Cottler L, Bucholtz K, et al: NIMH Diagnostic Interview Schedule for DSM-IV (NIMH DIS-IV), Bethesda, MD, National Institute of Mental Health, 1997

Rutter M: Relationships between mental disorders in childhood and adulthood. Acta Psychiatr Scand 91:73–85, 1995

Rutter M, Giller H, Hagell A: Antisocial Behavior by Young People. Cambridge, UK, Cambridge University Press, 1998, p 124

Rutter M, Kim-Cohen J, Maughan B: Continuities and discontinuities in psychopathology between childhood and adult life. J Child Psychol Psychiatry 47:276–295, 2006

van den Oord EJ, Boomsma DI, Verhulst FC: A study of problem behaviors in 10- to 15-year-old biologically related and unrelated international adoptees. Behav Genet 24:193–205, 1994

Verhulst FC, Akkerhuis GW, Althaus M: Mental health in Dutch children, I: a cross-cultural comparison. Acta Psychiatr Scand Suppl 323:1–108, 1985a

Verhulst FC, Berden GF, Sanders-Woudstra JAR: Mental health in Dutch children, II: the prevalence of psychiatric disorder and relationships between measures. Acta Psychiatr Scand Suppl 324:1–45, 1985b

Verhulst FC, van der Ende J, Koot HM: [Manual for the CBCL/4–18]. Rotterdam, the Netherlands, Sophia Children's Hospital/Erasmus University, Department of Psychiatry, 1996

Verhulst FC, van der Ende J, Koot HM: [Manual for the Youth Self-Report (YSR)]. Rotterdam, the Netherlands, Sophia Children's Hospital/Erasmus University, Department of Psychiatry, 1997

World Health Organization: Composite International Diagnostic Interview. Geneva, World Health Organization, 1992

Zoccolillo M, Pickles A, Quinton D, et al: The outcome of childhood conduct disorder: implications for defining adult personality disorder and conduct disorder. Psychol Med 22:71–986, 1992

Part 4

THE FUTURE OF
THE STUDY OF
DEVELOPMENTAL
PSYCHOPATHOLOGY
IN GENETICS AND
CLINICAL SETTINGS

Chapter 12

STATISTICAL AND MOLECULAR GENETIC APPROACHES TO DEVELOPMENTAL PSYCHOPATHOLOGY

The Pathway Forward

Stephen V. Faraone, Ph.D.

Family twin and adoption studies have unequivocally demonstrated that genes influence most if not all psychiatric disorders. As Figures 12–1A and 12–1B show, the relative contributions of genes and environment vary widely among these illnesses. These figures show that, as estimated from twin studies, the heritability of psychiatric disorder ranges from highs of 0.75 and greater for attention-deficit/hyperactivity disorder (ADHD), autism, schizophrenia, and bipolar disorder to lows less than 0.30 for many person-

This work was supported in part by grants to S.V. Faraone, Ph.D., from the National Institutes of Health (R01MH66877; R21MH/NS66191; R01MH62873).

ality disorders and phobias. Twenty years ago, many of us thought that applying the tools of molecular genetics to highly heritable disorders would yield disease genes and their underlying mechanisms in short order. We were wrong. Today, we know that most psychiatric disorders have a complex genetic architecture with a hidden blueprint that has been difficult to discover.

It is somewhat disconcerting that the field of psychiatric genetics might have saved valuable time if we had read more earnestly Gottesman and Shields's (1967) defense of the multifactorial model of schizophrenia. They realized four decades ago that the pattern of results from genetic epidemiology studies showed that many genes worked together to cause schizophrenia and that the single-gene model defended so eloquently by Paul Meehl (1962) simply did not fit the data. A decade after their work, more complex segregation analysis studies of schizophrenia (Faraone and Tsuang 1985) and other psychiatric disorders (Faraone et al. 1990) showed that Gottesman and Shield's multifactorial hypothesis was correct, not only for schizophrenia but also for other disorders.

These considerations suggest that for the complex psychiatric disorders the prospects for gene discovery are bleak. The goal of this chapter is to counter that view by examining the following questions: 1) What are the relative values of linkage and association studies? 2) Can meta-analysis clarify conflicting findings? 3) How can environmental risk factors facilitate molecular genetic studies? 4) Are endophenotypes useful for molecular genetic studies? 5) How should one address etiologic heterogeneity? and 6) Can we move beyond putative statistical significance to document the functional significance of DNA variants associated with psychopathology?

LINKAGE OR ASSOCIATION?

For decades, the two main molecular genetic methods applied to psychiatric research were association and linkage studies. Using the method of association, investigators would study specific genes relevant to the pathophysiology of disorders in the hopes of discovering variants that predisposed to illness. Because the DNA found in blood was, in the absence of epigenetic effects, the same as the DNA found in brain, studies of candidate genes seemed to open a window for studying the brain that had not previously been possible.

Unfortunately, candidate gene studies have, with some exceptions, produced conflicting and inconsistent results, which is likely due to the multifactorial nature of these disorders. When many genes cause a disorder their individual contributions to the heritability of the disorder are small, which

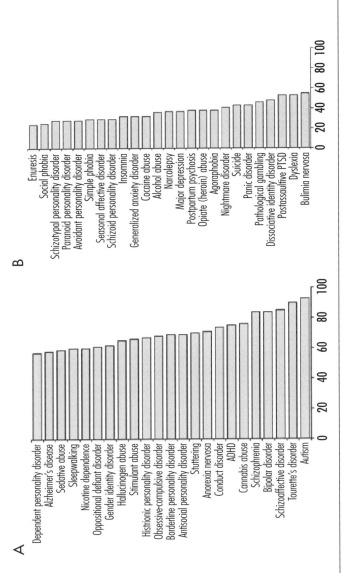

FIGURE 12–1. Heritabilities of psychiatric disorders.

(A) Disorders having higher heritabilities. (B) Disorders having lower heritabilities.
ADHD=attention–deficit/hyperactivity disorder; PTSD=posttraumatic stress disorder.

greatly reduces the statistical power of molecular genetic studies. This problem worsens in the presence of gene–environment interaction and epistasis and therefore leads to a paradoxical statistical fact: when a disease allele is detected in a modest sample size, the probability of replicating that finding in a second sample of the same size is very low, even if the disease allele detected is a causal allele in both samples (Suarez et al. 1994). To replicate the original finding, a much larger sample size would be needed. This leads to the counterintuitive prediction that in dealing with modest sample sizes, if we were to attempt an exact replication of a positive linkage or association study, we would not reproduce the positive finding. A corollary of this work is that a typical linkage or association study of a multifactorial disorder will have high power to detect one of many genes yet very low power to detect a specific gene. Put simply, when studying multifactorial conditions with modest sample sizes, we expect conflicting and inconsistent results.

The candidate gene method was also limited by the availability of true candidate genes. Crowe (1993) described most candidate genes as "lottery tickets," based on the observation that most were chosen on the basis of thin theoretical justifications rather than solid foundations of empirical work. Many candidate genes had been chosen based on prior knowledge of drug effects. For example, the effects of typical neuroleptics on the D_2 dopamine receptor generated many studies of D_2 in schizophrenia, although ultimately a meta-analysis suggested the gene was not associated with schizophrenia (Glatt et al. 2004). The effects of dopamine reuptake inhibitors (e.g., stimulants) led ADHD researchers to study the dopamine transporter gene (Cook et al. 1995), and the effects of norepinephrine reuptake inhibitors on the disorder led to the study of the norepinephrine transporter gene (Yang et al. 2004). These theories, in turn, motivated association studies of candidate genes in dopaminergic and serotonergic pathways. Similar patterns of psychopharmacology-driven genetic research were seen in studies of the serotonergic system in depression and obsessive-compulsive disorder.

Initially, the method of linkage analysis seemed to solve the problems posed by the method of association. By screening the entire genome, linkage analysis theoretically could detect genes without specifying beforehand the name of the gene or even how it might be involved in the etiology of a disorder. Although linkage analysis had been extremely successful for single-gene disorders, its shortcomings for multifactorial disorders soon became evident. Empirical evidence was seen in the many linkage studies of schizophrenia and mood disorders that did not yield clear results, even when studies were pooled through meta-analysis (Badner and Gershon 2002a; Lewis et al. 2003). Risch and Merikangas (1996) used simulated data to show that between 185 and 4,260 families (depending on the frequency of the disease allele) would be needed to detect a locus containing a gene that was responsible for a fourfold increase in the risk of disorder to relatives of patients having the disorder. The number of families required to detect a gene that only increases risk by 50% (between approximately 18,000 and 4.6 million families) is so excessive as to be practically impossible. This was a sobering analysis given that it now appears that most susceptibility genes for psychiatric disorders will increase risk by about 50%–100%.

These considerations have led the field to change course again so that currently the method of association is favored. According to Risch and Merikangas (1996), this method could detect a gene affording a 50% increased risk to relatives with as few as 949 parent–child trios. Fortunately, users of association methods can escape the limitations of the candidate gene approach. This has been made possible by the creation of the HapMap (Gibbs et al. 2003) and the advent of genotyping technologies that have made it feasible to screen the entire genome by using the method of association. With these commercially available genotyping platforms, researchers can be assured that nearly all the genes in the genome are close enough to a DNA marker so that any gene could be detected if causally involved in the disease. Because the method no longer requires users to specify candidate genes, it retains the potential for discovering new biological pathways to disease expression.

Whole-genome association studies face a serious multiple comparison problem. For example, one commonly used whole-genome association genotyping platform requires that 500,000 DNA markers be assayed to complete a whole genome scan. If we apply a Bonferroni correction to the entire panel of markers, we would need a P value of 0.0000001 to declare genome-wide statistical significance. The implications for statistical power and sample size are obvious. For a case–control study to maintain a power of 0.90 to detect a 5% versus 2.5% difference in allele frequencies, more than 5,000 cases and 5,000 control subjects would be required. For a difference of 15% versus 10%, nearly 4,000 cases and 4,000 control subjects would be needed.

There are numerous approaches to multiple comparisons that help reduce this problem, such as the sequential Bonferroni (Holm 1979), false discovery rate procedures (Benjamini and Hochberg 1995; Storey and Tibshirani 2001, 2003), and methods that address the intercorrelations among genetic markers (Nyholt 2004). Although these methods provide small increases in power, the only way to substantially increase power would be to find a way to reduce the number of statistical tests. Fortunately, such a reduction is possible with the family-based association test (FBAT)/power FBAT (PBAT) suite of analytic tools.

FBAT and PBAT are based on a unified approach to family-based association analysis that allows valid testing of association with any phenotype, sampling structure, and pattern of missing marker allele information (Horvath et al. 2001, 2004; Lange et al. 2004). The FBAT/PBAT approach provides an elegant solution to the very severe problem of multiple comparisons created by the many single nucleotide polymorphisms (SNPs) typed in a genome-wide association scan. By using information from families that are not informative for a given SNP, PBAT selects a set of SNPs with the most power to detect association in a manner that does not bias the statistical test of association in the informative families (Lange et al. 2003a, 2003b). This reduces the multiple comparison problem by focusing the analysis on a reduced set of SNPs. Simulations show that PBAT substantially outperforms other multiple testing strategies (Van Steen et al. 2005). PBAT has also been successful in finding disease SNPs in a genome-wide study of obesity, a complex genetic disorder, with successful replication of this finding in four additional studies spanning various age ranges and ethnic groups (Herbert et al. 2006).

MEGA-SAMPLES OR META-ANALYSES?

As illustrated previously, the power of most prior linkage and association studies has been woefully inadequate for detecting genes with realistic (i.e., very small) effects on disease risk. Thus, one of the greatest challenges to the successful implementation of these methods is their low power, limited by the typically low sample size of individual studies. Large collaborative studies of mega-samples can overcome this obstacle, and although some such studies have been completed (Lowe et al. 2004; McQueen et al. 2005) or are in progress, the cost of such studies can be prohibitive.

An alternative to the collection of a mega-sample is the use of meta-analysis to combine previously published results. For example, meta-analysis has been applied to linkage analyses of schizophrenia (Badner and Gershon 2002b; Lewis et al. 2003). Looking at each individual study would suggest that there is some, albeit modest, evidence for linkage to 16 chromosomal regions. In contrast, two meta-analyses of these data found evidence for only three strongly linked loci, one of which had not been strongly implicated in any of the individual linkage analyses (Badner and Gershon 2002a; Lewis et al. 2003). Meta-analyses of linkage studies have also helped clarify the genetics of bipolar disorder (Badner and Gershon 2002b; Segurado et al. 2003) and autism (Badner and Gershon 2002b).

Meta-analysis has also been successfully applied to the candidate gene literature. For example, Figure 12–2 gives the pooled odds ratios for genes that have been implicated in ADHD through meta-analysis (Faraone et al. 2005). As is evident from the figure, although each of these genes was statistically significant in the meta-analysis, all of the odds ratios were very low,

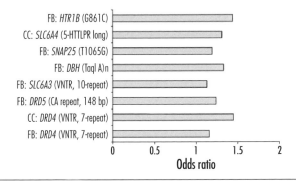

FIGURE 12–2. Pooled odds ratios from positive meta-analyses of attention-deficit/hyperactivity disorder.

VNTR = variable number of tandem repeats.

with none exceeding 1.5. Clearly, in the absence of meta-analysis, mega-samples will be needed to detect ADHD genes.

What Figure 12–2 does not show is how highly variable results can be among studies. We can see this in Figure 12–3, which presents the odds ratios for individual studies that examined the association of ADHD and the dopamine D_4 receptor gene (*DRD4*). This figure clearly shows a good deal of variability among studies, with few studies reporting relatively large effects (e.g., odds ratios greater than 2.5), most studies reporting small effects (e.g., odds ratios of about 1.5), and some studies suggesting no effect (e.g., odds ratios close to 1.0).

Although these examples show that meta-analysis can transform a confusing array of inconsistent results into firm conclusions, we must be alert to the potential drawbacks of this approach. Because meta-analysis relies on published studies, it cannot include unpublished work and cannot include studies that do not provide the data needed for the meta-analysis. If there is a bias against publishing negative studies, a meta-analysis can conclude that a linkage or association is positive when in fact it is not. Fortunately, statistical methods can detect and correct for publication biases (Duval and Tweedie 2000; Peters et al. 2006). For the case of the ADHD data presented, such analyses showed that the positive results could not be attributed to publication bias.

Whether one collects mega-samples, uses pooled mega-samples, or applies meta-analysis, the need for efficient collaboration among colleagues will arise. We usually need multiple sites to collect mega-samples, and multiple sites must agree on the methods and ground rules for publication for the analysis of pooled mega-samples. Although in principle meta-analyses can proceed without collaboration, it is often the case that the meta-analyst

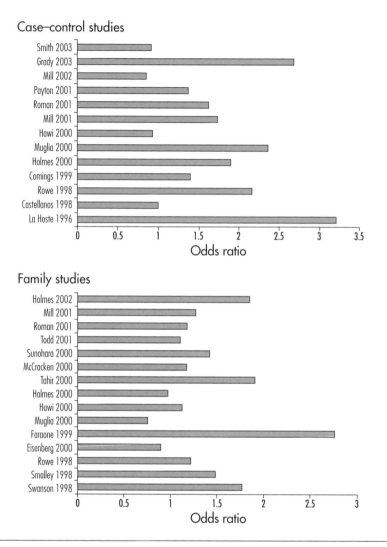

FIGURE 12–3.   Meta-analyses of the *DRD4*–attention-deficit/hyper-activity disorder association.

needs colleagues to provide a more detailed level of data than what is available in their published report.

There are many obstacles to collaboration. These include the use of different measures across sites, cultural differences in disease expression for international collaborations, how to fairly allocate authorship, how to assure that all sites can be assured that their data are appropriately used, and how to assure that junior scientists can benefit from working with a large number of collaborations. There are many examples to suggest that such obstacles can be overcome, yet large-scale collaboration seems to be the exception rather than the rule for psychiatric genetics research.

GENES OR ENVIRONMENT?

Although by definition molecular genetic studies focus on the search for genes, it may not be possible to find genes without also addressing environmental risk factors. This is not a new idea. Several authors have promoted "ecogenetics" as a method for better understanding how genes causes disease (Khoury et al. 1987, 1988; Ottman 1990), and Khoury et al. (1988) described an epidemiologic framework for ecogenetic studies.

The potential power of ecogenetic models has been shown by mathematical simulations. These indicate that when genes play a role in the onset of a disorder their effects will substantially dilute the apparent effects of environmental causes. This means that in the absence of genetic information, studies of environmental risk factors may erroneously conclude that such factors are not related to disease or have only a small impact on disease status (Khoury et al. 1987). Thus, an advantage of ecogenetic studies is that they can identify environmental risk factors and more accurately estimate their effects.

Another advantage of the ecogenetic framework is that it provides a comprehensive assessment of different types of biologically plausible gene–environment interactions. Following Khoury et al. (1988) and Ottman (1990), these patterns are summarized in Table 12–1. Each of these patterns assumes that both genes and environment play a role in pathogenesis and that the combination of adverse environments and pathogenic genes always leads to increased risk for adverse outcomes. The following section briefly describes these patterns along with examples given by Khoury et al. and Ottman.

Pattern 1 assumes that there is no main effect of either the pathogenic genotype or the environmental risk factor; both are needed for the disorder to occur. Here and elsewhere we use the term *genotype* to refer to the gene or set of genes that predisposes to illness. The effect of the environment is seen only among people with the pathogenic genotype, and the effect of the genotype is seen only among people exposed to the environmental risk factor. The classic example is phenylketonuria, which requires both the mutant gene that interferes with the metabolism of phenylalanine and the ingestion of that substance.

In pattern 2 the pathogenic genotype exacerbates the effects of the environmental risk factor but has no effect in the absence of that factor. In con-

TABLE 12–1. Ecogenetic patterns of gene–environment interaction

Pattern	Effect of genotype when environmental risk factor is not present	Effect of environment when pathogenic genotype is not present
1	None	None
2	None	Increases risk
3	Increases risk	None
4	Increases risk	Increases risk

Source. Adapted from Khoury et al. 1993.

trast, the environmental agent increases the risk for illness in the absence of the genotype, but its effects are more potent when the genotype is present. Pattern 2 is seen in the effects of sunlight on skin cancer. Anyone exposed to excessive sunlight increases their risk for skin cancer, but this increase in risk is much greater for some genetic types. Pattern 3 is the converse of pattern 2: the genotype increases risk regardless of the environmental risk factor; the environmental agent exacerbates the outcome of the pathogenic genotype but does not affect outcome in the absence of the genotype.

In pattern 4 both genes and environment increase risk in the absence of the other risk factor. The risk is greatest when both causes are present. An example of this pattern is the interaction between a genetic condition, alpha$_1$-antitrypsin deficiency, and cigarette smoking. Each increases the risk for emphysema, but the risk is greatest for smokers who also have alpha-antitrypsin deficiency.

As the ecogenetic paradigm predicts, studies implicating genes and environment in the etiology of psychiatric disorders have shown statistically significant effects, but none have been large enough to provide precise predictions of which children are at highest risk for adverse outcomes. The ecogenetic model predicts that our ability to predict adverse outcomes will increase dramatically if we use statistical models that incorporate gene–environment interactions.

This increase in predictability was shown by Khoury et al. (1988) with statistical simulations. One of their examples is as follows. Suppose that we are evaluating a gene and an environmental factor that interact in accordance with pattern one. Next assume that the environmental cause leads to a 100-fold increase in the risk for an adverse outcome when the susceptibility gene variant is also present. This 100-fold relative risk will be underestimated dramatically if the gene variant is infrequent. For example, if only 1% of the population has the variant, the estimated relative risk for the environmental cause would be only 2. At a gene frequency of 10%, the estimated relative risk would be 11. Thus, not accounting for relevant genetic variation diminishes our ability to accurately estimate the risk imparted by environmental causes. Similar effects are seen for the other patterns of interaction (Khoury et al. 1988).

DISORDERS OR ENDOPHENOTYPES?

In addition to the fact that most psychiatric disorders have multifactorial polygenic etiologies with multiple underlying risk genes of small effect, the heterogeneity of these disorders also contributes to the difficulties thus far experienced in isolating their risk genes. Two main types of heterogeneity can be delineated: clinical heterogeneity and causal heterogeneity (Faraone et al. 1999). Clinical heterogeneity exists when more than one condition can be brought about by the same cause, whereas causal heterogeneity exists when two or more causes independently can lead to the same condition. Through different means, both forms of heterogeneity serve to obscure the effects of risk genes, delaying and sometimes even preventing their identification.

Clinical heterogeneity is a problem for psychiatric genetics because it complicates the proper identification and ascertainment of individuals who may be carrying the same risk genes. For example, in a given family through which several risk genes for anxiety disorders are segregating, the individual family members may present with a wide range of illnesses, from one or more anxiety disorders through none at all. Between these extremes, other family members may express conditions that appear to be more or less related to anxiety. For example, behavioral inhibition to the unfamiliar—an observational measure of shy, inhibited behavior—is more common among the biological relatives of panic disorder patients than among the relatives of control subjects or in the general population, suggesting that behavioral inhibition shares some genetic basis with panic disorder (Rosenbaum et al. 1991; Smoller et al. 2001). Similarly, many studies have suggested that neuropsychological impairment and brain imaging measures assess conditions that are genetically related to disorders such as schizophrenia (Faraone et al. 1995b, 2000b; Seidman et al. 2002) and ADHD (Doyle et al. 2005a, 2005b; Durston et al. 2004).

Such conditions are frequently referred to as *endophenotypes*, which are defined as phenotypes that are closer to the biological etiology of a clinical disorder than their signs and symptoms suggest and that are influenced by one or more of the same genes that confer susceptibility to the condition (Almasy and Blangero 2001; Cornblatt and Malhotra 2001; Gottesman and

Gould 2003; Skuse 2001; Tsuang and Faraone 1990). Endophenotypes have been studied for two main reasons. First, because they are evident among the otherwise unaffected relatives of patients with a specific disorder, they provide a window on the pathophysiology of illness that cannot be confounded by treatment or the course of illness. Second, endophenotypes might provide greater statistical power for detecting genes. In considering Figures 12–1A and 12–1B, we can see that there are two ways in which endophenotypes might increase the power of molecular genetic studies. For disorders having low heritability (Figure 12–1B), a highly heritable phenotype would clearly be more suitable for study than the disorder itself. For disorders having high heritability (Figure 12–1A), the endophenotype would be useful if it were less genetically complex than the disorder. This distinction is crucial. For example, neuropsychological test scores have been proposed as endophenotypes for ADHD, a disorder having a heritability of about 0.75, yet most of the test scores proposed as endophenotypes have considerably lower heritabilities (Doyle et al. 2005b).

Several authors have proposed criteria for defining endophenotypes (see Almasy and Blangero 2001; Gottesman and Gould 2003; Leboyer et al. 1998; Skuse 2001). Although there is some variability among these criteria, most suggest that endophenotypes should 1) co-occur with the disorder being studied, 2) have good psychometric properties (i.e., reliability, concurrent validity), 3) be heritable (the higher the better), and 4) have an increased prevalence or expression among the unaffected relatives of patients who have the disorder being studied. This last point is crucial because, lacking such evidence, any genes discovered for the endophenotype might not be relevant to the disorder being studied. Because an endophenotype is conceptualized as an expression of the genetic liability for a disorder, it should appear in individuals who carry genes for a condition but do not express the disorder itself.

To assess the utility of endophenotypes for molecular genetic studies, I and my colleagues (Faraone et al. 1995a) suggested using a method developed by Risch (1990a, 1990b) that assesses the relative influence of genetic effects in subgroups of a disorder population. Risch proved that the statistical power of a linkage study increases with the magnitude of risk ratios computed by dividing the affection rate among each relative type to the rate of affection in the population. Following Risch's usage we refer to these ratios as *lambdas*. Risch also showed that power depends only on lambda and on no other genetic parameters. Given his mathematical analysis, Risch (1990a, 1990b) suggested that defining disease status in a manner that increased lambda would increase the power of linkage studies, and I and my colleagues (Faraone et al. 1995a) showed how this could be applied empirically in phenotype definition for molecular genetic studies of schizophrenia.

As another example, I and my colleagues (Faraone et al. 2000a) also found that two dimensions of genetic heterogeneity, comorbidity with conduct disorder and persistence of ADHD into adolescence, would be useful for selecting ADHD subjects for molecular genetic studies. These subphenotypes are useful for molecular genetic studies because 1) they have much higher empirical lambda values than the unstratified ADHD sample and 2) they affect a substantial minority of ADHD patients (Faraone et al. 2000a). Similarly, Purcell's method (Purcell et al. 2001) quantifies the informativeness of phenotypes as the χ^2 statistic that would be obtained in a test for linkage. Thus, when incorporated into genetic studies, endophenotypes that demonstrate strong familial transmission have the potential to afford enhanced statistical power for the detection of genes.

MANY GENES OR MANY DISORDERS?

The difficulties caused by the multifactorial etiology will be exacerbated in the presence of etiologic heterogeneity. It will be difficult enough to find genes if many cause a disorder, but should we consider the possibility that any one disorder can have several discrete causes? From the perspective of genetic heterogeneity, the work discussed earlier in this chapter in support of a multifactorial model rules out the possibility that an apparently multifactorial disorder comprises many single-gene disorders, with the exception of rare cases. Yet, it is possible that a given multifactorial disorder could be separated into at least two classes having different known etiologies and, perhaps, different pathophysiological signatures. This perspective contrasts with the homogeneity hypothesis, which asserts that there is a single necessary and sufficient cause or configuration of causes for each disorder.

Because the assumption of one etiologic class (i.e., homogeneity) is more parsimonious than the assumption of two or more, homogeneity is, in the absence of disconfirming data, our null hypothesis. To assert either etiologic heterogeneity or homogeneity implies that we can describe fully one or more mechanism of etiology. Although there are many clues to the etiologic puzzle of many psychiatric disorders, they do not allow a full description because the etiologic mechanisms have not been worked out in sufficient detail. Thus, we must also appeal to descriptive, phenotypic data and infer the presence of one or more etiologies.

Unfortunately, the correspondence between etiology and phenotype is not isomorphic. Differing etiologies may lead to similar phenotypes. For example, the clinical syndrome known as Alzheimer's disease can arise from either genetic or nongenetic factors. Mutations in any one of three different genes—those for amyloid-beta precursor protein, presenilin 1, or presenilin 2—will almost invariably cause Alzheimer's disease, independent of the presence of other risk genes or deleterious environmental circumstances. To further add to this complexity, the familial, early-onset forms of the disorder caused by mutations in any of these genes only account for a small fraction of the total cases of Alzheimer's disease. In fact, the vast majority of cases of the illness are probably attributable to an as-yet-unknown combination of genetic and environmental factors, although several specific risk genes are quickly becoming recognized, including those for α_2-macroglobulin, angiotensin I converting enzyme 1, and apolipoprotein E.

Although the observation of dissimilar phenotypes (clinical heterogeneity) may suggest etiologic heterogeneity, such inferences are also limited because a single disease entity with a homogeneous etiology can have variable expression due to moderating factors (Tsuang et al. 1993). In genetics the term *pleiotropy* describes the situation in which a pathogenic genotype can express more than one phenotype. Pleiotropy is not unusual for human genetic diseases (Vogel and Motulsky 1986).

Because the link between phenotypic and etiological heterogeneity is weak, using purely phenotypic data to infer etiologic heterogeneity must be viewed cautiously. Although it is tempting to use unimodal distributions of phenotypes to assert etiologic homogeneity and multimodal ones to assert heterogeneity, the utility of phenotypic distributions to inform nosological theory is limited by the need for large samples to detect modality and even larger samples to detect low-prevalence subtypes (Everitt 1981; Ghosh and Sen 1985; Hartigan 1985; Schork and Schork 1988). Thus, such data should be complemented by other data of biological or genetic relevance as they have for bipolar disorder, in which the observation of multimodal ages at onset (Leboyer et al. 2005) was followed by reports of meaningful clinical and genetic distinctions between early- and late-onset cases (Etain et al. 2006; Faraone et al. 2003, 2006).

From a conceptual perspective, it is of interest to note that a multifactorial disorder could masquerade as an etiologically heterogeneous disorder in some circumstances. For example, if there were 10 risk factors (e.g., 5 genes and 5 environmental experiences) that predisposed to ADHD and 9 were needed to express the disorder, there would be a considerable degree of similarity among ADHD cases as regards the presence or absence of the risk factors and their phenotypic expression. In contrast, if only 4 of the 10 risk factors (in any combination) were needed to reach the threshold for ADHD, there would be 210 different pathways to develop the disorder. Some of these etiologic pathways would overlap almost entirely, some only partially, and others not at all. Some of these pathways to ADHD would be entirely genetically determined, whereas others would be produced by a combination of genes and environmental factors. Other cases (called *phenocopies*) might be caused solely by environmental factors. Phenocopies are particularly problematic for genetic studies because they will be counted as affected individuals but will show no evidence implicating the risk genes that underlie the true genetic or partially genetic forms of the disease, with a net effect of reducing the strength of genetic linkage or association detected in the group of affected individuals.

The presence of multiple genetic paths to psychiatric illness will have clear detrimental effects on the power of both linkage and association studies. This suggests that statistical models for analyzing data incorporate heterogeneity, as has been proposed and implemented in several ways (Ott 1983, 1986; Smith and Stephens 1996).

STATISTICAL SIGNIFICANCE OR FUNCTIONAL RELEVANCE?

The main paradigm for gene discovery in psychiatric genetics has been the search for a DNA marker that shows a consistently replicated statistically significant association with the disorder of interest. Because of this, the approaches discussed above provide different approaches toward increasing the power of studies in the hopes that the small genetic effects we seek to detect will emerge. Although the search for genome-wide statistical significance will and should continue, we should also consider whether equal effort should be expended on paradigms that seek to establish functional relevance, because we hope ultimately to have in hand a sequence of DNA variation that has a well-understood function in the biological pathway leading to disease expression. Yet, after we have completed mega-analyses and meta-analyses, we are left with many variants that appear to be susceptibility variants. How can we separate the functionally relevant from the pack?

There are many ways to study the function of DNA variations. Such variations lead to variability in RNA transcripts and ultimately to their expression in the proteins used to build cells. With use of microarray technologies, it is now possible to assay the expression levels of thousands of genes to test hypotheses about altered gene expression in psychiatric disorders. Moreover, gene expression can be studied at the level of RNA or of proteins. When used in an exploratory fashion, such methods raise even more questions. Because of alternate splicing of transcripts and posttranslational modifications in proteins, the number of RNA transcripts and proteins we can assay with gene expression experiments is much greater than the number of genes in the genome. Therefore, just as we can become overwhelmed with the information provided by genotyping DNA markers on a genome-wide scan, so can we become overwhelmed with genome-wide studies of RNA transcripts or proteins.

One approach to this issue is the method of *convergent functional genomics*, which is a series of methods that combines multiple levels of information before concluding that a DNA variant is or is not involved in a disease (Niculescu and Kelsoe 2001; Niculescu et al. 2000). For example, consider the following data types that could be generated for a given disorder: 1) a chromosomal locus implicated by linkage analysis, 2) a positive association with a candidate gene, 3) dysregulated expression of a gene in postmortem brain tissue of patients, 4) dysregulated expression of a gene in postmortem brain tissue of a validated animal model, 5) dysregulation of a target protein in an in vitro assay, 6) dysregulation of a target protein in a transgenic animal, 7) a positive association of a candidate gene in a pharmacogenomic study, 8) demonstration that a known environmental risk factor for the disorder (e.g., exposure to nicotine) dysregulates the gene through epigenetic events, 9) functional imaging of patients with and without putative risk alleles, and 10) a host of other assays we might consider to examine disorders, their endophenotypes, or animal models.

Clearly, when a gene is implicated by multiple levels of evidence, we can have more confidence that it is truly involved in the disorder. Yet, what is not clear is how such studies might be conducted in a systematic manner that would be cost-effective while lending clarity to scientific inference. One idea would be to borrow a method that has been effective for another difficult problem, the development of safe and effective drugs. Because of the costs of drug development, much of pharmaceutical development follows the dictum "fail early and fail cheap" (Roses 2004). The general idea is that potential drug targets should be studied with many inexpensive assays to determine which targets have the most potential. These targets are then tested with a small set of more expensive assays to again determine which should proceed to another level of more expensive testing. This sequential process continues until one reaches the clinical trial stage.

This approach is sometimes referred to as the *drug development pyramid*, with the wide base of the pyramid formed by many inexpensive assays applied to many targets and the narrow peak formed by the few targets that reach human trials. Figure 12–4 shows a schematic of how this idea might be applied to the search for psychiatric disease genes. The base of the pyramid is formed by simple assays such as bioinformatic studies (which require no human or animal subjects) and studies in cell culture. These studies are relatively inexpensive but are less certain as regards their biological validity. The next level comprises studies of animal models, and the highest level uses relatively expensive studies in humans such as examining the effects of DNA variants on functional imaging measures that have very high levels of biological validity. Perhaps with such an approach we could make the needed transition from putative statistical significance to clear functional relevance.

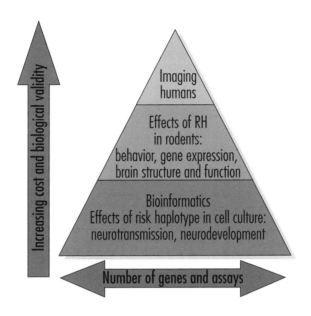

FIGURE 12–4. A translational hierarchy of biological significance.

Note. RH=risk haplotype.

REFERENCES

Almasy L, Blangero J: Endophenotypes as quantitative risk factors for psychiatric disease: rationale and study design. Am J Med Genet 105:42–44, 2001

Badner JA, Gershon ES: Meta-analysis of whole-genome linkage scans of bipolar disorder and schizophrenia. Mol Psychiatry 7:405–411, 2002a

Badner JA, Gershon ES: Regional meta-analysis of published data supports linkage of autism with markers on chromosome 7. Mol Psychiatry 7:56–66, 2002b

Benjamini Y, Hochberg Y: Controlling the false discovery rate: a practical and powerful approach to multiple testing. J R Stat Soc Ser B 57:289–300, 1995

Cook EH, Stein MA, Krasowski MD, et al: Association of attention deficit disorder and the dopamine transporter gene. Am J Hum Genet 56:993–998, 1995

Cornblatt BA, Malhotra AK: Impaired attention as an endophenotype for molecular genetic studies of schizophrenia. Am J Med Genet 105:11–15, 2001

Crowe RR: Candidate genes in psychiatry: an epidemiological perspective. Am J Med Genet 48:74–77, 1993

Doyle AE, Faraone SV, Seidman LJ, et al: Are endophenotypes based on measures of executive functions useful for molecular genetic studies of ADHD? J Child Psychol Psychiatry 46:774–803, 2005a

Doyle AE, Willcutt EG, Seidman LJ, et al: Attention-deficit/hyperactivity disorder endophenotypes. Biol Psychiatry 57:1324–1335, 2005b

Durston S, Hulshoff Pol H, Schnack HG, et al: Magnetic resonance imaging of boys with attention-deficit/hyperactivity disorder and their unaffected siblings. J Am Acad Child Adolesc Psychiatry 43:332–340, 2004

Duval S, Tweedie R: A nonparametric "trim and fill" method of accounting for publication bias in meta-analysis. J Am Stat Assoc 95:89–98, 2000

Etain B, Mathieu F, Rietschel M et al: Genome-wide scan for genes involved in bipolar affective disorder in 70 European families ascertained through a bipolar type I early onset proband: supportive evidence for linkage at 3p14. Mol Psychiatry 11:685–694, 2006

Everitt BS: A Monte Carlo investigation of the likelihood ratio test for the number of components in a mixture of normal distributions. Multivariate Behav Res 16:171–180, 1981

Faraone SV, Tsuang MT: Quantitative models of the genetic transmission of schizophrenia. Psychol Bull 98:41–66, 1985

Faraone SV, Kremen WS, Tsuang MT: Genetic transmission of major affective disorders: quantitative models and linkage analyses. Psychol Bull 108:109–127, 1990

Faraone SV, Kremen WS, Lyons MJ, et al: Diagnostic accuracy and linkage analysis: how useful are schizophrenia spectrum phenotypes. Am J Psychiatry 152:1286–1290, 1995a

Faraone SV, Seidman LJ, Kremen WS, et al: Neuropsychological functioning among the nonpsychotic relatives of schizophrenic patients: a diagnostic efficiency analysis. J Abnorm Psychol 104:286–230, 1995b

Faraone SV, Tsuang MT, Tsuang DW: Genetics and Mental Disorders: A Guide for Students, Clinicians, and Researchers. New York, Guilford, 1999

Faraone SV, Biederman J, Monuteaux MC: Toward guidelines for pedigree selection in genetic studies of attention deficit hyperactivity disorder. Genet Epidemiol 18:1–16, 2000a

Faraone SV, Seidman LJ, Kremen WS, et al: Neuropsychologic functioning among the nonpsychotic relatives of schizophrenic patients: the effect of genetic loading. Biol Psychiatry 48:120–126, 2000b

Faraone SV, Glatt S, Tsuang MT: The genetics of pediatric onset bipolar disorder. Biol Psychiatry 53:970–977, 2003

Faraone SV, Perlis RH, Doyle AE, et al: Molecular genetics of attention deficit hyperactivity disorder. Biol Psychiatry 57:1313–1323, 2005

Faraone SV, Lasky-Su J, Glatt SJ, et al: Early onset bipolar disorder: evidence for linkage to chromosome 9q34. Bipolar Disord 8:144–151, 2006

Ghosh JK, Sen PK: On the asymptotic performance of the log likelihood ratio statistic for the mixture model and related results, in Proceedings of the Berkeley Conference in Honor of Jerzy Neyman and Jack Kiefer, Vol 2. Edited by Le Cam LM, Olshen RA. Belmont, CA, Wadsworth, 1985, pp 789–806

Gibbs RA, Belmont J, Hardenbol TD, et al: The International HapMap Project. Nature 426:789–796, 2003

Glatt SJ, Faraone SV, Tsuang MT: DRD2-141C insertion/deletion polymorphism is not associated with schizophrenia: results of a meta-analysis. Am J Med Genet B Neuropsychiatr Genet 128:21–23, 2004

Gottesman I, Gould T: The endophenotype concept in psychiatry: etymology and strategic intentions. Am J Psychiatry 160:636–645, 2003

Gottesman II, Shields J: A polygenic theory of schizophrenia. Proc Natl Acad Sci U S A 58:199–205, 1967

Hartigan JA: A failure of likelihood asymptotics for normal mixtures, in Proceedings of the Berkeley Conference in Honor of Jerzy Neyman and Jack Kiefer, Vol 2. Edited by Le Cam LM, Olshen RA. Belmont, CA, Wadsworth, 1985, pp 807–810

Herbert A, Gerry NP, McQueen MB, et al: A common genetic variant is associated with adult and childhood obesity. Science 312:279–283, 2006

Holm S: A simple sequentially rejective multiple test procedure. Scandinavian Journal of Statistics 6:65–70, 1979

Horvath S, Xu X, et al: The family based association test method: strategies for studying general genotype–phenotype associations. Eur J Hum Genet 9:301–306, 2001

Horvath S, Xu X, Lake SL, et al: Family-based tests for associating haplotypes with general phenotype data: application to asthma genetics. Genet Epidemiol 26:61–69, 2004

Khoury MJ, Stewart W, Beaty TH: The effect of genetic susceptibility on causal inference in epidemiologic studies. Am J Epidemiol 126:561–567, 1987

Khoury MJ, Adams MJ Jr, Flanders WD: An epidemiologic approach to ecogenetics. Am J Hum Genet 42:89–95, 1988

Khoury MJ, Beaty TH, Cohen BH: Fundamentals of Genetic Epidemiology. New York, Oxford University Press, 1993

Lange C, DeMeo D, Silverman EK, et al: Using the noninformative families in family based association tests: a powerful new testing strategy. Am J Hum Genet 73:801–811, 2003a

Lange C, Lyon H, DeMeo D, et al: A new powerful non-parametric two-stage approach for testing multiple phenotypes in family based association studies. Hum Hered 56:10–17, 2003b

Lange C, DeMeo D, Silverman EK, et al: PBAT: tools for family based association studies. Am J Hum Genet 74:367–369, 2004

Leboyer M, Bellivier F, Nosten-Bertrand M, et al: Psychiatric genetics: search for phenotypes. Trends Neurosci 21:102–105, 1998

Leboyer M, Henry C, Paillere-Martinot ML, et al: Age at onset in bipolar affective disorders: a review. Bipolar Disord 7:111–118, 2005

Lewis CM, Levinson DF, Wise LH, et al: Genome scan meta-analysis of schizophrenia and bipolar disorder, part II: schizophrenia. Am J Hum Genet 73:34–48, 2003

Lowe N, Kirley A, Hawi Z, et al: Joint analysis of DRD5 marker concludes association with ADHD confined to the predominantly inattentive and combined subtypes. Am J Hum Genet 74:348–356, 2004

McQueen MB, Devlin B, Faraone SV, et al: Combined analysis from eleven linkage studies of bipolar disorder provides strong evidence of susceptibility loci on chromosomes 6q and 8q. Am J Hum Genet 77:582–595, 2005

Meehl PE: Schizotaxia, schizotypy, schizophrenia. American Psychologist 17:827–838, 1962

Niculescu AB 3rd, Kelsoe JR: Convergent functional genomics: application to bipolar disorder. Ann Med 33:263–271, 2001

Niculescu AB 3rd, Segal DS, Kuczenski R, et al: Identifying a series of candidate genes for mania and psychosis: a convergent functional genomics approach. Physiol Genomics 4:83–91, 2000

Nyholt DR: A simple correction for multiple testing for single-nucleotide polymorphisms in linkage disequilibrium with each other. Am J Hum Genet 74:765–769, 2004

Ott J: Linkage analysis and family classification under heterogeneity. Ann Hum Genet 47:311–320, 1983

Ott J: Linkage probability and its approximate confidence interval under possible heterogeneity. Genet Epidemiol Suppl 1:251–257, 1986

Ottman R: An epidemiologic approach to gene-environment interaction. Genet Epidemiol 7:177–185, 1990

Peters JL, Sutton AJ, Jones DR, et al: Comparison of two methods to detect publication bias in meta-analysis. JAMA 295:676–680, 2006

Purcell S, Cherny SS, Hewitt JK, et al: Optimal sibship selection for genotyping in quantitative trait locus linkage analysis. Hum Hered 52:1–13, 2001

Risch N: Linkage strategies for genetically complex traits, I: multilocus models. Am J Hum Genet 46:222–228, 1990a

Risch N: Linkage strategies for genetically complex traits, II: the power of affected relative pairs. Am J Hum Genet 46:229–241, 1990b

Risch N, Merikangas K: The future of genetic studies of complex human diseases. Science 273:1516–1517, 1996

Rosenbaum JF, Biederman J, Hirschfeld DR, et al: Further evidence of an association between behavioral inhibition and anxiety disorders: results from a family study of children from a nonclinical sample. J Psychiatr Res 25:49–65, 1991

Roses AD: Pharmacogenetics and drug development: the path to safer and more effective drugs. Nat Rev Genet 5:645–656, 2004

Schork NJ, Schork MA: Skewness and mixtures of normal distributions. Communications in Statistics 17:3951–3969, 1988

Segurado R, Detera-Wadleigh SD, Levinson DF, et al: Genome scan meta-analysis of schizophrenia and bipolar disorder, part III: bipolar disorder. Am J Hum Genet 73:49–62, 2003

Seidman LJ, Faraone SV, Goldstein JM, et al: Left hippocampal volume as vulnerability indicator for schizophrenia: a magnetic resonance imaging morphometric study of nonpsychotic first-degree relatives. Arch Gen Psychiatry 59:839–849, 2002

Skuse DH: Endophenotypes and child psychiatry. Br J Psychiatry 178:395–396, 2001

Smith CAB, Stephens DA: Estimating linkage heterogeneity. Ann Hum Genet 60:161–169, 1996

Smoller JW, Rosenbaum JF, Biederman J, et al: Genetic association analysis of behavioral inhibition using candidate loci from mouse models. Am J Med Genet 105:226–235, 2001

Storey JD, Tibshirani R: Estimating False Discovery Rates Under Dependence With Applications to DNA Microarrays. Technical Report 2001–28. Palo Alto, CA, Stanford University, Department of Statistics, 2001

Storey JD, Tibshirani R: Statistical significance for genomewide studies. Proc Natl Acad Sci U S A 100:9440–9445, 2003

Suarez BK, Hampe CL, Van Eederwegh P: Problems of replicating linkage claims in psychiatry, in Genetic Approaches in Mental Disorders. Edited by Gershon ES, Cloninger CR, Barrett JE. Washington, DC, American Psychiatric Press, 1994, pp 23–46

Tsuang MT, Faraone SV: The Genetics of Mood Disorders. Baltimore, MD, Johns Hopkins University Press, 1990

Tsuang MT, Faraone SV, Lyons MJ, et al: Identification of the phenotype in psychiatric genetics. Eur Arch Psychiatry Clin Neurosci 243:131–142, 1993

Van Steen K, McQueen MB, Herbert A, et al: Genomic screening and replication using the same data set in family based association testing. Nat Genet 37:683–691, 2005

Vogel F, Motulsky AG: Human Genetics: Problems and Approaches. Berlin, Springer-Verlag, 1986

Yang L, Wang Y, Li J, et al: Association of norepinephrine transporter gene with methylphenidate response. J Am Acad Child Adolesc Psychiatry 43:1154–1158, 2004

GENETIC AND ENVIRONMENTAL INFLUENCES ON WELLNESS, RESILIENCE, AND PSYCHOPATHOLOGY

A Family-Based Approach for Promotion, Prevention, and Intervention

James J. Hudziak, M.D.
Meike Bartels, Ph.D.

It is a difficult job for a child to grow up. This job comes with few choices. Your genetic makeup has been determined; you do not get to choose your parents or how many brothers and sisters you will have. You do not get to choose your environment—for example, the town in which you will live, the school to which you will go, and, in most instances, the peer group to which you are exposed. Similarly, you typically do not get to choose whether you will be raised in a religious environment, whether you will be encouraged to play sports, what languages you will be taught, or whether you will be offered the chance to play a musical instrument. Lastly, you have little control over what life events (good or bad) to which you will be exposed. Taken together, kids do not have a lot of choices about the early trajectory of their lives.

The job of growing up becomes more difficult if you suffer from an emotional-behavioral illness while trying to negotiate the business of growing up. Perhaps most germane to this chapter, growing up is even more difficult if the environment you grow up in is chaotic, particularly if you and your parents both struggle with emotional-behavioral problems. A similar argument can be made from a parental point of view (although there are more choices available to the adult). It is tough to be a parent; it is even tougher to be a parent if your child has an emotional-behavioral illness. Perhaps most important to this discussion, it is terribly difficult to be a good parent if both you and your children suffer from emotional-behavioral illness. It is well known that children's temperaments and psychopathology directly affect their environments and their relations with their parents (Rettew et al. 2006). Similarly, parents' temperament and psychopathological profile will affect their relationships and the environment of the home. Simply put, a child who suffers from severe psychopathology can quickly overwhelm a parent who has otherwise adequate parenting skills.

The interaction between the parents and offspring, as originally discussed by Thomas and Chess (1977) and elaborated by others (Rettew et al. 2006), can either be protective from illness or represent a marked risk for illness. The perspective that all of the conditions that we study (e.g., attention problems, aggressive behavior, anxiety disorders, obsessive-compulsive disorder [OCD], juvenile bipolar disorder) are influenced by multiple genetic and environmental factors is now generally accepted (Althoff et al. 2006; Boomsma et al. 2005; van Grootheest et al. 2007; Rietveld et al. 2003; van Beijsterveldt et al. 2003). The fact that most of these illnesses run in families is also fully accepted.

In this chapter it will be argued that by taking a family-based gene–environment approach (FBA) in the developmental psychopathology (FBA/DP) perspective, researchers and clinicians alike will be able to better understand etiopathology and ultimately treatment. We offer that the FBA/DP perspective is the ideal approach for general medicine to embrace. It should be the goal of all involved in the care and well-being of children and families that we embrace the following strategy. We should aim to devise strategies to keep well children well, prevent at-risk children from developing psychopathology, and intervene on behalf of those who are ill. This movement toward health promotion and prevention is fully supported by the FBA/DP perspective. We argue that in light of recent discoveries it is prudent to once again embrace a full family approach to the assessment and treatment of emotional-behavioral disorders. Further, we will argue that strategies that can be learned from the FBA/DP perspective can already be useful in the promotion, prevention, and intervention approach simply by embracing the clinical mandate of "do no harm."

GENOMIC MEDICINE AND THE FBA/DP PERSPECTIVE

In the era of genomic medicine we are treated daily to new discoveries relating specific emotional-behavioral problems to specific genetic and environmental influences. Such discoveries are becoming commonplace yet are often misunderstood in the context of their complexity. Typically both the genetic and environmental influences identified in these studies are of small to modest effect and thus only explain a very small part of the story. However, the results are often so intoxicating that the public overvalues the findings in the search for a single diagnostic test or gene treatment. These discoveries doubtless portend a period of rapid discovery that could well lead to new diagnostic, treatment, and prevention strategies for children who suffer from common psychopathologies.

However, in order to ensure proper progression in our field, we must protect these findings from overgeneralization and misuse. Simply put, the experts in our field need to prepare to teach practitioners, families, and patients the lessons that common psychopathologies are best described in the context of complex illnesses, for which complex solutions and approaches will be necessary to ensure that children and their families are receiving the best of care. On the other hand, despite the fact that we are not likely ever to be able to use genetic tests that are diagnostic (e.g., "If you carry this gene you will have a disorder") or even predictive (e.g., "If you carry this gene it is likely that you will have a disorder"), our testing may yield information on relative risk (e.g., "You carry one—or more—of the genes that confer risk for a disorder"). As we move toward discussion of relative risk with our families, this may help change the history of psychiatric treatment by diminishing resistance to treatment because of the stigma and shame often associated with psychiatric illness. In other words, clinical use of relative risk genetic testing may yield advances with patients by "biologizing" and "validating" psychiatric illness, which practitioners have long known to be both biological and valid.

Nonetheless, perhaps the most important lessons of the past 10 years that have emerged have demonstrated that genotypes associated with psychiatric illness are correlated with some environmental stressors but not others. Thus therapeutic avenues of the "environmental type" can be revisited. In this book you will have read a number of examples that provide evidence of the importance of the FBA/DP perspective. As a result, we focus this chapter on an alternative strategy—the study and implementation of FBA/DP wellness and resilience strategies for both research and clinical medicine.

THE CONCEPTS OF WELLNESS AND RESILIENCE

Societies, cultures, and families have often struggled to promote wellness in children. It is easy to forget that educational programs for children are a relatively recent development in the course of human existence. As with providing an education to all children (see, e.g., *Guns, Germs, and Steel,* by Jared Diamond [1997]), cultures also have spent a great deal of energy trying to make participation in sports a right to all children. Similarly it has long been believed that there are benefits of a musical education (see *The Mozart Effect,* by Don Campbell [1997]), a healthy diet, and religious upbringing. What has been so baffling is the question of why these factors are protective in only some children. Why do some families value these elements of living and others ignore them? We argue that one of the values of using genomically informative designs in family-based research paradigms is the possibility of understanding which children are likely to benefit from one program versus another. To do this properly, we think an emphasis on the study of the environmental and genetic influences on wellness and resilience may be even more important than previously argued. In the study of developmental psychopathology, little attention is paid to the well and the very well child and family. Psychiatry and clinical psychology have focused largely on psychopathology rather than on positive behavior or wellness. This focus has led to a definition of wellness as the absence of emotional and/or behavioral problems. However, we are convinced that variance at the "positive" side of the normal distribution (see Figure 13–1) is as common as variance in psychopathology.

We believe that by studying children, adolescents, and families who are well, happy, and satisfied with their lives in addition to resilient children who once showed psychopathology but have recovered, we can develop new strategies for intervention and prevention.

FBA/DP AND WELLNESS AND RESILIENCE

Unfortunately, bad things happen to all children, but fortunately only some go on to develop psychiatric illness. Pathways into and out of psychopathology need to be better studied using the DP approach. We argue that using the FBA approach will be even more illustrative, because children's problems and family's problems often coexist. One such example is the well-

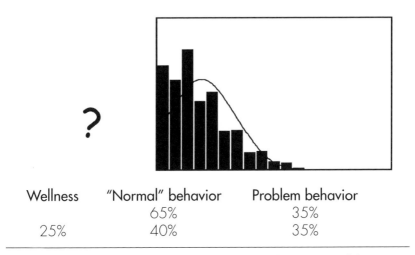

Wellness	"Normal" behavior	Problem behavior
	65%	35%
25%	40%	35%

FIGURE 13–1. **Gaussian distribution from wellness to problem behavior.**

known data on the effects of maternal well-being on the child. Failure to consider the effects of maternal absence or maternal illness when conceptualizing DP pathways will likely lead to spurious findings. Weissman et al. (2006) have nicely demonstrated that in some cases measures of child psychopathology can change with improvement in maternal depression. Similarly, failure to consider genetic factors as playing a role in negative outcomes can also lead to spurious findings. Elegant primate research, detailed elsewhere in this book (see Chapter 7, "Genetic and Environmental Modifiers of Risk and Resiliency in Maltreated Children"), has demonstrated the key role of maternal interaction and offspring genotypes in outcomes in behavior and stress response (Barr et al. 2004; Suomi 2005). Thus, to discover why some children are always well, some children apparently suffer from emotional-behavioral problems from conception through adulthood, and others are sometimes affected and other times well, it may be essential to also understand the family's health and genetic makeup together. Epidemiologic studies show that the majority of the children are free of emotional-behavioral problems at any given time. Emerging evidence from longitudinal studies suggests that within this group of "well" children, many have always been well, whereas others may have been ill at one point but are relatively well at others.

To date, it is not clear what factors influence the shift from illness to wellness or why some children recover from illness and remain well ever afterwards. Suspected factors include life events and risk factors as well as genetic and epigenetic factors.

We believe that in order to study wellness and resilience (i.e., the ability to recover from a prior illness or the capacity to remain well in the face of extraordinary genetic and/or environmental risk factors) in the domain of developmental psychopathology, it is necessary to study children longitudinally using genetically informative strategies. Thus, twin, family, adoption, and molecular genetic studies that measure environmental mediators and modifiers in a longitudinal fashion are needed in order to estimate genetic and environmental factors that put children at risk for or protect them from psychopathology.

To study the factors that promote resilience, we must understand the factors contributing to change and stability in developmental psychopathology. However, when we are examining the etiology of developmental stability and underlying factors for resilience, one caveat is that the mechanisms responsible could differ for genetic and environmental influences (Bartels et al. 2004; Bishop et al. 2003; Haberstick et al. 2005). Bartels et al. (2004), for example, found that stability in internalizing (INT) and externalizing (EXT) behaviors, based on maternal ratings, was accounted for by genetic and shared environmental influences. The genetic contribution to stability (INT: 43%; EXT: 60%) resulted from the fact that a subset of genes expressed at an earlier age was still active at the next time point. Further, a common set of shared environmental factors operated at all ages (INT: 47%; EXT: 34%). The more general conclusion that genetic factors contribute primarily to stability whereas nonshared environments contribute largely to change has also been supported with findings for other phenotypes such as attention problems (Rietveld et al. 2003) and aggression (van Beijsterveldt et al. 2003). The finding of distinct developmental patterns for genetic and environmental influences is important for scientific as well as clinical purposes. The shared environmental influences, for instance, exert a continuous influence from their time of onset. So the children who continue to experience adverse shared environments are at risk for later maladjustment. For additive genetic influences, parts of previous effects are transmitted to later ages. However, the genetic influence is less static owing to new genetic influences that come into play at each age. Nonshared environmental influences seem to be important for age-specific behavior problems and have almost no developmental significance.

Combining these findings from longitudinal studies with knowledge of measured environmental risk and protective factors supports the study of wellness and resilience, which may well yield insight into a wide variety of complex questions. Why for instance do some children benefit from exposure to sports participation, music, nutritious diet, and other widely implemented social programs? Why is it that these social programs, which common sense would indicate should benefit all children, often help only a small percentage of children? Why do prevention programs work for only some children and families? Why do pharmacotherapies and psychotherapies not work in all children with the same "diagnosis"? Although the answers are doubtless so complex that many approaches will be needed to dissect the relative contribution of a wide variety of factors, it is suggested that the study of the genetic and environmental influences on wellness and resilience in families may lead to a clearer understanding of which children will respond to which interventions, as well as to design more effective prevention programs.

Such research may lead to strategies that will change the way we assess children with emotional-behavioral illness. To review all of the potential protective strategies is beyond the scope of this chapter, however in order to present some relative simple yet provocative exemplars, we summarize here findings for protective and risk factors known to be mostly environmentally mediated (sports participation, religiosity, and life events).

EXERCISE BEHAVIOR AND SPORTS PARTICIPATION

In our research clinic at the Vermont Center for Children, Youth, and Families (VCYFF), it is not uncommon for parents to leave with a prescription for "team sports" for a child. We have taken this rather atypical approach because it is our contention that participating on sports teams is protective for children, particularly children at risk. There is research that indicates that children who carry genes of risk for attention-deficit/hyperactivity disorder (ADHD) and cigarette smoking are likely to be protected against smoking initiation if they are able to participate on a team (Audrain-McGovern et al. 2006). Just what is the protective value of sports?

Our group has reported results from a large adolescent twin study that found that individual differences in sport participation between ages 13 and 16 years are mainly accounted for by shared environmental factors (78%–84%). In other words, it is the family who is responsible for getting their children to participate in sports (or not). At the ages of 17–18 years, genetic influences begin to appear (36%), and the role of shared environment decreases (Stubbe et al. 2005). This study provides evidence that at one stage of development a mediator may be primarily environmental, but at other stages genetic effects appear.

The relation between exercise behavior and mental health has been described by many researchers (Byrne and Byrne 1993; Folkins and Sime 1981; Gauvin and Spence 1996; North et al. 1990; Salmon 2000; Scully et al. 1998). However, population studies on the association between exercise and mental health are harder to find. Recently, our group (De Moor et al. 2006) studied the association of exercise with anxiety, depression, and personality in a large population-based adult sample. The primary findings from this investigation are that exercisers are on average less anxious and depressed (effect sizes −0.18 to −0.29 SD), less neurotic (effect size −0.14 SD), more extraverted (effect size +0.32 SD), higher in thrill and adventure seeking (effect size +0.47), and higher in disinhibition (effect size +0.25 SD) than nonexercisers. The differences between exercisers and nonexercisers, although small (Cohen 1969), are very consistent across gender and age and with the previous reports on depression and anxiety.

Further, lack of exercise was found to be cross-sectionally associated with depression in population samples with a broad age range (Farmer et al. 1988; Weyerer 1992) and in samples consisting of young (Steptoe and Butler 1996; Steptoe et al. 1997) or older adults (Kritz-Silverstein et al. 2001; Strawbridge et al. 2002). In a sample of adolescents, however, Allison et al. (2005) found that regular exercise was associated with better social functioning. The latter shows that sports participation might be a moderator of clinical and scientific interest, because besides the significant effects of its absence on depression and anxiety, positive or protective effects are also found. In line with these findings our group found that exercise participation is associated with higher levels of life satisfaction and happiness (Stubbe et al. 2007). It was further found that exercise participation correlates moderately ($r=0.20$) with self-rated health (De Moor et al. 2007). The genetic characteristics of the latter study provide evidence for overlapping genes influencing both phenotypes ($r_g=0.36$).

Cross-sectional analyses, as presented here, *cannot* inform us on the causal structure between exercise, personality, anxiety, and depression. An approach to study causality, therefore, is the use of prospective analyses in large longitudinal population-based samples. A prospective association between lack of exercise at baseline and depression or anxiety at follow-up was found in some population studies (Camacho et al. 1991; Farmer et al. 1988; Strawbridge et al. 2002) but was absent in other studies (Allison et al. 2005; Cooper-Patrick et al. 1997; Kritz-Silverstein et al. 2001; Weyerer 1992). These studies did not, unfortunately, examine the reverse causality, where depression or anxiety at baseline may predict reduced exercise participation at follow-up. Further, most of the previously mentioned studies are based on adult samples. Future studies involving children and adolescents are essential to gain insight into the association between sports participation and wellness and psychopathology.

Moreover, since it has been found that variance in exercise behavior in adolescents is accounted for by shared environment, sports participation in itself is a likely target for intervention. Expansion of the previous results that show significant genetic overlap between exercise behavior and self-rated health and satisfaction with life and happiness should be replicated in children and adolescents. To this end we have completed preliminary analyses in our sample of more than 1,000 adolescent twin pairs and their nontwin siblings. Our data, in which 70% of 13-year-old boys and girls are on sports teams, reveal that in both genders, adolescents who participate in sport on a regular basis generally feel healthier ($P=0.000$) and happier ($P=0.020$) and report a higher quality of life ($P=0.006$).

Given the low risk and potential high return of aiming to include sports participation in a child's life, particularly when at earlier ages the influences are primarily of the shared environmental type, we aim to have more families get their at-risk children to participate in sports (and as a result of these and other studies, other activities such as music training, clubs, and other social programs).

RELIGIOSITY

The concept that being raised in a religious household is protective has long been a staple belief of religious disciplines. Our group has analyzed large sets of twin data revealing that differences between individuals in religious upbringing, affiliation, and participation in church activities are environmentally mediated. The familial resemblance for different aspects of religion is high but can be explained entirely by environmental influences common to family members (Boomsma et al. 1999). In a study of Finnish twins, low heritabilities (11%–22%) and large shared environmental influences (45%–60%) were found (Winter et al. 1999). High levels of religious involvement predict a reduced risk of substance misuse (Gorsuch 1995; Koenig et al. 1994; Larson et al. 1980; Payne et al. 1991). A protective effect of religious involvement and values against adolescent alcohol use was found by Heath et al. (1999).

Furthermore, associations between religiosity and the lower levels of psychopathology and substance use behavior have been suggested. Using data from the National Longitudinal Study of Adolescent Health, Nonnemaker et al. (2003) found religiosity to be protective against cigarette, alcohol, and marijuana use. It has also been found that for boys, low religiosity predicted progression to regular smoking and failure to quit regular smoking (van den Bree et al. 2004).

Spirituality has also been conceptualized by some as a component of personality (Luby et al. 1999). In a population-based adult twin sample, it was found that general religiosity was inversely and significantly linked to nicotine dependence, alcohol dependence, drug misuse and dependence, and adult antisocial behavior. However, general religiosity was significantly related to panic disorder (Kendler et al. 2003a).

Maes et al. (1999) found that genetic factors account for the association between church attendance and alcohol use in males, but in females the association is primarily due to shared environmental factors and genotype–environment covariance. In the Netherlands Twin Register adult twin sample, Koopmans et al. (1999) reported that in females who scored high on religiosity, genetic factors explained 0% of the variance of initiation of drinking. Conversely, in females who scored low on religiosity, genetic factors accounted for 40% of the variance. Subjects with a religious upbringing and who participate in church activities score lower on Sensation Seeking Questionnaire scales, with religiosity being associated with reduced genetic influence on disinhibition, especially in males (Boomsma et al. 1999).

Further, there is a wealth of psychiatric research studying the relationship between OCD, culture, and religious identity and practice (Abramowitz et al. 2002; Chia 1996; Greenberg and Shefler 2002; Greenberg and Witztum 1994; Raphael et al. 1996; Rassin and Koster 2003; Shooka et al. 1998; Sica et al. 2002; Tek and Ulug 2001; Tezcan and Millet 1997). A tentative summary of these studies is that in the normal population there are relations between religiosity and obsessive-compulsive ideation and behavior. However, the literature on OCD and religiosity across a variety of religions, cultures, and ethnic groups shows no proof that religion causes OCD or any other psychopathology.

These data inform the FBA/DP approach. For example, they lead us to ask the question: Are there clinical implications and lessons for family-based activities that extend beyond religion and may relate to other measures of family cohesion (and adversely, family conflict)? Although it is too provocative to imagine recommending participation in religion or religious groups as a "therapeutic intervention," our group and others have been struck by what appears to be the protective qualities of family-based activities and wonder whether the data are already strong enough to support a greater role for family-based approaches aimed at increasing family cohesion as a role for health promotion and prevention strategies.

LIFE EVENTS

A recent study on genetic effects on life events in adolescent and young adult twins and their nontwin siblings reveals no differences in prevalence of life events between monozygotic twins, dizygotic twins, and their siblings. The results indicate familial aggregation of life events, except for traffic accidents in women. Familial resemblance of illness and death of a significant other was mainly due to common environment. For the other life events, it was not possible to distinguish between genetic and common environmental effects (Middeldorp et al. 2005). Kendler et al. (1993) also reported moderate influences of genes (20%) and shared environment (20%), and relatively large effects of nonshared environment (60%) on life events.

Life event research has shown that both major life events and accumulated daily hassles may serve as stressors with negative implications for mental health. For example, it has been found that stressful life events influence the onset and course of depression (Kendler et al. 1999; Kessler 1997; Pine et al. 2002). However, there is no linear and direct relation (Goodyer 1990), and we are not aware of any study that directly tests the direction of causation. It has also been reported that adolescents initiate smoking to cope with stressful life events (Koval and Pederson 1999; Koval et al. 2000). For example, job loss for a household member is a risk factor for adolescents' involvement in problem behaviors (Unger et al. 2004). Groundbreaking work by Caspi et al. (2003) showed that individual differences in the development of depression caused by stressful life events depend on genetic makeup.

Again, although direction of causation research is under way in many groups around the world using genetically informative designs, it is not clear if genetic predisposition to negative life events is at the root cause of the above relations. However, it can be argued that it is clear that family chaos, conflict, and negative life events, in the genetically informative studies done to date, are associated with higher rates of psychopathology in adults and children. Clearly a strategy aimed modifying the environments of the genetically at risk seems a thoughtful approach that may bring clarity to the questions of why some events lead to impairment in only some of the people. Similarly, why do supportive strategies only help some who have endured negative life events (Kaufman et al. 2004)? Again, studies using the FBA/DP approach are likely to yield important diagnostic and therapeutic advances.

FAMILY CONFLICT

Using data from the large longitudinal database of the Netherlands Twin Register (Boomsma et al. 2006), we are currently investigating the role of familial factors on adolescent wellness and problem behavior. Large studies in our samples of twin children showed moderate to large genetic influences on aggressive behavior during childhood. This classical twin study however, does not reveal information on the possible interacting effects of genes and environment on aggressive behavior. In our new project, "A Twin-Sibling Study of Adolescent Wellness," we have tested the effects of familial conflict, measured with the 11-item Conflict scale from the Family Environment Scale (Moos and Moos 1974), on the etiology of aggressive behavior from the Youth Self-Report (YSR). The Dutch Health and Behavior Questionnaire has been collected in adolescent twins ($n = 1,000$ pairs) and their nontwin siblings ($n = 500$ individuals).

A main effect of familial conflict on adolescent aggressive behavior (AGG) has been found, with significantly higher levels of AGG in families with high levels of familial conflict ($P = 0.00$). Preliminary analyses based on twin correlations indicate gene–environment interaction effects, because a higher heritability estimate for AGG is found for the adolescents with low familial conflict in comparison to heritability estimates for the group with moderate familial conflict and the group who reports high familial conflict. Sophisticated model fitting, which will include tests for gender effects and possible effects of gene–environment correlations, will be conducted to gain more insight into the role of familial conflict in AGG. In this way we can begin to estimate the measured genetic and environmental influences on resilience by determining factors that move children into wellness or illness or identifying factors that seem to be protective against inferred genetic and environmental risk factors. Again, these data seem to cry out for family-based intervention approaches (that have long been advocated by a variety of experts) that will reduce family conflict. With a genetically informative approach, these interventions may be tailored more accurately to families who are more likely to respond to them. We argue that while we wait for that evidence it is prudent to move ahead with these strategies now.

OTHER EXAMPLES OF THE FAMILY-BASED GENE–ENVIRONMENT APPROACH

Recent studies reveal the complex interplay between genes and environment when studying family dysfunction in the context of childhood psychopathology. Kendler et al. (2003b), for example, investigated whether dysfunction in the family of origin moderates the impact of genetic factors on liability for psychiatric disorders. They found no evidence for this effect. Furthermore, McGue and Lykken (1992) found that divorce risk was largely caused by genetic influences. An association between genes and environment is also found when neighborhood characteristics (based on zip code) are studied as predictors of adolescent psychopathology. For example, genetic factors account for more individual differences in drinking patterns among adolescents residing in urban areas, whereas shared environmental influences were larger in rural settings (Rose et al. 2001). Similar effects of neighborhood were found for aggressive behavior. Adolescents in high socioeconomic status (SES) neighborhoods were significantly less likely than their counterparts in low-SES neighborhoods to engage in serious and violent delinquency. Results indicated that risk factors for later repeated violence among adolescents in high-SES neighborhoods, such as physical aggression, may be caused by genetic influences, whereas risk factors for later violence among adolescents in low-SES neighborhoods, such as poor parent–adolescent communication and early intercourse, appeared to be context-dependent (Beyers et al. 2001).

THE GENE–ENVIRONMENT FAMILY-BASED APPROACH AT WORK

Our clinical approach at the VCCYF is inspired by the FBA/DP perspective. We argue that it is no longer sufficient to assess and treat a child's emotional-behavioral problems as if they occur in a vacuum. Put in simple terms, does it really make sense to only treat a 6-year-old boy's anxious depression (with medication and or psychotherapy) when the boy's mother is suffering from panic disorder and his father from alcohol abuse? In this pedigree, for example, all three individuals suffer from disorders that have been identified to be influenced by genetic and environmental factors. We argue that each then contributes to the environmental influences that further can exacerbate the psychopathology. Rather than simply treat the child, we think it prudent to assess the entire family's emotional well-being, health, risk, and protective behavior, and to consider approaches that intervene at the family level and that are developmentally appropriate. While we wait for genetic testing and other promises of our genomic era of medicine, we feel the research to date has already provided us with enough evidence to know that the family-based approach should be implemented in child clinics now.

To operationalize the VCCYF approach, we obtain 1) Child Behavior Checklist (CBCL) data from mothers and fathers and 2) Teacher's Report Forms (TRF) and YSR forms on all children. (We also use DSM interviews, but rely heavily on the CBCL family of instruments because they provide a developmental and gender sensitive perspective absent in the DSM.) These data provide us with a multi-informant, quantitative, developmentally sensitive description of the child's emotional-behavioral health. The CBCL family of instruments generate data on eight syndromes (Attention Problems, Aggressive Behavior, Rule Breaking Behavior, Withdrawn Behavior, Social Problems, Thought Problems, Anxious Depression, and Somatic Complaints) as well as two broadband scales (Internalizing Problems and Externalizing Problems) (Achenbach and Rescorla 2001) and phenotypic markers for obsessive-compulsive behavior and the broad phenotype of juvenile bipolar disorder. Our group has published findings on the genetic and environmental influences on each of these syndromes. Simply put, in every single instance there is evidence for both genetic and environmental influences on each of these syndromes. We use these data to fuel our family-based explanation of the child's psychopathology. We know each of these child psychopathologic conditions is highly heritable yet influenced by environmental factors. Because children inherit their genes from their parents, and because it is widely known that children with psychopathology often have parents with psychopathology, we considered it prudent to develop an assessment protocol that considered the possibility that parents of children with psychopathology may be struggling against the yoke of their own genetics and the environment that exists in the family. As a result, we also collect emotional-behavioral data on all parents in our clinic.

We obtain the Adult Self-Report on both parents, in which parents describe their own emotions and behaviors on the same syndromes studied in childhood but modified and normed in a developmentally sensitive approach for adults (ages 18–54) and for older adults (ages 55–68 years, Older Adult Self-Report). In addition, we collect the Adult Behavior Checklist, in which partners report on each other's emotions and behaviors, again using the developmental perspective. In addition we collect the Vermont Health Behavior Questionnaire (VHBQ) from parents and children. These data provide us with a detailed description of the child and family's environment with an emphasis on known risk and protective factors, such as happiness (Lyubomirsky and Lepper 1999), life satisfaction (Horley 1984), self-esteem (Kajita et al. 2002), sports participation/physical activity (Babyak et al. 2000), diet/eating habits (Stokes and Frederick-Recascino 2003), academic performance and leisure time (Wilens et al. 2002), and religiosity. We collect data on zip code/SES, medication history, peer smoking/drinking, family relation and family conflict, family structure, cohesion, conflict, life events, parenting styles, and activities such as membership in musical groups, time spent on computers, TV, and electronic games.

The resulting data set forms the foundation for our clinical approach. We have dimensional, developmentally sensitive data on related psychopathological syndromes in the children and their parents (and, in cases in which grandparents are involved, data on the grandparents as well). We can relate a child's anxious depression and inattention syndromes to parental anxiety and inattention. In this way, the child escapes being the identified patient, and the family becomes the focus of treatment. We offer to treat every member of the family who has treatable psychopathology. In addition, we use the data from the VHBQ to identify factors such as family chaos and conflict (see above), which generates a family-based intervention aimed at reducing chaos and conflict in families. With the VHBQ we also learn that many children and families do not participate in sports programs, music programs, or have healthy diet and exercise programs. Many children leave our clinic with prescriptions to join sports teams, to begin Suzuki violin, to see a dietician, to begin a fitness regimen, or to turn off their TVs, iPods, and computer games. Each of these therapeutic interventions is aimed at modifying the environment and, it is hoped, mediating the genetic expression of these illnesses. Using the CBCL approach as an outcome measure, Weissman et al. (2006) demonstrated that by successfully treating maternal depression, childhood Internalizing and Externalizing scores improved by a full standard deviation, *without* treating the children. Although this remarkable study needs to be replicated, it provides another bit of evidence for the family-based approach. In the near future—indeed, we have a proposal to do this project in review at this time—we would like to provide family genotyping as part of our approach so that we may begin to build a database on which families will benefit from which types of intervention, whether they be of the health promotion, prevention, or intervention (treatment) types. The end game of this approach is to bridge the gap between research findings in the genetic and environmental influences on developmental psychopathology by developing a real-world application. Each of these interventions at worst does no harm and at best may prove to be the types of approaches that will move child psychiatry into the overall family of medical disciplines that embrace health promotion and disease prevention as well as intervention.

CONCLUSIONS

By assessing a child's (and indeed a family's) relative risk for psychopathology using family and molecular genetic approaches, in concert with an assessment of the risk and protective environmental factors, we may be able better to design the complex interventions that are doubtless needed for the complex problems of developmental psychopathology. Although it is clear that molecular genetic testing is a long way from being implemented in clinical settings, it is not too early to learn from the research presented in this book. A more thorough assessment of the child's developmental trajectory, family, and unique environmental risk and protective factors, and, possibly the estimation of the contribution of relative risk genes, may help in the design of more effective treatment and prevention strategies for at-risk children. Indeed, the work of Kaufman et al. (2004), in which children with one relative risk genotype (S/S allele of the serotonin transporter gene [*SERT*]) were more likely to benefit from social support in the face of extreme environmental disadvantage, offers us the promise of potentially understanding which children will respond to supportive therapies (see Chapter 7, "Genetic and Environmental Modifiers of Risk and Resiliency in Maltreated

Children," this book). Such an advance could well benefit patients, their families, and the clinical teams who serve them. One of the great disappointments of the practice of clinical child psychiatry is the inability to help children achieve wellness despite using all of the methods available in our clinical formulary. It is our contention that the study of resilience, as long as it includes both well and suffering children, while assessing both genetic and environmental factors, is likely to lead to more effective treatments for children and their families and thus improve the efficiency of our clinical efforts.

Routine use of genotyping in clinical practice is probably still decades away. It may well be that through the use of genetic testing, and debunking of damaging misconceptions about etiopathology of child psychiatric illness, families and children will be more likely to seek and accept psychiatric health care. In so doing, we may be able to encourage families to embrace wellness strategies aimed at the family, rather than the child alone. We envision a future that includes assessment of genetic and environmental strengths and weaknesses of the entire family, married to a family-based treatment approach partnered with wellness and therapeutic strategies. It is in this context that we hope to see a reduction in those environmental factors that can be changed in the lives of children and families that contribute to negative outcomes for common psychiatric illnesses. The overall aim is to contribute to healthier, happier families and communities using the research generated by the FBA/DP perspective.

REFERENCES

Abramowitz JS, Huppert JD, Cohen AB, et al: Religious obsessions and compulsions in a non-clinical sample: The Penn Inventory of Scrupulosity (PIOS). Behav Res Ther 40:825–838, 2002

Achenbach TM, Rescorla LA: Manual for the ASEBA School-Age Forms & Profiles. Burlington, University of Vermont Research Center for Children, Youth, & Families, 2001

Allison KR, Adlaf EM, Irving HM, et al: Relationship of vigorous physical activity to psychological distress among adolescents. J Adolesc Health 37:164–166, 2005

Althoff RR, Rettew DC, Faraone SV, et al: Latent class analysis shows strong heritability of the Child Behavior Checklist-juvenile bipolar phenotype. Biol Psychiatry 60:903–911, 2006

Audrain-McGovern J, Rodriguez D, Wileyto EP, et al: Effect of team sport participation on genetic predisposition to adolescent smoking progression. Arch Gen Psychiatry 63:433–441, 2006

Babyak M, Blumenthal JA, Herman S, et al: Exercise treatment for major depression: maintenance of therapeutic benefit at 10 months. Psychosom Med 62:633–638, 2000

Barr CS, Newman TK, Shannon C: Rearing condition and rh5-HTTLPR interact to influence limbic-hypothalamicpituitary-adrenal axis response to stress in infant macaques. Biol Psychiatry 55:733–738, 2004

Bartels M, van den Oord EJCG, Hudziak JJ, et al: Genetic and environmental mechanisms underlying stability and change in problem behaviors at ages 3, 7, 10, and 12. Dev Psychol 40:852–867, 2004

Beyers JM, Loeber R, Wikstrom PO, et al: What predicts adolescent violence in better-off neighborhoods? J Abnorm Child Psychol 29:369–381, 2001

Bishop EG, Cherny SS, Corley R, et al: Developmental genetic analysis of general cognitive ability from 1 to 12 years in a sample of adoptees, biological siblings, and twins. Intelligence 31:31–49, 2003

Boomsma DI, de Geus EJ, van Baal GC, et al: A religious upbringing reduces the influence of genetic factors on disinhibition: evidence for interaction between genotype and environment on personality. Twin Res 2:115–125, 1999

Boomsma DI, van Beijsterveldt CEM, Hudziak JJ: Genetic and environmental influences on Anxious/Depression during childhood: a study from the Netherlands Twin Register. Genes Brain Behav 4:466–481, 2005

Boomsma DI, de Geus EJC, Vink JM, et al: Netherlands Twin Register: from twins to twin families. Twin Res Hum Genet 9:849–857, 2006

Byrne A, Byrne DG : The effect of exercise on depression, anxiety and other mood states—a review. J Psychosom Res 37:565–574, 1993

Camacho TC, Roberts RE, Lazarus NB, et al: Physical activity and depression: evidence from the Alameda County Study. Am J Epidemiol 134:220–231, 1991

Campbell D: The Mozart Effect: Tapping the Power of Music to Heal the Body, Strengthen Mind, and Unlock the Creative Spirit. New York, HarperCollins, 1997

Caspi A, Sugden K, Moffitt TE, et al: Influence of life stress on depression: moderation by a polymorphism in the 5-HTT gene. Science 301:386–389, 2003

Chia BH: A Singapore study of obsessive–compulsive disorder. Singapore Med J 37:402–406, 1996

Cohen J: Statistical Power Analysis for the Behavioral Sciences. New York, Academic Press, 1969

Cooper-Patrick L, Ford DE, Mead LA, et al: Exercise and depression in midlife: a prospective study. Am J Public Health 87:670–673, 1997

De Moor MHM, Stubbe JH, Boomsma DI, et al: Exercise participation and self-rated health: do common genes explain the association? Eur J Epidemiol 22:27–32, 2007

De Moor MHM, Beem AL, Stubbe JH, et al: Regular exercise, anxiety, depression and personality: a population-based study. Prev Med 42:273–279, 2006

Diamond J: Guns, Germs, and Steel: The Fates of Human Societies. New York, WW Norton, 1997

Farmer ME, Locke BZ, Moscicki EK, et al: Physical activity and depressive symptoms: NHANES I epidemiologic follow-up study. Am J Epidemiol 128:1340–1351, 1988

Folkins CH, Sime WE: Physical fitness training and mental health. Am Psychol 36:373–389, 1981

Gauvin L, Spence JC: Physical activity and psychological well-being: knowledge base, current issues, and caveats. Nutr Rev 54 (4, part 2):s53–s65, 1996

Goodyer IM: Life Experiences, Development, and Childhood Psychopathology. Chichester, UK, Wiley, 1990

Gorsuch RL: Religious aspects of substance abuse and recovery. J Soc Issues 5:65–83, 1995

Greenberg D, Shefler G: Obsessive-compulsive disorder in ultra-orthodox Jewish patients: a comparison of religious and non-religious symptoms. Psychol Psychother 75 (part 2):123–130, 2002

Greenberg D, Witztum E: Influence of cultural factors on OCD: religious symptoms in a religious society. Isr J Psychiatry Relat Sci 31:211–220, 1994

Haberstick BC, Schmitz S, Young SE, et al: Contributions of genes and environments to stability and change in externalizing and internalizing problems during elementary and middle school. Behav Genet 35:381–96, 2005

Heath AC, Madden PAF, Grant JD, et al: Resiliency factors protecting against teenage alcohol use and smoking: influences of religion, religious involvement and values, and ethnicity in Missouri Adolescent Female Twin Study. Twin Res 2:145–155, 1999

Horley J: Life satisfaction, happiness, and morale: two problems with the use of subjective well-being indicators. Gerontologist 24:124–127, 1984

Kajita M, Takahashi T, Hayashi K, et al: Self-esteem and mental health characteristics especially among lean students surveyed by University Personality Inventory. Psychiatry Clin Neurosci 56:123–129, 2002

Kaufman J, Yang BZ, Douglas-Palumberi H, et al: Social supports and serotonin transporter gene moderate depression in maltreated children. Proc Natl Acad Sci U S A 101:17316–17321, 2004

Kendler KS, Neale MC, Kessler R, et al: A twin study of recent life events and difficulties. Arch Gen Psychiatry 50:789–796, 1993

Kendler KS, Karkowski LM, Prescott CA: Causal relationship between stressful life events and the onset of major depression. Am J Psychiatry 156:837–841, 1999

Kendler KS, Aggen SH, Jacobson KC, et al: Does the level of family dysfunction moderate the impact of genetic factors on the personality trait of neuroticism? Psychol Med 33:817–825, 2003a

Kendler KS, Liu XQ, Gardner CO, et al: Dimensions of religiosity and their relationship to lifetime psychiatric and substance use disorders. Am J Psychiatry 160:496–503, 2003b

Kessler RC: The effects of stressful life events on depression. Annu Rev Psychol 48:191–214, 1997

Koenig H, George L, Meador K, et al: Religious practices and alcoholism in a southern adult population. Hosp Community Psychiatry 45:225–231, 1994

Koopmans JR, Slutske WS, van Baal GCM, et al: The influence of religion on alcohol initiation: evidence for genotype X environment interaction. Behav Genet 29:445–453, 1999

Koval JJ, Pederson LL: Stress-coping and other psychosocial risk factors: a model for smoking in grade 6 students. Addict Behav. 24(2):207–18, 1999

Koval J, Pederson L, Mills C, et al: Models of the relationship of stress, depression, and other psychosocial factors to smoking behavior: a comparison of a cohort of students in grades 6 and 8. Prev Med 30:463–477, 2000

Kritz-Silverstein D, Barrett-Connor E, Corbeau C: Cross-sectional and prospective study of exercise and depressed mood in the elderly—the Rancho Bernardo study. Am J Epidemiol 153:596–603, 2001

Larson D, Wilson WP: Religious life of alcoholics. South Med J 73:723–727, 1980

Luby JL, Svrakic DM, McCallum K, et al: The Junior Temperament and Character Inventory: preliminary validation of a child self-report measure. Psychol Rep 84 (3, part 2):1127–1138, 1999

Lyubomirsky S, Lepper HS: A measure of subjective happiness: preliminary reliability and construct validation. Soc Indic Res 46:137–155, 1999

Maes HH, Neale, MC Martin NG, et al: Religious attendance and frequency of alcohol use: same genes or same environment: a bivariate extended twin kinship model. Twin Res 2:169–179, 1999

McGue M, Lykken D: Genetic influence on divorce. Psychol Sci 3:368–373, 1992

Middeldorp CM, Cath DC, Vink JM, et al: Twin and genetic effects on life events. Twin Res Hum Genet 8:224–231, 2005

Moos RH, Moos BS: Manual for the Family Environment Scale. Palo Alto, CA, Consulting Psychologists Press, 1974

Nonnemaker JM, McNeely CA, Blum RW: Public and private domains of religiosity and adolescent health risk behaviors: evidence from the National Longitudinal Study of Adolescent Health. Soc Sci Med 57:2049–2054, 2003

North TC, McCullagh P, Tran ZV: Effect of exercise on depression. Exerc Sport Sci Rev 18:379–415, 1990

Payne I, Bergin A, Bielema K, et al: Review of religion and mental health: prevention and enhancement of psychosocial functioning. Prev Hum Serv 9:11–40, 1991

Pine DS, Cohen P, Johnson JG, et al: Adolescent life events as predictors of adult depression. J Affect Disord 68:49–57, 2002

Raphael FJ, Rani S, Bale R, et al: Religion, ethnicity and obsessive-compulsive disorder. Int J Soc Psychiatry 42:38–44, 1996

Rassin E, Koster E: The correlation between thought-action fusion and religiosity in a normal sample. Behav Res Ther 41:361–368, 2003

Rettew DC, Stanger C, McKee L, et al: Interactions between child and parent temperament and child behavior problems. Compr Psychiatry 47:412–420, 2006

Rietveld MJ, Hudziak JJ, Bartels M, et al: Heritability of attention problems in children; I: cross-sectional results from a study of twins, age 3–12 years. Am J Med Genet B Neuropsychiatr Genet 117:102–113, 2003

Rose RJ, Dick DM, Viken RJ, et al: Gene-environment interaction in patterns of adolescent drinking: regional residency moderates longitudinal influences on alcohol use. Alcohol Clin Exp Res 25:637–643, 2001

Salmon P: Effects of physical exercise on anxiety, depression, and sensitivity to stress: a unifying theory. Clin Psychol 21:33–61, 2000

Scully D, Kremer J, Meade MM, et al: Physical exercise and psychological well being: a critical review. Br J Sports Med 32:111–120, 1998

Sica C, Novara C, Sanavio E: Religiousness and obsessive-compulsive cognitions and symptoms in an Italian population. Behav Res Ther 40:813–823, 2002

Shooka A, al-Haddad MK, Raees A: OCD in Bahrain: a phenomenological profile. Int J Soc Psychiatry 44:147–154, 1998

Steptoe A, Butler N: Sports participation and emotional wellbeing in adolescents. Lancet 347:1789–1792, 1996

Steptoe A, Wardle J, Fuller R, et al: Leisure-time physical exercise: prevalence, attitudinal correlates, and behavioral correlates among young Europeans from 21 countries. Prev Med 26:845–854, 1997

Stokes R, Frederick-Recascino C: Women's perceived body image: relations with personal happiness. J Women Aging 15:17–29, 2003

Strawbridge WJ, Deleger S, Roberts RE, et al: Physical activity reduces the risk of subsequent depression for older adults. Am J Epidemiol 156:328–334, 2002

Stubbe JH, Boomsma DI, Geus de EJC: Sports participation during adolescence: a shift from environmental to genetic factors. Med Sci Sports Exerc 37:563–570, 2005

Stubbe JH, Moor de MHM, Boomsma DI, et al: The association between exercise participation and well-being: a co-twin study. Prev Med 44:148–152, 2007

Suomi SJ: Aggression and social behaviour in rhesus monkeys. Novartis Found Symp 268:216–226, 2005

Tek C, Ulug B: Religiosity and religious obsessions in obsessive-compulsive disorder. Psychiatry Res 104:99–108, 2001

Tezcan E, Millet B: Phenomenology of obsessive-compulsive disorders. Forms and characteristics of obsessions and compulsions in East Turkey [in French]. Encephale 23:342–350, 1997

Thomas A, Chess S: Temperament and development. Brunner/Mazel, 1977

Unger JB, Hamilton JE, Sussman S: A family member's job loss as a risk factor for smoking among adolescents. Health Psychol 23:308–313, 2004

van Beijsterveldt CE, Bartels M, Hudziak JJ, et al: Causes of stability of aggression from early childhood to adolescence: a longitudinal genetic analysis in Dutch twins. Behav Genet 33:591–605, 2003

van den Bree MB, Whitmer MD, Pickworth WB: Predictors of smoking development in a population-based sample of adolescents: a prospective study. J Adolesc Health 35:172–181, 2004

van Grootheest DS, Bartels M, Cath DC, et al: Genetic and environmental contributions underlying stability in childhood obsessive-complusive behavior. Biol Psychiatry 61:308–315, 2007

Weissman MM, Pilowsky DJ, Wickramaratne PJ, et al: Remissions in maternal depression and child psychopathology: a STAR*D-child report. JAMA 25:1389–1398, 2006

Weyerer S: Physical inactivity and depression in the community: evidence from the upper Bavarian field study. Int J Sports Med 13:492–496, 1992

Wilens TE, Biederman J, Brown S, et al: Psychiatric comorbidity and functioning in clinically referred preschool children and school-age youths with ADHD. J Am Acad Child Adolesc Psychiatry 41:262–268, 2002

Winter T, Kaprio J, Viken RJ, et al: Individual differences in adolescent religiosity in Finland: familial effects are modified by sex and region of residence. Twin Res 2:108–114, 1999

INDEX

*Page numbers printed in **boldface** type refer to tables or figures.*